Medicines Reuse

Medicines Reuse

Editor

Parastou Donyai

MDPI • Basel • Beijing • Wuhan • Barcelona • Belgrade • Manchester • Tokyo • Cluj • Tianjin

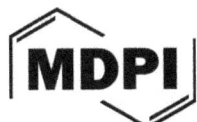

Editor
Parastou Donyai
Pharmacy
University of Reading
Reading
United Kingdom

Editorial Office
MDPI
St. Alban-Anlage 66
4052 Basel, Switzerland

This is a reprint of articles from the Special Issue published online in the open access journal *Pharmacy* (ISSN 2226-4787) (available at: www.mdpi.com/journal/pharmacy/special_issues/Medicines_Reuse).

For citation purposes, cite each article independently as indicated on the article page online and as indicated below:

LastName, A.A.; LastName, B.B.; LastName, C.C. Article Title. *Journal Name* **Year**, *Volume Number*, Page Range.

ISBN 978-3-0365-4090-0 (Hbk)
ISBN 978-3-0365-4089-4 (PDF)

Cover image courtesy of Parastou Donyai

© 2022 by the authors. Articles in this book are Open Access and distributed under the Creative Commons Attribution (CC BY) license, which allows users to download, copy and build upon published articles, as long as the author and publisher are properly credited, which ensures maximum dissemination and a wider impact of our publications.

The book as a whole is distributed by MDPI under the terms and conditions of the Creative Commons license CC BY-NC-ND.

Contents

About the Editor vii

Preface to "Medicines Reuse" ix

Abdullah Alshemari, Liz Breen, Gemma Quinn and Uthayasankar Sivarajah
Can We Create a Circular Pharmaceutical Supply Chain (CPSC) to Reduce Medicines Waste?
Reprinted from: *Pharmacy* 2020, 8, 221, doi:10.3390/pharmacy8040221 1

Hamza Alhamad, Nilesh Patel and Parastou Donyai
Towards Medicines Reuse: A Narrative Review of the Different Therapeutic Classes and Dosage Forms of Medication Waste in Different Countries
Reprinted from: *Pharmacy* 2020, 8, 230, doi:10.3390/pharmacy8040230 23

SuHak Lee and Jon C. Schommer
Medication Use and Storage, and Their Potential Risks in US Households
Reprinted from: *Pharmacy* 2022, 10, 27, doi:10.3390/pharmacy10010027 63

Parastou Donyai, Rachel McCrindle, Terence K. L. Hui and R. Simon Sherratt
Stakeholder Views on the Idea of Medicines Reuse in the UK
Reprinted from: *Pharmacy* 2021, 9, 85, doi:10.3390/pharmacy9020085 83

David McRae, Abigail Gould, Rebecca Price-Davies, Jonathan Tagoe, Andrew Evans and Delyth H. James
Public Attitudes towards Medicinal Waste and Medicines Reuse in a 'Free Prescription' Healthcare System
Reprinted from: *Pharmacy* 2021, 9, 77, doi:10.3390/pharmacy9020077 91

Hamza Alhamad and Parastou Donyai
The Validity of the Theory of Planned Behaviour for Understanding People's Beliefs and Intentions toward Reusing Medicines
Reprinted from: *Pharmacy* 2021, 9, 58, doi:10.3390/pharmacy9010058 107

Hamza Alhamad and Parastou Donyai
Intentions to "Reuse" Medication in the Future Modelled and Measured Using the Theory of Planned Behavior
Reprinted from: *Pharmacy* 2020, 8, 213, doi:10.3390/pharmacy8040213 119

Monica Chauhan, Hamza Alhamad, Rachel McCrindle, Terence K. L. Hui, R. Simon Sherratt and Parastou Donyai
Medicines as Common Commodities or Powerful Potions? What Makes Medicines Reusable in People's Eyes
Reprinted from: *Pharmacy* 2021, 9, 88, doi:10.3390/pharmacy9020088 139

Terence K. L. Hui, Bilal Mohammed, Parastou Donyai, Rachel McCrindle and R. Simon Sherratt
Design of pharmaceutical packaging to facilitate the reuse of medicines and reduce medicinal waste
Reprinted from: *Pharmacy* 2020, 8, 58, doi:10.3390/pharmacy8020058 151

Yasmin Lam, Rachel McCrindle, Terence K. L. Hui, R. Simon Sherratt and Parastou Donyai
The Effect of Quality Indicators on Beliefs about Medicines Reuse: An Experimental Study
Reprinted from: *Pharmacy* 2021, 9, 128, doi:10.3390/pharmacy9030128 169

About the Editor

Parastou Donyai

Prof. Parastou Donyai is Professor of Social and Cognitive Pharmacy in the Department of Pharmacy at the University of Reading. She is a qualified pharmacist and registrant of the General Pharmaceutical Council (GPhC), a member of the Royal Pharmaceutical Society (RPS), a fellow of the Higher Education Academy, a graduate member of the British Psychological Society and an associate member of the College of Mental Health Pharmacy. She studied pharmacy at King's College London (1990-1993), and after her pre-registration training in hospital returned to King's to complete a PhD in pharmacy (1994-1998). Inspired by her experiences as a pharmacist, she began studying people within healthcare settings. She completed a postgraduate diploma in psychological research methods in 2007 and obtained a second full degree in psychology in 2014. She researches the practical and behavioural aspects of medicines use, from the time of their prescribing to their disposal and potential for reuse, including patient and practitioner education and training. She has explored medication usage in a range of conditions including dementia, psychosis, attention deficit hyperactivity disorder, and following myocardial infarction and breast cancer. Her research on Continuing Professional Development provided the basis for revalidating pharmacy professionals in Great Britain and she has also developed training for pre-registration pharmacists. She is a co-director of the Interdisciplinary Research Centre for Health Humanities at the University of Reading, promoting projects on health and illness that combine the traditional and social sciences with the humanities. Her research on reducing medicines wastage has created in-depth understandings of the psychology of drug holidays, medication use reviews and beliefs about medication reuse, facilitating the interdisciplinary ReMINDS (Reuse of Medicines though Informatics, Networks and Digital Sensors) collaboration.

Preface to "Medicines Reuse"

This is a book about 'medicines reuse'. In a pharmacy setting, medicines reuse is about re-dispensing unused medication returned by one patient for use by another. The 'reuse' of dispensed medicines instead of the disposal of the medication as waste is preferable where possible. Disposal as waste is the current practice that takes place in many parts of the world, including in the UK. A number of related or alternative terminologies also exist to describe the concept of medicines reuse, including re-dispensing, recycling, redistributing and reverse flow. Medicines reuse is gaining popularity around the world, either as an existing scheme or as an idea to be explored for implementation in the future. The contributing authors were motivated to write this book because medicines reuse has the potential to help reduce the waste and environmental pollution created by unused medicines, reduce the depletion of material resources and/or help save money and provide medicines to people who cannot otherwise afford them. Medicines reuse might also help deal with the problem of drug shortages or assist with the creation of new medicines using extracted and repurposed pharmaceutical ingredients. This can facilitate greater responsiveness and recovery in times of supply chain disruption when shortages occur. Yet, perhaps for historical reasons, this subject remains under-investigated. Our aim was to bring together leading authors in the field to help create a comprehensive and contemporary account of medicines reuse research. The intended audience for this book includes academics, health professionals, policy-makers, researchers and students, and indeed anyone else with an interest in making medicines use more sustainable by learning from research within the emerging field of medicines reuse. This book brings together over 20 authors from graduate students to Professors from the UK and the US working within a breadth of specialisms including Biomedical Engineering, Biosensors, Computer and Human Interaction, Health Psychology, Health Service Operations, Pharmacy Practice, and Technology Management and Circular Economy.

Paper one outlines a Circular Pharmaceutical Supply Chain and explains how it could be considered and tested as a sustainable supply chain proposition.

Paper two examines the different therapeutic classes and dosage forms making up medication waste around the world, to inform potential reuse practice.

Paper three describes medications stored in US households, gauging their risk to minors, pets, and the environment, while estimating the costs of unused medications.

Paper four draws on stakeholder meetings to detail the range of views expressed on medication waste and the potential for medicines reuse within a UK context.

Paper five reports on public attitudes towards medicinal waste and medicines reuse within a 'free prescription' healthcare system in Wales, UK.

Paper six examines the validity of the Theory of Planned Behaviour (TPB) for understanding people's intentions to engage in medicines reuse as a behaviour.

Paper seven reports on a TPB model which predicts behavioural intentions showing how people could embrace medicines reuse via practical measures.

Paper eight illustrates people's perceptions of medicines as common commodities to explain their pro-medicines-reuse beliefs and desire for these to be recycled.

Paper nine shows how sensing technologies applied to pharmaceutical packaging could enlist medicines to the Internet of Things to facilitate medicines reuse.

Paper ten gauges the effect of quality indicators, including sensing technology applied to packaging, on people's beliefs about medicines reuse in an experiment.

This is a unique, indispensable collection of papers whose publication coincides with the NHS's ambition to be the world's first net-zero national health service. With medicines accounting for 25% of the carbon emissions within the NHS (20% rooted in the medicines manufacturing and freight within the supply chain), medicines reuse could be the key to reducing emissions and helping the NHS and other health services globally to reach net zero status.

We are grateful to Elsa Wang at MDPI for facilitating the publication of this collection. We are indebted to all research participants and to all workplaces hosting the contributors.

Parastou Donyai
Editor

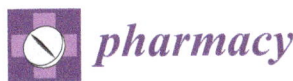

Review

Can We Create a Circular Pharmaceutical Supply Chain (CPSC) to Reduce Medicines Waste?

Abdullah Alshemari [1,*], Liz Breen [2], Gemma Quinn [2] and Uthayasankar Sivarajah [1]

1. School of Management, Faculty of Management, Law and Social Sciences, University of Bradford, Bradford BD7 1DP, UK; U.Sivarajah@bradford.ac.uk
2. School of Pharmacy and Medical Sciences, University of Bradford, Bradford BD7 1DP, UK; L.Breen@bradford.ac.uk (L.B.); G.Quinn@bradford.ac.uk (G.Q.)
* Correspondence: a.alshemari@bradford.ac.uk

Received: 31 August 2020; Accepted: 16 November 2020; Published: 18 November 2020

Abstract: Background: The increase in pharmaceutical waste medicines is a global phenomenon and financial burden. The Circular Economy, as a philosophy within the pharmaceutical supply chain, aims to promote waste reduction, maximise medicines value, and enable sustainability within this supply chain (increasing circularity). Circularity strategies for pharmaceuticals are not currently implemented in many countries, due to quality and safety barriers. The aim of this study was to determine whether the application of circular economy principles can minimise pharmaceutical waste and support sustainability in the pharmaceutical supply chain; Methods: a detailed narrative literature review was conducted in order to examine pharmaceutical waste creation, management, disposal, and the application of circular economy principles; Results: the literature scrutinised revealed that pharmaceutical waste is created by multiple routes, each of which need to be addressed by pharmacists and healthcare bodies through the Circular Economy 9R principles. These principles act as a binding mechanism for disparate waste management initiatives. Medicines, or elements of a pharmaceutical product, can be better managed to reduce waste, cost, and reduce negative environmental impacts through unsafe disposal. Conclusions: the study findings outline a Circular Pharmaceutical Supply Chain and suggests that it should be considered and tested as a sustainable supply chain proposition.

Keywords: waste; reuse; reduce; pharmaceutical; medicines; hospital; circular economy

1. Introduction

The World Health Organization (WHO) defines pharmaceutical waste as undesirable pharmaceuticals, including expired, unused, spilled, and infected pharmaceutical products, medications, vaccines, and sera that are not required and should be disposed of appropriately [1]. The volume of pharmaceutical waste has increased primarily due to growth in the number of patients and prescriptions and the use and overproduction of medicines. The increase in unused, expired, and misplaced medicines contributes to medicine shortages, higher percentages of pharmaceuticals waste, and increased medicine disposal costs, and it is a growing concern globally requiring a systemic approach to its resolution [2]. According to the Pharmaceutical Services Negotiating Committee (PSNC), prescribing pharmaceuticals represents the second-highest cost in the United Kingdom (UK), after medical staff [3]. As of 2019, around $1.25 trillion USD had been spent on medicines globally, up from only $887 billion in 2010. The spending on medicines is anticipated to increase to $1.59 billion by 2024 [4]. By 2019, the UK had around £127 billion spent in healthcare [5]. Such figures indicate an extensive waste of resources in the healthcare system. This waste includes inappropriately prescribed medication, which results in the overstocking of medications. Gebremariam et al. [6] reported that supply chain management and related variables were principal contributors to the generation of pharmaceutical waste. Likewise, poor storage conditions, storing medicines on the floor, the absence of specific stocking plans, poor climate control, and overstocking expired medicines can lead to significant medication spoilage [6].

The last phase of the pharmaceutical waste is disposal, traditional burning or non-burning technique utilized. It is essential to note that, out of all pharmaceutical waste, only 15% is hazardous, whilst the remaining 85% is general [7]. Large amounts of prescribed pharmaceutical waste are found in the waterways, streams and groundwater, and it has similarly been shown that a percentage of these are affecting the water and the climate [8]. The WHO classification of different types of healthcare waste is [7]:

- pathological; this includes body parts, body fluids, human waste, and tissue waste and animal corpses that are contaminated;
- pharmaceutical; this is either unused, contaminated medicine or medicine which has expired;
- cytotoxic; genotoxic waste (highly hazardous);
- sharps; includes syringes, needles, and blades, etc.;
- infectious; this usually contains blood or any bodily fluid which is contaminated and could, therefore, infect other people when they come into contact;
- non-hazardous; these waste materials can not cause any chemical, radioactive, biological, or physical dangers; and,
- radioactive; products that are infected by radionuclides.

These different types of waste require differing methods of disposal and/or new approaches in order to reduce or eliminate waste. It is important to determine the most suitable method to help preventing/reducing the negative consequences of the disposing methods on the environment, specifically on water, soil, air, and on human well-being [7,8].

The circular economy (CE) is a holistic philosophy that is conveyed through a system for managing and preserving resources 'in use as long as possible through recovery and reuse', hence circularity [9]. The CE approach closes the gap between production and the life cycle of the natural ecosystem upon which individuals rely for business and physical survival. It signposts practical ways of eliminating waste, transforming biodegradable and non-biodegradable waste, and promoting reuse and recycling. In CE, a distinction is made amongst different choices of circularity, represented as the R-model of 3R, 4R, or even 9R models (the 9R model being the optimal application of CE incorporating Refuse, Rethink, Reduce, Reuse, Repair, Refurbish, Remanufacture, Repurpose, Recycle, and Recover) [10,11]. Kirchherr et al. [12] claimed that the CE is 'the combination of reduce, reuse and recycle activities' to ensure systematic change. The CE has been rapidly growing to realise the United Nation Sustainable Development Goals (SDGs) and as an alternative strategy for business advancement. In the CE, products and services operate in closed loops (being produced and then recycled for further use) and they are intended to work in harmony with the environment. The Ellen MacArthur Foundation, which was founded in 2010 and aims to accelerate progress towards a regenerative CE [13], defines the CE as a move from a linear model of resource consumption, which pursues a take-make-dispose design, to an economy that is restorative by intention. The CE associates the supply and demand of supply chain industries in order to increase resource efficiency and help achieve sustainable production and consumption [11].

Sufficiency economy philosophy (SEP) is another approach that has been considered in academic circles as contributing to the sustainability agenda. SEP is defined by the United Nations [14] as "an innovative method for development that is designed for practical application over a wide range of problems and situations". The objective of SEP is to improve planning procedures in order to ensure sustainability, manage changes in the world and utilise natural resources in a capable way while preserving nature. SEP is a sustainable development approach that was introduced by the late king of Thailand and implemented through three different components; moderation, which aims for the effective consumption of resources; reasonableness, which concerns objectively choosing the degree of products adequacy while considering the elements that are involved and the normally expected results; and, risk management, which entails adapting that is based on reasonable effects and changes that are projected by considering the likelihood of future circumstances from different viewpoints [15].

A key objective of the CE is to promote and facilitate greater sustainability. A sustainable supply chain is defined as a supply chain, in which operations, assets, data, and funds are managed to increase supply chain production while simultaneously reducing environmental effects and improving social wellbeing [16]. As mentioned by the European Union (EU) parliament [17], the application of CE practices for waste management in general could help to save EU organisations nearly €600 billion through, for example, waste avoidance, eco-friendly products and reuse programmes. It could also help minimise yearly greenhouse gas emissions by 4%. The benefits of the CE include improvement of the environment, improvement of the safety of raw materials, acceleration of innovation, and improvement of economic growth [18,19].

An example of the CE in practice can be seen in closed-loop supply chains, in which recyclers and manufacturers collaborate and work closely to realise resource and cost savings. Many sectors have adopted closed-loop supply chains in their processes. In the medical field, GE Motors and Philips [20,21] have started to refurbish medical products, including magnetic resonance imaging (MRI), computed tomography (CT), ultrasound, and X-ray machines, by obtaining full control to guarantee that all exchanged materials are repurposed or reused and produced with high quality to ensure the efficiency of the products.

The aim of this study was to determine whether the application of CE principles reduce pharmaceutical waste and support sustainability in the Pharmaceutical Supply Chain (PSC). The rationale of the aim of this research was to identify ways to decrease the negative environmental impact, costs and promote sustainable supply chain and eco-design through the application of CE principles in the PSC. By identifying how the CE principles and the R-strategies can be used in the pharmaceutical supply chain it will be possible to determine how the negative impact of pharmaceutical waste be reduced in terms of costs, sustainability, and increasing circularity. To achieve this aim, the following objectives were posited: (1) to ascertain how pharmaceuticals waste is created, (2) to better understand how this waste is managed, (3) to outline how it is safely disposed, and (4) to determine how pharmaceuticals waste can be reduced and better managed through the adoption of CE principles.

2. Materials and Methods

A review of current pharmaceutical waste management studies was undertaken to document how pharmaceuticals be reused and whether implementation of the CE philosophy and associated principles could help to reduce waste. The following keywords were used for the primary search: 'Medicines' AND 'Pharmaceutical' AND 'Pharmaceutical Waste' OR 'Drugs' OR 'Pharmaceutical Return' OR 'Disposal' OR 'Hospitals' OR 'Pharmaceutical Supply Chain' OR 'Medicines Reuse' OR 'Circular Economy' OR 'Circular Economy Principles'.

First, the titles and abstracts of each article were screened, and the most significant articles were selected. Second, the related abstracts were chosen, and the full form of each selected article was retrieved. A few papers were eliminated after their selection, as described below. Journals and papers published in English were chosen. Articles, papers, and studies published before July 2020 were explored while using Elsevier, Google Scholar, MDPI, PubMed, SAGE, and Science Direct.

To be included in the review, articles/papers had to be related to pharmaceuticals, medicine reuse, waste management, and/or CE, and they had to present new and/or relevant information. Articles/papers on approaches to waste management improvement, legislation, the PSC, waste generation minimisation, and CE application were also included. Excluded papers are not explicitly relate to the keywords highlighted above.

The search was conducted while using electronic databases, avoiding manual exploration. Duplications were eliminated. Non-academic grey literature was also searched in Google utilising similar keywords. These sources included journalistic articles, reports, and webpages on pharmaceuticals waste and CE. A conventional quality examination was not utilised, as one of the goals of this study was to gather a broad base of proof, including all of the procedures and studies related to gathering in-depth literature data. Figure 1 shows the areas of the literature that were reviewed to meet the aim of this study.

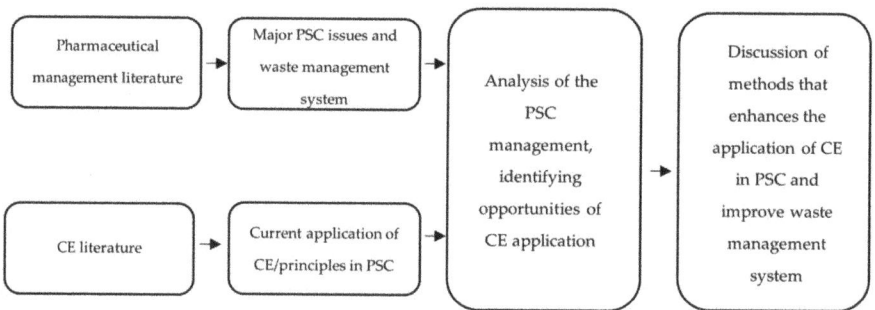

Figure 1. Areas of literature discovery.

3. Results

3.1. Pharmaceutical Waste Management

The literature review identified three clearly defined areas of focus when examining pharmaceutical waste management. These are discussed individually below.

3.1.1. Waste Creation

Instances of pharmaceuticals waste may be caused by patients who are unable to utilise all of their administered pharmaceuticals due to unfavourable impacts (side effects), daily dosage modifications, health improvements, the expiry of medicines, doctors' prescribing practices, or dispensers' practices. Non-adherence to prescriptions can also cause stockpiling of leftover medications in the home. According to the WHO, half of the patients neglect to take medication effectively [22]. As such, families and patients around the world are in possession of unused or terminated prescriptions, and the associated dangers have prompted research interest. Many individuals who stockpile undesirable, unused, or expired pharmaceuticals in their homes dispose of them through waste containers or sinks or by flushing them down the toilet. It is important to realise that discarding unused or terminated pharmaceuticals through non-permitted methods affects the environment and individual wellbeing [6,23].

Table 1 shows the different waste creation of pharmaceuticals.

Table 1. Waste creation point and issues associated.

Waste Creation Point	Issue	Current Resolution/Practice
Manufacturing	Overproduction of stock based on forecasted demand.	Secure accurate demand based on transparency and sharing of information across the supply chain facilitated by government bodies [24,25]
	Overproduction of stock based on actual demand, e.g., a medicines shortage (but short lived so excess stock is created).	Ensure the transparency of stock production and use and effective reporting of medicines shortages between pharmacies, wholesalers, and manufacturers [24] Distinguish the cause of the shortage and focus efforts there to increase or use on-hand supply [24,25]
Pharmacy	Overordering of stock by pharmacy.	Implement effective procurement training and inventory management systems [26]
	Insufficient storage conditions by pharmacy.	Conduct regular checks ensure suitable conditions of light, humidity, ventilation, temperature, and security [26]
Hospital Wards/Clinics/Estates	Excess stock requested and held by wards or clinics.	Create stock lists at the ward level with the support of pharmacy store teams to manage stock levels of wards effectively [27]
	Incorrect medication prescribed for patient and not enough or unclear information given.	Enact effective processes to process and dispense prescriptions supported by accurate information from a consultant to avoid irrational medication. Also, ensure that clarification is offered to the patients regarding the dosage, use, and advantages and disadvantages of the recommended pharmaceutical [28–30]
	Patient is deceased but medication is in their name and cannot be used by anyone else.	Reuse prescribed medications if the patient is deceased. This applies if, for example, there is no available stock, no available alternatives, and there is no risk associated with other patients using the medicines [31,32]
	Medicines not rotated or used effectively (manual intervention based on expiry dates) or inventory management systems not utilized effectively to reduce stock obsolescence.	Provide effective training for staff and use of inventory management systems [26]
	Patient's own medicine lost on admission and, therefore, are not available for use.	Encourage patients to bring their own medicines. Design system to ensure patients' own medicines stay with them using green bags, e.g., the green bag scheme for improving the utilization of prescriptions for better results and decreased waste [29,30]
	Inadequate resources to support effective management of pharmaceuticals waste segregation and disposal.	Create dedicated resources to support pharmaceuticals waste management and safe disposal [33] Both small-scale (e.g., training programs) and large-scale (e.g., legislative and administrative) solutions are needed to ensure safe waste management [34]

Table 1. Cont.

Waste Creation Point	Issue	Current Resolution/Practice
General Practitioner (GP)/Consultants	Overprescribing by GPs/consultants.	Undertake informed prescribing in relation to quantity and frequency, guided by current data on stock availability provided by government bodies [35,36] Develop a system to permit patients to improve their overstocking and ordering of medication [35,36]
	Remote prescribing by GPs.	Remote prescribing are applied care home. But is being addressed with the introduction of pharmacists to manage prescriptions more effectively [37–39]
Care Homes	Excess stock received and held for patients.	Educate staff to contact GP regarding prescribing patterns and use a pharmacist to support medicines use [31–40]
Patients	Repeating prescriptions requested by patients.	Educate and facilitate patients to request stock when needed and approved by GP without overstocking [34–36,40]
	Advising GP or healthcare professional when they cannot take medicines and no longer needed.	Educate and facilitate medicines returns to pharmacy, GP, or another reliable repository [38]

Unused pharmaceuticals could be the result of changes in the recommended treatment. Such practices lead to the expiration of prescriptions, which are then put away or discarded by household members who flush them down toilets instead of returning them to pharmacies [39]. Analysis indicates that £300 million worth of prescription pharmaceuticals that are authorised by the UK National Health Services (NHS) are wasted every year [41]. Such wastage accounts for a significant percentage of pharmaceutical-related expenditures in the UK. For every £25 spent on pharmaceutical products, £1 is wasted. The £300 million includes £90 million worth of unused prescriptions in people's homes at any one time. An estimated £110 million worth of prescriptions are returned to pharmacies every year. Approximately £50 million worth of unused pharmaceuticals from care homes are disposed of every year by NHS [41].

The UK government funds its healthcare system through taxation of its citizens and businesses. Pharmaceutical waste increases the cost to the government of meeting the healthcare needs of the country. At the same time, pharmaceutical waste that results from non-adherence to prescribed medications increases the cost of treatment, because patients subsequently require additional treatment [42]. An increase in unused and expired medicine contributes to pharmaceutical waste and increases the use of financial resources [43–45]. Although unused pharmaceuticals have been studied extensively worldwide, there are obstacles to decreasing the number of unused pharmaceuticals. Leftover medicines in hospitals may expire and remain unused, because of a lack of proper controls [44,45]. Most hospitals experience increased pharmaceutical waste as a result of poor dispensing strategies by the pharmacy, which contributes to the overflow of pharmaceuticals [45].

Another reason for increased pharmaceutical waste is a lack of knowledge regarding medication usage and disposal [46,47]. Patients may not be educated as how best to safely dispose of their medicines. Another reason for unused medicine may be changes in treatment, meaning that the unused medications become a source of waste [46].

3.1.2. Waste Management

Current pharmaceutical waste management and disposal methods and related social, economic, and environmental burdens must be understood from different points of view [48]. The lack of awareness of proper waste management in hospitals, particularly those in developing countries, has made these institutions a focal point in the spread of disease and infection, rather minimising and eliminating waste [48,49]. Research on hospitals in Kuwait found that pharmacists lacked knowledge about the consequences of sub-optimal/unsafe pharmaceutical disposal methods and often did not follow guidelines that were issued by the Ministry of Health [49]. A similar study [47] on Iraqi hospitals found that pharmacists needed programmes to improve their knowledge of appropriate disposal methods for pharmaceuticals waste. Inadequate training and a lack of awareness among hospital staff, such as nurses and pharmacists, contribute to the increase in pharmaceutical waste in many countries. Control and visibility are crucial in the reduction of losses due to expiry. When the inventory system is functioning at optimal levels, inventories could be redistributed within the system in order to enable a quick workflow.

Johnson et al. [50] found that the inadequate segregation of waste increases costs to hospitals already under significant budget constraints. There is much misunderstanding regarding the best possible methods of medication disposal, and several countries do not have standard medication disposal requirements. For decades, there have been various reports about the presence of pharmaceuticals in groundwater, lakes, waterways and drinking water due to improper disposal [22]. These pharmaceutical disposal methods negatively affect natural ecosystems and human health.

Against this backdrop, there is a need to effectively manage waste and focus on avenues to control or decrease waste creation. Waste management practices are currently undergoing significant changes from a simplified collection and sorting procedure to a sustainable smart waste management system, as per Zhang et al. [51]. This is achieved by effectively managing and focusing on product/service system designs, resource and energy recovery and end-of-life management of currently wasted resources through initiatives, such as waste reduction practices, biological and thermal processes, and material recycling techniques.

Significant efforts are underway in order to reduce pharmaceutical waste, not just for financial reasons but also to address issues related to current pharmaceutical waste disposal methods, such as landfills [52]. Returned medications are treated as waste and disposed of or destroyed [53]. Reuse and recycling remain generally unexplored, because, under current regulations, many countries, including the UK, do not allow for unused or returned medications to be reused or to enter the PSC [54].

Better waste management can be achieved by focusing on improving the efficiency throughout the value chain in terms of the production, inventory management, usage/consumption, and performance of resources. There is also a need to change the waste management approach by introducing waste management plans that enable facilities to plan for all necessary resources, including staff training; to monitor and evaluate the waste generated from the facilities; and, to take charge of all activities that are likely to generate waste [55]. In addition, waste management also requires effective segregation of waste, which is key to reducing the volume of waste that needs attention and ensuring that each treatment process only receives compatible waste [55]. The introduction of a digital track and trace system would provide timely information to support the production and distribution of medicines in order to optimise medicine production and reduce overproduction, which leads to the generation of waste [55–57].

A large amount of waste is generated when there is lack of visibility of waste generation by the hospital management. Capturing data usage and using that in supply chain management is critical for reducing waste [58]. Tracking utilisation ensures that a facility only has what it needs without excesses or wastage. A balance must also be maintained between what gets produced, ordered, and distributed. Forecasting is critical in maintaining a balance in the healthcare management system. Pharmaceuticals waste is currently managed and processed in multiple ways, and all stakeholders, e.g., manufacturers, general practitioners (GPs), pharmacy, care homes, and patients, in the pharmaceuticals waste management context play roles in waste management, treatment, and disposal.

3.1.3. Waste Disposal

Studies on household pharmaceuticals in Ethiopia [59], Kuwait [60], Poland [61], Saudi Arabia [62], Qatar [63], the UK [64], and the United States [65] concluded that most unused and expired pharmaceuticals are disposed of in the garbage, as there is no clear guidance for patients on the proper disposal of medications. The causes of medication wastage are different in each household. The death of a patient, changing from one medication to another, stopping treatment and lack of consistent use by patients all contribute to pharmaceutical waste [59–65]. Continued pharmaceutical waste over time significantly impacts the environment [8].

The Basel Convention recommends that all healthcare organisations follow waste treatment methods that reduce the release of chemicals or hazardous waste [66]. Likewise, the WHO recommends following waste treatment methods that help to reduce the release of chemicals while recognising the differences in local conditions and availability. To a large extent, poor disposal practices are often due to an absence of adequate training for clinical staff. Insufficient hospital funding also leads to improper waste disposal [60–62]. Table 2 shows the advantages and disadvantages of different pharmaceuticals waste disposal methods.

Table 2. Medicines waste disposal methods.

Treatment	Advantages	Disadvantages
Incineration [67]	Low cost, accepts different waste types, minimises the waste volume	Not environmentally friendly, increases pollution, high cost
Autoclaving [68]	Environmentally friendly, used for infectious waste and sharps	Does not minimise the volume and is not cost effective
Microwave Irradiation [69]	No combustion or gasification, minimal emissions	Not applicable for all waste, high cost
Pyrolysis [69]	Environmentally friendly, disposes of all kinds of waste, minimises the waste volume	High cost, requires certified professional workers
Landfill [68]	Low cost	Not environmentally friendly, increases health risks
Recycling [70]	Environmentally friendly, reduces cost	Not all types of waste can be recycled

Landfills and incineration are the two most utilised disposal strategies [71]; these alternatives for the final removal of waste are utilised to various extents worldwide. In every country, geographical, economic, social, technical, and other factors must be considered when selecting preferred waste disposal methods. In the EU and Japan, incineration is viewed as the preferable method of pharmaceutical waste disposal, and landfills are considered to be a last resort.

Final safe disposal of pharmaceuticals waste is critical, given the potential public health risks that are associated with this type of waste. The most effective way to minimise and dispose of pharmaceuticals waste is to separate waste at the generation stage [72]. It is important to separate waste streams in the workplace to protect people and the environment, regardless of the disposal and treatment strategy. Separation involves sorting various types of waste while using liners with different coloured codes or original packaging in which they are produced. This has regularly been the main task of pharmaceuticals waste disposal. The lack of adequate separation of pharmaceuticals waste increases the risk of workplace accidents and blood-borne viral infections [73].

Pharmaceutical disposal methods need to be adhered to properly, and pharmaceuticals should be returned to a predetermined pharmacy controlled by the health ministry [31]. Pharmaceutical waste disposal frameworks are available in certain nations, and many countries follow the same framework in dealing with returned or expired medications. In the UK and New Zealand, individuals are advised to return expired and unused medications to the pharmacy for safe disposal and they are advised never to dispose of them down toilets [31,33]. In the United States, a system for managing pharmaceuticals waste removal has been developed under the regulations of the Food and Drug Administration (FDA) and the Environmental Protection Agency (EPA) [74]. Australia has implemented a programme (NATRUM) that accepts returned and unwanted medicines for free [75].

3.1.4. Waste Reuse and Recycling

Current methods of disposing of unused pharmaceuticals, including expired pharmaceuticals, have become a global issue. Take-back programmes for pharmaceuticals are eco-friendly and they have been implemented in many countries, as discussed by Alnahas et al. [48]. The objective of these programmes is to safely dispose of pharmaceuticals returned by patients who no longer need them. Many countries do not permit returned medications to be re-dispensed. For example, the UK requires disposal, even if the medications are in good condition and have not been used. However, a study of pharmaceutical reuse in the UK concluded that, based on the findings of the interviews data, reusing unused medicines would reduce NHS spending and lower manufacturing costs [46].

The United States and Greece allow for medications to be reused to make medicine more affordable for people who would not otherwise be able to pay for them [76]. These programmes involve the collection and reintroduction of medicines to the original processing location to be recycled or reused by the government, retailers, or manufacturers. For instance, SMARXT Disposal, a partnership between the American Pharmacists Association, Pharmaceutical Research and Manufacturers of America and Fish and Wildlife services, has developed awareness campaigns for take-back initiatives that involve a collaborative structure for pharmaceuticals waste reuse [77]. This programme helps to reduce the cost of pharmaceuticals and improve the efficiency of the supply chain. Similar programmes have been initiated around the world: in Canada, the ENVIRx programme accepts unused and expired medication for proper disposal; New Zealand adopted the Disposal of Unwanted Medicines Properly (DUMP) programme to encourage individuals to return unused and expired pharmaceuticals; and, in Australia, the Return Unwanted Medicines (RUM) programme was adopted for proper disposal [78,79].

When medicines are returned to physicians, they are destroyed according to guidelines that operate on the assumption that these end-of-life items are useless, as mentioned by Breen [80]. This process could be improved by collecting information about the returned products from GPs, pharmacists, administration improvement managers, and commissioners. Information, such as the amount prescribed, to whom it was prescribed and when it was administered, could be utilised in order to improve prescribing, minimise waste and improve medicine optimisation [80].

Open medicines return events can be jointly held by pharmacies and local councils to help spread awareness in communities about the importance of returning medicines so that they can be destroyed according to government guidelines. These events can help to minimise pharmaceutical waste and increase recycling and the proper disposal of medication [81]. They can also help to increase awareness regarding how following appropriate procedures helps minimise environmental effects [81]. Raja et al. [82] proposed that governments develop and implement a national medication return programme to gather unused or terminated medications at each hospital, so that they can be disposed of properly. Improving the pharmaceutical waste management system and achieving a green PSC requires the cooperation of the entire supply chain from the manufacturers and wholesale suppliers to the GPs, community pharmacies, and patients.

Research that was conducted by Hsieh et al. [83] indicates that the lifespan of specific Active Pharmaceutical Ingredients (API) can be extended where APIs from medicines can be recovered and reused for new formulation development if they do not contain excipients. The recovery process can be done using green engineering, a technique that uses water for the separation process and mechanical energy to provide the power for membrane separation. The process used are tablet milling and dissolution, solid-liquid separation, diafiltration by ultrafiltration, reverse osmosis membrane operation, and crystallization. The recovery process helps to reuse of the API and minimize the cost of API production [83]. Some important points need to be considered for the recovery process [84]. The purity of the reused API should be close to that of a new API, which includes, for example, its density and flowability, while the concentration of the polymer that is recovered should be insignificant, making sure that chemical degradation is avoided by using a suitable temperature during the process, and avoiding any harmful chemicals in order to ensure a low-cost green process [84]. The API recovery cycle is considered to be green because any solvents from waste are completely recovered and reused.

3.1.5. Obstacles to the Safety and Quality of Returned Pharmaceuticals

Regulatory agencies must have strict quality control and safety monitoring measures in order to affirm the appropriateness of medications for reuse. Such procedures include monitoring by specialists to confirm the capacity and limit any risk of damage, contamination, or infection. Moreover, the proper reuse and recycling of medications can reduce the environmental impacts of improper or illegal disposal of pharmaceuticals and reduce the associated carbon footprint.

Table 3 identifies some barriers to the safety and quality of returned medications, which may affect redistribution. The safe disposal of medicines determines the standards of quality in the PSC. Health and safety are essential factors to consider in the PSC in order to protect consumers from infections, complications, and side effects from medications, as well as death due to improper medication usage.

Table 3. Obstacles to the safety and quality of returned pharmaceuticals.

Issues	Obstacles
Safety [2,31,76,85]	Returned medicines may have been subject to intentional tampering, e.g., incorrect packaging. Some presently utilised seals on external medication packaging lack careful designs and effectiveness. Packaging may be unsealed. Packaging may have been contaminated while in a patient's possession.
Quality [2,31,76,85]	Medicines may have been stored in undesirable conditions, e.g., temperature, moisture, light. Medicines may have an undesirable smell. Counterfeit medicines via a redistribution scheme. The dispensing and expiration dates may affect the quality of the medication.

The decision to reuse returned pharmaceuticals depends on a safety confirmation process, whereby devoted analysers at pharmacies can process unopened, intact, and authentic pharmaceuticals. Using technology and engaging arranged networks in smart pharmaceutical packaging will help to determine whether returned, unused, and unexpired medications are safe for reuse [57].

Huge strides have been made in the design of secure pharmaceutical packaging in ensuring trust and confidence in the integrity of medication [2,86–88]. This advances further support the global Falsified Medicines Directive launched in 2019, which ensures product integrity within the supply chain from the point of production through to customer sales [89]. Product protection within the supply chain was reinforced in 2018 when the International Organization for Standardization (ISO) published the new ISO standard 21976:2018, entitled "Packaging-Tamper verification features for medicinal product packaging", and again in 2019, when pharmaceutical companies that have prescription medicine in their portfolio were required in order to provide additional security features in accordance with the Anti-Counterfeiting Directive 2011/62/EU [90]. Stakeholders within the pharmaceutical supply chain need to know that medication has not been tampered with or affected by transportation/storage conditions. These developments in policy, along with high-tech tamper proof solutions and innovative pharmaceutical packaging that provides patients with clear instructions, prevents harm to the environment and conforms to government guidelines and strategies, support the premise that medication could be reused [2,91,92].

3.2. Circular Economy and the Management of Pharmaceutical Waste

When considering the application of CE principles to the PSC, the best methods for reducing pharmaceutical waste include reducing, reusing, and recycling disposable instruments and materials. CE offers several advantages to healthcare services, including cost savings, high quality of life, and continual service improvement [93]. Pachauri et al. [94] found that the CE promotes the use of sustainable products by replacing nonbiodegradable raw materials. The entire operational process is interlinked to accomplish sustainability, as the waste and products of one phase become the raw materials for other products or procedures.

As stated earlier in this discussion, the basic principles of CE are the three Rs; Reduce, Reuse, and Recycle. Examples of the application of these principles can be seen within the PSC. However, the more advanced principles of CE extend past the 3Rs and they present a stronger proposition, which are the 9Rs (see Table 4) [95]. Each R prompts product owners to focus on their creation, use, and disposal, in order to expend their lifespan, but where feasible also maximise the use of materials. This, is turn, contributes to the United Nations Sustainable Development Goals, to end poverty, protect the planet and ensure that all people enjoy peace and prosperity by 2030 [96].

Table 4. 9Rs Circularity strategies [95] (adapted by author).

		R-Strategies	Aim
Increasing Circularity ↑	Better Use of Products and Manufacture	(0) Refuse	Make product redundant by abandoning its function or by offering the same function with a radically different product.
		(1) Rethink	Make product use more intensive (e.g., by sharing product).
		(2) Reduce	Increase efficiency in product manufacture or use by consuming fewer natural resources and materials.
	Expanding the Lifecycle of Product and Elements	(3) Reuse	Reuse by another consumer of discarded product which is still in good condition and fulfils its original function.
		(4) Repair	Repair and maintenance of defective product so it can be used with its original function.
		(5) Refurbish	Restore an old product and bring it up to date.
		(6) Remanufacture	Use parts of discarded product in a new product with the same function.
	Useful Application of Material	(7) Repurpose	Use discarded product or its parts in a new product with a different function.
		(8) Recycle	Process materials to obtain the same (high grade) or lower (low grade) quality.
		(9) Recover	Incineration of material with energy recovery.

There are a number of excellent examples in the pharmaceutical supply chain where innovative practices are in place in order to promote the reduction of waste creation (reduce), to enhance the reuse of medication where legal and possible (reuse), and recycle products or product components where legal and feasible (recycle). These clearly support the CE ethos. Table 5 illustrate some examples of the practices.

Table 5. Examples of current pharmacy medicines waste management practice that endorses the circular economy (CE) ethos.

Product/Practice	Action
Drug Donations [9,94,95,97,98]	Consideration of how medicine donations from medicinal services and patients could help reduce waste and increase the reuse and recycling of medicines. These medicines could be used for individuals who cannot afford their medication.
Epinephrine Injection (EpiPen) [99,100]	Extension of the product's lifecycle, as prompted by medicine shortages.
Falsified Medicines Directive (FMD) and Support of Anti Counterfeit Technologies [101]	The introduction of FMD and the adoption of technologies to reduce counterfeit drug presence in the supply chain. This increases the transparency of stock, increases confidence in stock integrity and reduces risk of patient harm.
Inhalers [102,103]	Promotion of more environmentally friendly inhalers and recycling of outer packaging/cartridges for reuse.
Medication Dosing—Cancer Treatments [31]	Based on group volume, offering clinics to share vials of medications, ensuring maximum utilisation of stock and reducing waste and cost. This also positively impacts stock creation and holding within the supply chain due to the reduced risk of obsolescence.
Prescribing (quantity/frequency) [26,41,48,52]	Consideration of a practice of prescribing medicines in specific quantities and frequencies, which can smooth out the demand for specific medications, reducing the risk of shortage and domestic stockpiling. This practice could also promote the equity of access to medication.
Return Schemes for Medication Reuse [46,104]	Verifying the safety and quality of returned medications and ensuring that medicines have tamper evident packaging to help endorse the reuse of medication scheme.
Return Schemes for Safe Disposal [79]	For example, DUMP schemes, where patients are encouraged to remove unwanted products from their homes to reduce risks to patient and family safety and reduce potential environmental harm.
API Recovery for Reuse	Green engineering technology to recover and reuse the API (extracting, purifying, and repacking) can help to minimize waste and provide it value again [48,83].

At present, the used substances are considered to be obsolete, infectious, and harmful to society and the environment [105]. However, easing strict guidelines in pharmaceutical reuse could pave the way for strengthening circular principles in the healthcare economy [105]. Connelly [76] argued that this could also help pharmacists re-dispense returned medicine to other patients who need treatment, helping to reduce pharmaceutical waste in health facilities.

Recently, in response to the COVID-19 pandemic, the NHS in the UK released guidance for reusing medications in assisted care homes and hospices [106]. The government choice to reuse pharmaceuticals under strict governing criteria is an attempt to manage medical deficiencies and shortages during this period only. All of the prescriptions not required by the individual for whom they were initially prescribed can be reused under the management of registered healthcare professionals and proper recordkeeping [32]. However, some patients may not accept returned medication, citing concerns regarding the proper storage of unused medicines, e.g., room temperature, humidity or sanitation [8]. The reuse of medications to treat different patients during pandemic is especially feasible in cases where patients no longer need the drug, e.g., if they have died, or the provision of their medicine has been interrupted. Reuse applies to all medications—including fluid prescriptions, injections (analgesics, insulin), creams, and inhalers—that are in sealed or closed packs [9,32].

When contemplating the adoption of the CE into the PSC, key factors that should be considered are presented in the Political, Economic, Social, Technological, Legal, and Environmental (PESTLE) model, which supports or challenges practice change. The following PESTLE analysis is proposed based on the literature reviewed in this study (Table 6).

Table 6. Political, Economic, Social, Technological, Legal, and Environmental (PESTLE) analysis of the adoption of the Circular Economy in the Pharmaceutical Supply Chain (PSC).

Criteria PESTLE	Enablers	Barriers	Importance
(P) [107–109]	Tax incentives in the PSC positively support the CE. International agreements and collaborations lead to the enforcement of effective policies in the PSC. Government funding exists for CE projects.	There is inadequate government funding to shift the PSC to the CE. There is no effective enforcement strategy to shift the pharmaceutical sector to the CE. The discriminatory implementation and establishment of PSC policies discourage the shift to the CE.	Political factors help to set the directions and encourage innovation through funding.
(E) [80–82]	Reduction in the use of pharmaceuticals leads to minimised costs. An increase in household healthcare expenditures creates a need to reduce the cost of production.	There are pricing pressure in the PSC between different suppliers. The high cost of establishing the CE is challenged by the low revenues of the pharmaceutical industry. The current medicine taxation system is a barrier to the transition to the CE.	The economy is a significant determinant of the running of the PSC because it guides supply and demand.
(S) [46,109,110]	New preferences in the population regarding the form of medications that are administered enable the shift towards the CE. Suppliers in the sector have a shared CE vision, which facilitates achieving it.	There is resistance from internal PSC and society to change from linear production to the CE in the PSC. Insufficient information on the recycling and reuse of medicine and related benefits results in hesitation to change. There is an absence of technical skills in applying the CE in the PSC while saving on costs.	Social factors determine the demand for medications by consumers of pharmaceutical products and their medication disposal behaviours.
(T) [2,92,110]	Secure information sharing systems are needed within medication tracking systems. Technology makes it easier to engage with patients. Technology helps minimise the stockpile of medications on the shelf and efficiently manage the stock. Advanced medicine manufacturing technology supports the transition to CE.	The cost of developing and applying a new advanced technology to transition to the CE is high. There is inadequate expertise in running the technical equipment needed for the CE in the PSC.	The PSC relies on technology for production and efficiency in its operations.
(L) [82,111,112]	Proposals concerning the reduction of waste produced by pharmaceutical manufacturers support the CE. Regulations on standards of pharmaceutical distribution process support the CE.	There is a lack of systems to measure and assess the CE in the PSC. There is a lack of effective legislation on poor waste management. The existing laws are not clear about pharmaceutical producers' responsibility for waste management.	The PSC requires legal regulations to guide supply chain operations.
(E) [62–64]	Pharmaceutical and biotech companies' high levels of energy consumption drive them to seek more eco-friendly means of operation. Emphasis that is placed on the benefits of recycling, reusing and reducing medicines supports the production of medicines in a CE. Needs to change the poor management of pharmaceutical disposal methods.	There is a lack of adequately set strategies on the recycling and reuse of medicine in an environmentally friendly way. Existing laws are not clear about the responsibility of the producers regarding waste management. Individuals' awareness of proper medicine disposal is low.	The PSC is a sector that must meet high standards of quality, which are achieved by improving existing environmental conditions.

In CE implementation, a definitive objective is to hold the essential value of items using an item for as long as might be feasible and in a closed loop, such as reuse and recycle. The most suitable path must be explored in terms of approaches and legislation in order to set up circular material dissemination in a closed circle and ensure the sufficiency of the production and consumption of pharmaceuticals. Progress towards CE implementation requires interactions between specialists, the legislation, the supply chain, production frameworks, and utilisation, which are controlled and characterised through authoritative, financial, and instructive instruments.

4. Discussion

It is clear from the literature presented above that there is a discerning focus on pharmaceutical waste management across multiple channels; however, what is not evident is a binding mechanism, a home for the disparate initiatives and practices to come together and make sense for the users to adopt when tackling pharmaceutical waste. We posit that the Circular Economy philosophy offers this.

Officially, pharmaceutical waste management is an exceptionally specialised field that must be managed by qualified, skilled, and experienced staff at the administrative and ground levels. A large amount of waste is generated in healthcare institutions, due to a lack of proper systems, inadequate training, and a lack of balance between supply and demand within the healthcare inventory management system, which can increase financial and environmental issues. Proper measures should be taken, especially medicinal stock management, evaluation, quantification, procurement, and utilisation, in order to improve the supply chain and minimise waste. There are many examples of excellent practice that aspire to reduce, reuse, and recycle medicines, as noted in this study, but more needs to be done to maximise these efforts and offer clear steering on standardised methods that can be adopted and built into pharmacy practice. We see clear reference in this work to the basic 3Rs of CE, Reduce, Reuse, and Recycle, but endorsing CE in its entirety would prompt pharmacy, pharma, and healthcare professionals to consider the use of green product design, production, logistics, and dispensing to patients to move closer to the optimal 9Rs of CE.

Pharmaceutical waste management can also be both exacerbated and more effectively managed by the actions of healthcare providers and patients by inappropriate prescribing, repeat medication requests, lack of compliance to medication regimes, and stockpiling, as highlighted earlier in the paper. Measures can be taken in order to identify sources of waste creation and take steps to address these to maximise product utilisation when in the system as a finished product, but also reduce additional risk to the patient, their families in their homes (by returning unwanted stock to pharmacies), and also the environment (using safe disposal methods). The role of the patient in supporting effective pharmaceutical waste management should not be underestimated.

From a systemic approach, the adoption of the CE and associated principles can support waste reduction across the entire pharmaceutical supply chain. While reusing and recycling medicine helps to reduce pharmaceutical waste from environmental and economic perspectives, their application needs further improvement and approval by economic and government authorities and endorsement from all supply chain stakeholders. Moreover, it is important to redesign the current pharmaceutical product life cycle to facilitate medication reuse and minimise waste.

Four key aspects of creating a Circular PSC (CPSC) related to the internal mechanisms of associations and the duties of various PSC actors have been identified. Figure 2 shows how these aspects are interconnected and how they affect the implementation of the CPSC.

A set of legislative guidelines regarding the reuse of medicines must be set in order to limit wastage and introduce CE principles throughout the PSC, endorsed by all stakeholders. By resolving conflicting goals and involving all stakeholders, including packaging manufacturers, recyclers, decision makers, society, and consumers, pharmacists can legitimately and supportively influence patients' understanding of proper medicine use and commitment to reducing waste generation through proper use and disposal. They can also educate their patients on medicine-related issues, such as proper medicine use, pharmaceuticals waste, and appropriate disposal and return methods for unused and expired medications.

Thus, the use of the CE as a binding mechanism for existing and potential waste reduction practices can improve pharmaceutical waste management. Table 6 shows the changes needed related to moving from a linear chain (take, make, dispose) to a circular (proposed practice) PSC under an analytical level. Table 7 shows a systemic multi-level appraisal of practice changes that can be undertaken to move from a linear chain (take, make, dispose) to a circular PSC (proposed practice to expand product lifespan and material reuse).

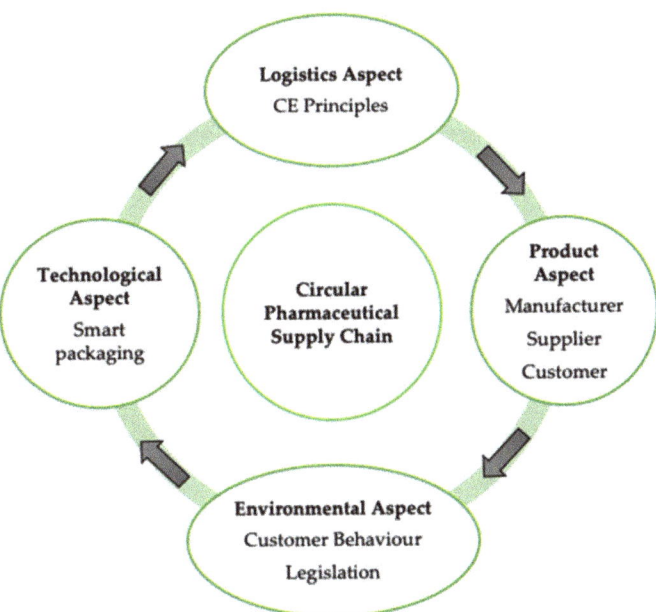

Figure 2. Aspects of the Circular Pharmaceutical Supply Chain (CPSC).

Table 7. Proposed changes needed to move toward a Circular PSC.

Level of Analysis	Focus Area	Consideration for Change
Meta Level (Global) E.g., WHO, UN, International Federation of Pharmacists	Recognition and endorsement Policy generation	Global recognition of pharmaceutical waste levels. Inclusion of waste reduction targets in global sustainability policy
Macro Level (National) E.g., government, suppliers/wholesalers, healthcare bodies, pharma advisory bodies	Recognition and endorsement Resource allocation CE philosophy acknowledgment Financial support Adoption of innovative technologies Awareness and education	Endorsement of CE agenda in the pharmaceutical supply chain. Agreement to provide resources to target pharmaceuticals waste reduction Acknowledgment of the value of CE philosophy in the design of waste reduction policies and practices Financial support for innovative technologies to deliver green design/logistics Building awareness of the 3Rs of CE (reduce, reuse, recycle) into pharmacist education Design and delivery of awareness campaigns to healthcare professionals and patients (co-designed output)
Meso Level (Organisational) E.g., hospitals, community pharmacies, GP, healthcare professionals	System design and delivery Patient education delivery and support Facilitation of medicine returns/design of collection channels Resource allocation Champion identification Strategic organisational approach to waste reduction	Creation of efficient medicine management systems to minimize waste creation and ensure safe disposal Engage in patient education to raise awareness of medicine use and waste creation channels Design effective channels for medicine returns/collections Dedicate time for medicine management training regarding ordering, storage, reuse/recycling Build teams to facilitate medicine stock management/retrieval from wards, conduct returns audits and safe disposal Identify champions to support pharmaceuticals waste reduction practices

Table 7. Cont.

Level of Analysis	Focus Area	Consideration for Change
Micro Level (Individual) E.g., pharmacy staff, manufacturers, suppliers wholesaler, distributors, patients	Awareness of pharmaceuticals waste creation Awareness of medicine returns Facilitation of returns Civic responsibility Engagement in educational campaigns	Engage in an educational campaign on the scale of pharmaceuticals waste and the financial, social and environmental repercussions associated with poor medicine management Adopt a personal responsibility to reduce pharmaceuticals waste as part of civic duty Work with stakeholders to design simple mechanisms to prompt medicine returns (e.g., text messages, flyers).

The proposition is based on moving from the linear traditional approach of making products, use, and dispose, to (1) designing for potential future re-use (having components that can be remanufactured/reconfigured to be part of a new product e.g., inhaler cartridges); (2) making only what is needed; (3) using in a thrifty manner (both support SEP philosophy); (4) reusing products/components where possible (e.g., API extraction); (5) disposing in an environmentally safe capacity; and, (6) offering growth capacity in order to promote greener practices and a 9R agenda. Figure 3 shows the changes factors needed for CPSC.

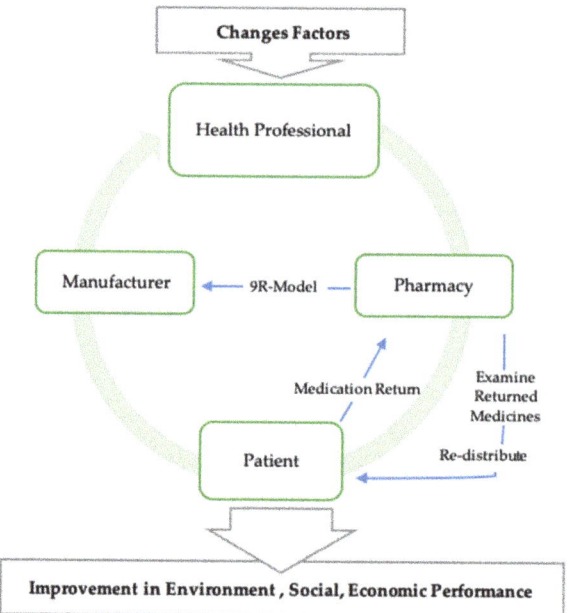

Figure 3. Circular Pharmaceutical Supply Chain (CPSC).

The limitations of this study are that it is theoretical and as such the conceptual model developed does need to be considered further and tested. Further research would be to undertake qualitative analysis with stakeholders in the PSC in order to determine their views on current waste management practices and the application of CE principles to the PSC and the adoption of CPSC.

5. Conclusions

This study aimed to determine whether the application of circular economy principles can minimise pharmaceuticals waste and support sustainability in the pharmaceutical supply chain. The results show that there are a multitude of practices that are used in order to reduce pharmaceuticals waste, but these are not always targeted or informed by any guiding principles or strategies. The CPSC as designed advocates that all stakeholders in the supply chain should contribute to effective management of medicines which includes design, production, use, reuse, and recycling (at its optimal level incorporating 9R practices). The following conclusions are proposed.

In our exploration of the application of CE to the PSC and the conceptual model produced, the CPSC, we acknowledge that there are existing examples of CE in this supply chain, but these reflect the application of the 3Rs as opposed to the wider remit of CE, the 9Rs. How the 9Rs can be applied throughout the PSC is unclear at present.

The success of the embodiment of the CPSC relies on both government and professional body endorsement and the recognition of pharmaceuticals waste management in pharmacist training and development. It also requires the inclusion of skills from other disciplines, e.g., engineering and management (for product/technology/systems development), in order to ensure greener thinking from product conception through to use and safe disposal by the patients.

Author Contributions: A.A. conceived, conducted the literature review and prepared the manuscript. L.B., conceived, critically reviewed and revised the manuscript. G.Q. reviewed and revised the manuscript from a pharmaceutical perspective. U.S. reviewed and revised the manuscript from a management/circular economy perspective. All authors have read and agreed to the published version of the manuscript.

Funding: This research received no external funding.

Conflicts of Interest: The authors declare no conflict of interest.

References

1. WHO. Guidelines for Safe Disposal of Unwanted Pharmaceuticals in and After Emergencies. 1999. Available online: https://www.who.int/water_sanitation_health/medicalwaste/unwantpharm.pdf (accessed on 1 March 2020).
2. Hui, T.; Mohammed, B.; Donyai, P.; McCrindle, R.; Sherratt, R. Enhancing Pharmaceutical Packaging through a Technology Ecosystem to Facilitate the Reuse of Medicines and Reduce Medicinal Waste. *Pharmacy* **2020**, *8*, 58. [CrossRef]
3. PSNC. Essential Facts, Stats and Quotes Relating to Prescriptions. 2014. Available online: https://psnc.org.uk/services-commissioning/essential-facts-stats-and-quotes-relating-to-prescriptions/ (accessed on 7 June 2020).
4. Statista. Global Spending on Medicines 2024 Forecast|Statista, Statista. 2020. Available online: https://www.statista.com/statistics/280572/medicine-spending-worldwide/ (accessed on 27 May 2020).
5. Clark, D. Regional Expenditure on Health 2019 Statistic|Statista. 2019. Available online: https://www.statista.com/statistics/651514/identifiable-expenditure-on-health-by-region-united-kingdom/ (accessed on 24 October 2020).
6. Gebremariam, E.T.; Gebregeorgise, D.T.; Fenta, T.G. Factors contributing to medicines wastage in public health facilities of South West Shoa Zone, Oromia Regional State, Ethiopia: A qualitative study. *J. Pharm. Policy Pract.* **2019**, *12*, 1–7. [CrossRef]
7. WHO Health-Care Waste. 2018. Available online: https://www.who.int/news-room/fact-sheets/detail/health-care-waste (accessed on 23 October 2020).
8. Bungau, S.; Tit, D.M.; Fodor, K.; Cioca, G.; Agop, M.; Iovan, C.; Nistor-Cseppento, D.C.; Bumbu, A.; Bustea, C. Aspects Regarding the Pharmaceutical Waste Management in Romania. *Sustainability* **2018**, *10*, 2788. [CrossRef]
9. Kane, G.; Bakker, C.; Balkenende, A. Towards design strategies for circular medical products. *Resour. Conserv. Recycl.* **2018**, *135*, 38–47. [CrossRef]
10. Delahaye, R.; Hoekstra, R.; Ganzevles, J.; Lijzen, J.; Potting, J.; Hanemaaijer, A. *Circular Economy: What we Want to Know and Can Measure Framework and Baseline Assessment for Monitoring the Progress of the Circular Economy in the Netherlands*; PBL: Hague, The Netherlands, 2018.
11. Manavalan, E.; Jayakrishna, K. An Analysis on Sustainable Supply Chain for Circular Economy. *Procedia Manuf.* **2019**, *33*, 477–484. [CrossRef]

12. Kirchherr, J.; Reike, D.; Hekkert, M. Conceptualizing the circular economy: An analysis of 114 definitions. *Resour. Conserv. Recycl.* **2017**, *127*, 221–232. [CrossRef]
13. MacArthur. Towards the Circular Economy, Ellenmacarthurfoundation.org. 2020. Available online: https://www.ellenmacarthurfoundation.org/assets/downloads/publications/Ellen-MacArthur-Foundation-Towards-the-Circular-Economy-vol.1.pdf (accessed on 3 March 2020).
14. United Nation. Sufficient Economy Philosophy—United Nations Partnerships for SDGs Platform. 2012. Available online: https://sustainabledevelopment.un.org/partnership/?p=2126 (accessed on 17 August 2020).
15. Mongsawad, P. The philosophy of the sufficiency economy: A contribution to the theory of development. *Asia Pac. Dev. J.* **2012**, *17*, 123–143. [CrossRef]
16. Gupta, S.; Palsule-Desai, O.D. Sustainable Supply Chain Management: Review and Research Opportunities. *IIMB Manag. Rev.* **2011**, *23*, 195. [CrossRef]
17. European Parliament. Circular Economy: Definition, Importance and Benefits|News|European Parliament. 2018. Available online: https://www.europarl.europa.eu/news/en/headlines/economy/20151201STO05603/circular-economy-definition-importance-and-benefits (accessed on 27 July 2020).
18. Grdic, Z.S.; Nizic, M.K.; Rudan, E. Circular Economy Concept in the Context of Economic Development in EU Countries. *Sustainability* **2020**, *12*, 3060. [CrossRef]
19. Smol, M.; Marcinek, P.; Duda, J.; Szołdrowska, D. Correction: Smol, M., et al. Importance of Sustainable Mineral Resource Management in Implementing the Circular Economy (CE) Model and the European Green Deal Strategy. Resource 2020, 9, 55. *Resources* **2020**, *9*, 78. [CrossRef]
20. GE Healthcare. GoldSeal Refurbished Imaging Systems Reliable Quality. Certified Confidence. www3.gehealthcare.com. 2012. Available online: http://www3.gehealthcare.in/~{}/media/documents/us-global/products/goldseal-refurbished/brochures/gehealthcare-brochure_goldseal_refurbished-imaging-systems.pdf (accessed on 12 August 2020).
21. Philips. Addressing Healthcare Challenges Through Innovation. 2018. Available online: https://www.philips.com/static/annualresults/2017/PhilipsFullAnnualReport2017-English.pdf (accessed on 12 August 2020).
22. WHO. The World Medicines Situation 2011 Rational Use of Medicines. 2011. Available online: https://www.who.int/medicines/areas/policy/world_medicines_situation/WMS_ch14_wRational.pdf (accessed on 23 May 2020).
23. Narwat, A.; Sindhu, A. Practice towards disposal of medicines (unused/expired drugs) among the patients visiting tertiary care teaching hospital in Haryana, India. *Int. J. Res. Med. Sci.* **2019**, *7*, 3050. [CrossRef]
24. FDA. Drug Shortages: Root Causes and Potential Solutions. 2020. Available online: https://www.fda.gov/media/131130/download (accessed on 1 August 2020).
25. Bohmer, R.; Pisano, G.; Sadun, R.; Tsai, T. How Hospitals Can Manage Supply Shortages as Demand Surges. 2020. Available online: https://hbr.org/2020/04/how-hospitals-can-manage-supply-shortages-as-demand-surges (accessed on 2 August 2020).
26. Ali, A. Inventory Management in Pharmacy Practice: A Review of Literature. *J. Pharm. Pract.* **2011**, *2*, 151–156.
27. Khan, S.A.; Arora, D.S.; Mey, A.; Maganlal, S. Provision of pharmaceutical care in patients with limited English proficiency: Preliminary findings. *J. Res. Pharm. Pract.* **2015**, *4*, 123–128. [CrossRef] [PubMed]
28. Shafaat, K.; Yadav, V.; Kumar, B. An overview: Storage of Pharmaceutical Products. *J. Pharm. Pharm. Sci.* **2013**, *2*, 2499–2513.
29. Mayimele, N.; Meyer, H.; Schellack, N. What role does the pharmacist play in medicine management at ward level? *SA Pharm. J.* **2015**, *82*, 33–36.
30. Ofori-Asenso, R.; Agyeman, A.A. Irrational Use of Medicines—A Summary of Key Concepts. *Pharmacy* **2016**, *4*, 35. [CrossRef]
31. Makki, M.; Hassali, M.A.; Awaisu, A.; Hashmi, F.K. The Prevalence of Unused Medications in Homes. *Pharmacy* **2019**, *7*, 61. [CrossRef]
32. NHS. Medicines Re-use Pathway. 2020. Available online: https://www.leeds.gov.uk/docs/medicines%20reuse%20pathway%20and%20FAQs.pdf (accessed on 2 August 2020).
33. NHS. Medicines Policy Version 17. 2019. Available online: https://www.google.com/url?sa=t&rct=j&q=&esrc=s&source=web&cd=&ved=2ahUKEwjuw-WRkYLrAhVNqxoKHQ5qBe8QFjAAegQIBRAB&url=https%3A%2F%2Fwww.southernhealth.nhs.uk%2F_resources%2Fassets%2Fattachment%2Ffull%2F0%2F44372.pdf&usg=AOvVaw3WfBxx01PpYUC1uJmq8OI8 (accessed on 1 August 2020).

34. NHS. Moving Medicines Safely: Implementing and Sustaining a 'Green Bag' Schem. 2020. Available online: https://www.sps.nhs.uk/wp-content/uploads/2015/12/Moving_Meds_Safely-Imp_a_Green_Bag_Scheme_Vs-2.2.pdf (accessed on 1 August 2020).
35. NICE. Recommendations|Controlled Drugs: Safe Use and Management|Guidance|NICE. 2016. Available online: https://www.nice.org.uk/guidance/ng46/chapter/recommendations (accessed on 1 August 2020).
36. NHS. Stopping Managed Repeats. 2019. Available online: https://midessexccg.nhs.uk/livewell/your-medicines-your-nhs/reducing-medicines-waste/increasing-erds-and-stopping-managed-repeats/3531-1-practice-frequently-asked-questions-stopping-managed-repeats-december-2019/file (accessed on 1 August 2020).
37. Royal College of Nursing. COVID-19 Remote Prescribing|Medicines Management|Royal College of Nursing. 2020. Available online: https://www.rcn.org.uk/clinical-topics/medicines-management/covid-19-remote-prescribing (accessed on 1 August 2020).
38. Amaral, M.; Fop, L. Unused Pharmaceuticals Where Do They End up? 2013. Available online: https://noharm-europe.org/sites/default/files/documents-files/4646/2013-12%20Unused%20pharmaceuticals.pdf (accessed on 4 August 2020).
39. Michael, I.; Ogbonna, B.O.; Sunday, N.; Anetoh, M.; Matthew, O. Assessment of disposal practices of expired and unused medications among community pharmacies in Anambra State southeast Nigeria: A mixed study design. *J. Pharm. Policy Pract.* **2019**, *12*, 12. [CrossRef]
40. Dyer, C. Coroner warns about poor drug reviews after patient dies from tramadol overdose. *BMJ* **2020**, *370*. [CrossRef]
41. Hazell, B.; Robson, R. Pharmaceutical waste reduction in the NHS. *Rep. Version* **2015**, *1*, 6–23.
42. McGuire, M.J.; Iuga, A.O. Adherence and health care costs. *Risk Manag. Healthc. Policy* **2014**, *7*, 35–44. [CrossRef] [PubMed]
43. York Health Economics Consortium. Evaluation of the Scale Causes and Costs of Waste Medicines. 2010. Available online: https://discovery.ucl.ac.uk/id/eprint/1350234/1/Evaluation_of_NHS_Medicines_Waste__web_publication_version.pdf (accessed on 14 May 2020).
44. Royal College of Physicians. Less Waste, more Health: A Health Professional's Guide to Reducing Waste, RCP London. 2016. Available online: https://www.rcplondon.ac.uk/projects/outputs/less-waste-more-health-health-professionals-guide-reducing-waste (accessed on 19 May 2020).
45. Dilokthornsakul, P.; Chaiyakunapruk, N.; Nimpitakpong, P.; Jeanpeerapong, N.; Jampachaisri, K.; Lee, T.A. Understanding medication oversupply and its predictors in the outpatient departments in Thailand. *BMC Health Serv. Res.* **2014**, *14*, 408. [CrossRef] [PubMed]
46. Alhamad, H.; Patel, N.; Donyai, P. How do people conceptualize the reuse of medicines? An interview study. *Int. J. Pharm. Pract.* **2017**, *26*, 232–241. [CrossRef] [PubMed]
47. Albaroodi, K. Pharmacists' Knowledge Regarding Drug Disposal in Karbala. *Pharmacy* **2019**, *7*, 57. [CrossRef] [PubMed]
48. Alnahas, F.; Yeboah, P.; Fliedel, L.; Abdin, A.Y.; Alhareth, K. Expired Medication: Societal, Regulatory and Ethical Aspects of a Wasted Opportunity. *Int. J. Environ. Res. Public Health* **2020**, *17*, 787. [CrossRef] [PubMed]
49. Abahussain, E.; Waheedi, M.; Koshy, S. Practice, awareness and opinion of pharmacists toward disposal of unwanted medications in Kuwait. *Saudi Pharm. J.* **2012**, *20*, 195–201. [CrossRef]
50. Johnson, K.M.; González, M.L.; Dueñas, L.; Gamero, M.; Relyea, G.; Luque, L.E.; Caniza, M.A. Improving waste segregation while reducing costs in a tertiary-care hospital in a lower–middle-income country in Central America. *Waste Manag. Res.* **2013**, *31*, 733–738. [CrossRef]
51. Zhang, A.; Venkatesh, V.; Liu, Y.; Wan, M.; Qu, T.; Huisingh, D. Barriers to smart waste management for a circular economy in China. *J. Clean. Prod.* **2019**, *240*, 118198. [CrossRef]
52. White, K. UK interventions to control medicines wastage: A critical review. *Int. J. Pharm. Pract.* **2010**, *18*, 131–140.
53. Boxall, A.B.A. The environmental side effects of medication. *EMBO Rep.* **2004**, *5*, 1110–1116. [CrossRef]
54. McRae, D.; Allman, M.; James, D. The redistribution of medicines: Could it become a reality? *Int. J. Pharm. Pract.* **2016**, *24*, 411–418. [CrossRef] [PubMed]
55. Mbongwe, B.; Mmereki, B.T.; Magashula, A. Healthcare waste management: Current practices in selected healthcare facilities, Botswana. *Waste Manag.* **2008**, *28*, 226–233. [CrossRef] [PubMed]

56. Da Silva, R.B.; De Mattos, C.A. Critical Success Factors of a Drug Traceability System for Creating Value in a Pharmaceutical Supply Chain (PSC). *Int. J. Environ. Res. Public Health.* **2019**, *16*, 1972. [CrossRef] [PubMed]
57. Hui, T.K.L.; Donyai, P.; McCrindle, R.; Sherratt, R.S. Enabling Medicine Reuse Using a Digital Time Temperature Humidity Sensor in an Internet of Pharmaceutical Things Concept. *Sensors* **2020**, *20*, 3080. [CrossRef]
58. WHO Safe Management of Wastes from Health-Care Activities. 2014. Available online: https://www.euro.who.int/__data/assets/pdf_file/0012/268779/Safe-management-of-wastes-from-health-care-activities-Eng.pdf (accessed on 1 August 2020).
59. Ayele, Y.; Mamu, M. Assessment of knowledge, attitude and practice towards disposal of unused and expired pharmaceuticals among community in Harar city, Eastern Ethiopia. *J. Pharm. Policy Pract.* **2018**, *11*, 27. [CrossRef]
60. Abahussain, E.A.; Ball, D.E. Disposal of unwanted medicines from households in Kuwait. *Pharm. World Sci.* **2007**, *29*, 368–373. [CrossRef]
61. Rogowska, J.; Zimmermann, A.; Muszyńska, A.; Ratajczyk, W.; Wolska, L. Pharmaceutical Household Waste Practices: Preliminary Findings from a Case Study in Poland. *Environ. Manag.* **2019**, *64*, 97–106. [CrossRef]
62. Abdallah, Q.M.A.; Al-Haddad, M.S.M.; Al-Khathami, O.H.M.; Al-Kherish, O.H.H.; Al-Marri, K.M.T.; Al-Matani, M.F.K.; Al-Rashed, A.M.N. Knowledge, Attitude and Practice towards Discarding Unwanted Household Medicines among Univerisity Students in Western Region, KSA. *Int. J. Pharm.* **2014**, *4*, 14–21.
63. Kheir, N.; El Hajj, M.S.; Wilbur, K.; Kaissi, R.M.L.; Yousif, A. An exploratory study on medications in Qatar homes. *Drug Healthc. Patient Saf.* **2011**, *3*, 99–106. [CrossRef]
64. Bound, J.P.; Voulvoulis, N. Household Disposal of Pharmaceuticals as a Pathway for Aquatic Contamination in the United Kingdom. *Environ. Health Perspect.* **2005**, *113*, 1705–1711. [CrossRef]
65. Law, A.V.; Sakharkar, P.; Zargarzadeh, A.; Tai, B.W.B.; Hess, K.; Hata, M.; Mireles, R.; Ha, C.; Park, T.J. Taking stock of medication wastage: Unused medications in US households. *Res. Soc. Adm. Pharm.* **2015**, *11*, 571–578. [CrossRef] [PubMed]
66. UNEP. Basel Convention on the Control of Transboundary Movements of Hazardous Wastes and Their Disposal. 2014. Available online: https://www.basel.int/portals/4/basel%20convention/docs/text/baselconventiontext-e.pdf (accessed on 1 June 2020).
67. WHO. 8 Treatment and Disposal Technologies for Health-Care Waste. 1999. Available online: https://www.who.int/docstore/water_sanitation_health/wastemanag/ch10.htm (accessed on 19 May 2020).
68. Bujak, J. Thermal treatment of medical waste in a rotary kiln. *J. Environ. Manag.* **2015**, *162*, 139–147. [CrossRef]
69. Askarany, D.; Franklin-Smith, A.W. Cost benefit analyses of organic waste composting systems through the lens of time driven activity-based costing. *J. Appl. Manag. Account. Res.* **2014**, *12*, 59–73.
70. Lopez, G.; Artetxe, M.; Amutio, M.; Bilbao, J.; Olazar, M. Thermochemical routes for the valorisation of waste polyolefinic plastics to produce fuels and chemicals. A review. *Renew. Sustain. Energy Rev.* **2017**, *73*, 346–368. [CrossRef]
71. Albu, A. Landfilling or Incineration of Waste? Practices for Choosing the Appropriate Solution for Waste Management. Quality—Access to Success. *Calitatea* **2014**, *15*, 189.
72. Janagi, R.; Shah, J.; Maheshwari, D. Scenario of management of medical waste in US and UK: A review. *J. Glob. Trends Pharm. Sci.* **2015**, *6*, 2328–2339.
73. Almuneef, M. Effective medical waste management: It can be done. *Am. J. Infect. Control.* **2003**, *31*, 188–192. [CrossRef]
74. United States Environmental Protection Agency. Medical Waste. 2017. Available online: https://www.epa.gov/rcra/medical-waste (accessed on 17 November 2020).
75. Australian Government. Safe Disposal of Unwanted Medicines. 2019. Available online: https://www.tga.gov.au/safe-disposal-unwanted-medicines (accessed on 1 August 2020).
76. Connelly, D. Should pharmacists be allowed to reuse medicines? *Pharm. J.* **2018**. [CrossRef]
77. Lubick, N. Drugs in the Environment: Do Pharmaceutical Take-Back Programs Make a Difference? *Environ. Health Perspect.* **2010**, *118*, A210–A214. [CrossRef]
78. Tong, A.Y.C.; Peake, B.M.; Braund, R. Disposal practices for unused medications in New Zealand community pharmacies. *J. Prim. Health Care* **2011**, *3*, 197–203. [CrossRef]

79. Alberta Emerald Foundation. ENVIRx|RxA—Alberta Pharmacists' Association. 2015. Available online: https://rxa.ca/member-benefits/envirx/ (accessed on 1 August 2020).
80. Breen, L. Medicines Optimisation—Extracting the Last Vestiges of Value from Your Medicines. 2016. Available online: https://www.pharman.co.uk/uploads/imagelib/pdfs/Journal_articles_by_issue/JoMO_Sep_2016/Medicines%20Optimisation.pdf (accessed on 14 May 2020).
81. Xie, Y.; Breen, L. Greening community pharmaceutical supply chain in UK: A cross boundary approach. *Supply Chain Manag. Int. J.* **2012**, *17*, 40–53. [CrossRef]
82. Raja, S.; Mohapatra, S.; Kalaiselvi, A.; Rani, R.J. Awareness and Disposal Practices of Unused and Expired Medication among Health Care Professionals and Students in a Tertiary Care Teaching Hospital. *Biomed. Pharmacol. J.* **2018**, *11*, 2073–2078. [CrossRef]
83. Hsieh, D.S.; Lindrud, M.; Lu, X.; Zordan, C.; Tang, L.; Davies, M. A Process for Active Pharmaceutical Ingredient Recovery from Tablets Using Green Engineering Technology. *Org. Process. Res. Dev.* **2017**, *21*, 1272–1285. [CrossRef]
84. FDA. Chapter 56 Drug Quality Assurance 2015. Available online: https://www.fda.gov/media/75201/download (accessed on 24 October 2020).
85. Gould, H. 7 Things we Learned About Healthcare and the Circular Economy. *The Guardian*. 24 February 2016. Available online: https://www.theguardian.com/sustainable-business/2016/feb/24/opportunities-challenges-circular-economy-healthcare-live-chat-highlights (accessed on 14 April 2020).
86. Urciuoli, L.; Sternberg, H.; Ekwall, D.; Nyquist, C. Exploring security effects on transport performance. *Int. J. Shipp. Transp. Logist.* **2013**, *5*, 303. [CrossRef]
87. Agrawal, Y.K.; Shah, R.Y.; Prajapati, P. Anticounterfeit packaging technologies. *J. Adv. Pharm. Technol. Res.* **2010**, *1*, 368–373. [CrossRef]
88. Kumar, K.; Gupta, V.; Lalasa, P.; Sandhil, S. A Review on Packaging Materials with Anti-Counterfeit, Tamper-Evident Features for Pharmaceuticals. *Int. J. Drug Dev. Res.* **2013**, *5*, 26–34.
89. UK Government. Implementing the Falsified Medicines Directive: Safety Features. 2019. Available online: https://www.gov.uk/guidance/implementing-the-falsified-medicines-directive-safety-features (accessed on 28 August 2020).
90. ISO. Packaging—Tamper Verification Features for Medicinal Product Packaging. 2018. Available online: https://www.iso.org/obp/ui/#iso:std:iso:21976:ed-1:v1:en (accessed on 28 August 2020).
91. Snell, E. Benefits, Challenges of Secure Healthcare Data Sharing. 2017. Available online: https://healthitsecurity.com/features/benefits-challenges-of-secure-healthcare-data-sharing (accessed on 2 July 2020).
92. WHO. WHO Guidelines on Transfer of Technology in Pharmaceutical Manufacturing. 2011. Available online: https://www.who.int/medicines/areas/quality_safety/quality_assurance/TransferTechnologyPharmaceuticalManufacturingTRS961Annex7.pdf?ua=1 (accessed on 1 July 2020).
93. WHO. Circular Economy and Health: Opportunities and Risks. 2018. Available online: https://www.euro.who.int/__data/assets/pdf_file/0004/374917/Circular-Economy_EN_WHO_web_august-2018.pdf?ua=1 (accessed on 3 August 2020).
94. Pachauri, A.; Shah, P.; Almroth, B.C.; Sevilla, N.P.M.; Narasimhan, M. Safe and sustainable waste management of self-care products. *BMJ* **2019**, *365*, l1298. [CrossRef]
95. Potting, J.; Hekkert, M.; Worrell, E.; Hanemaaijer, A. *Circular Economy: Measuring Innovation in the Product Chain*; PBL Netherlands Environmental Assessment Agency: The Hague, The Netherlands, 2017.
96. UNDP Sustainable Development Goals. 2020. Available online: https://www.undp.org/content/undp/en/home/sustainable-development-goals.html#:~{}:text=The%20Sustainable%20Development%20Goals%20(SDGs,peace%20 (accessed on 28 August 2020).
97. Toh, M.R.; Chew, L. Turning waste medicines to cost savings: A pilot study on the feasibility of medication recycling as a solution to drug wastage. *Palliat. Med.* **2016**, *31*, 35–41. [CrossRef]
98. Viegas, C.V.; Bond, A.; Vaz, C.R.; Bertolo, R.J. Reverse flows within the pharmaceutical supply chain: A classificatory review from the perspective of end-of-use and end-of-life medicines. *J. Clean. Prod.* **2019**, *238*, 117719. [CrossRef]
99. FDA. Coronavirus (COVID-19) Supply Chain Update. 2020. Available online: https://www.fda.gov/news-events/press-announcements/coronavirus-covid-19-supply-chain-update (accessed on 28 August 2020).
100. Mylan. EpiPen Supply Information. 2020. Available online: https://www.epipen.com/about-epipen-and-generic/supply-information (accessed on 28 August 2020).

101. Ogden, J. Implementing the EU Falsified Medicines Directive. *Prescriber* **2019**, *30*, 30–33. [CrossRef]
102. NHS UK. Principles on the Disposal of Waste Pharmaceuticals Used Within Community Health Services. Version 3.1. 2013. Available online: https://www.sps.nhs.uk/wpcontent/uploads/2012/08/Disposal20of20Waste20Pharmaceuticals20used20within20CHS.pdf (accessed on 25 June 2019).
103. GSK Complete the Cycle|GSK UK. 2018. Available online: https://uk.gsk.com/en-gb/responsibility/our-planet/complete-the-cycle (accessed on 19 July 2019).
104. Crews, J. Prescription Drug Reuse and Recycling. *Oncol. Issues* **2019**, *34*, 2. [CrossRef]
105. Settanni, E.; Harrington, T.S.; Srai, J.S. Pharmaceutical supply chain models: A synthesis from a system view of operations research. *Oper. Res. Perspect.* **2017**, *4*, 74–95. [CrossRef]
106. NHS Novel Coronavirus (COVID-19) Standard Operating Procedure Running a Medicines Re-Use Scheme in a Care Home or Hospice Setting. 2020. Available online: https://www.gov.uk/government/publications/coronavirus-covid-19-reuse-of-medicines-in-a-care-home-or-hospice/novel-coronavirus-covid-19-standard-operating-procedure-running-a-medicines-re-use-scheme-in-a-care-home-or-hospice-setting (accessed on 1 June 2020).
107. Taylor, D. The Impact of Politics on UK Pharmacy and the Economics of Medicines Supply. 2007. *Pharm. J.* **2007**, *279*, 308.
108. WHO. WHO Guideline on Country Pharmaceutical Pricing Policies. 2015. Available online: https://apps.who.int/iris/bitstream/handle/10665/153920/;jsessionid=DD2BEA983D83DD818AA64A81F3BA3B28?sequence=1 (accessed on 5 July 2020).
109. European Commission. Leading the Way to a Global Circular Economy: State of Play and Outlook. 2020. Available online: https://ec.europa.eu/environment/circular-economy/pdf/leading_way_global_circular_economy.pdf (accessed on 5 July 2020).
110. De Groene Zaak. Governments Going Circular. 2015. Available online: http://www.govsgocircular.com/media/1354/governments-going-circular-dgz-feb2015.pdf (accessed on 9 July 2020).
111. Briguglio, M.; Spiteri, J. Enablers and Barriers to a Circular Economy. 2018. Available online: http://www.r2piproject.eu/wp-content/uploads/2018/08/R2pi-stakeholders-report-sept-2018.pdf (accessed on 6 July 2020).
112. Goodwin, E. Opinion: Circular Economy in Pharmaceutical Production Plants. 2020. Available online: https://www.cleanroomtechnology.com/news/article_page/Opinion_Circular_economy_in_pharmaceutical_production_plants/162646 (accessed on 5 July 2020).

Publisher's Note: MDPI stays neutral with regard to jurisdictional claims in published maps and institutional affiliations.

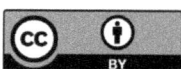

© 2020 by the authors. Licensee MDPI, Basel, Switzerland. This article is an open access article distributed under the terms and conditions of the Creative Commons Attribution (CC BY) license (http://creativecommons.org/licenses/by/4.0/).

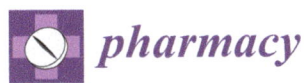

Review

Towards Medicines Reuse: A Narrative Review of the Different Therapeutic Classes and Dosage Forms of Medication Waste in Different Countries

Hamza Alhamad [1,2,*], **Nilesh Patel** [1] and **Parastou Donyai** [1]

[1] Department of Pharmacy, University of Reading, Reading RG6 6AP, UK; nilesh.patel@reading.ac.uk (N.P.); p.donyai@reading.ac.uk (P.D.)
[2] Department of Pharmacy, Zarqa University, 132222 Zarqa, Jordan
* Correspondence: halhamad@zu.edu.jo

Received: 2 September 2020; Accepted: 27 November 2020; Published: 1 December 2020

Abstract: Background: Medicines reuse, the idea of re-dispensing returned medicines to others following quality control, is yet to be implemented in the UK. This practice is potentially a sustainable way of dealing with returned medicines, which are otherwise classed as medication waste and destroyed. To inch towards medicines reuse, it is important to know more about the different therapeutic classes and dosage forms that make up medication waste. For example, it is helpful to know if medicines being returned are mostly solid-dosage forms and thus have the potential to be reused or are from therapeutic classes that would make medicines reuse cost-effective. Little is known about the therapeutic classes and the dosage forms of wasted medicines. This study aimed to narratively review and report findings from the international literature on the different therapeutic classes and the dosage forms of medicines that are returned by patients to community pharmacies, hospitals, general practitioners' clinics, or collected through waste campaigns. Studies based on surveys without physically returning medicines were also included where relevant. Methods: A comprehensive electronic search of databases, including PubMed and Google Scholar, was carried out over one month in 2017 and updated by 5 November 2020, using a combination of carefully created keywords. Results: Forty-five studies published in English between 2002 and 2020, comprising data from 26 countries were included and reviewed. Oral solid dosage forms (mostly tablets) were the commonly reported dosage form of all wasted medicines in 14 studies out of the 22 studies (64%) that described the dosage form, with percentages ranging from 40.6% to 95.6% of all wasted medicines. Although there was variability among the levels of medication waste reported in different countries, findings from the UK and Ethiopia were relatively consistent; in these, medicines for the cardiovascular system and anti-infective medicines, respectively, were the most common therapeutic classes for medication waste. Conclusion: This narrative review provides insights about the different therapeutic classes and dosage forms of medication waste either returned by patients, collected through waste campaigns, or indicated in survey responses. The findings could help policy makers understand the potential implications of treating most unused medicines as medication waste and whether therefore pursuing a medicines reuse scheme could be environmentally or financially logical. The quality and the safety of these returned medicines using criteria related to the storage conditions (such as heat and humidity), physical shape (such as being sealed, unopened, unused, and in blister packaging), and tampering are other important considerations for a medicines reuse scheme.

Keywords: medicines reuse; medication waste; therapeutic class; dosage form; sustainability; waste management

1. Introduction

Waste can be referred to as any substance or object the holder discards, intends to discard, or is required to discard [1]. The World Health Organisation (WHO) defines pharmaceutical or medication waste as "expired, unused, spilt, and contaminated pharmaceutical products, drugs, vaccines and sera" [2]. Medication waste is a growing problem in the UK and different parts of the world in terms of its negative impact on governmental expenditures, the environment, and human health [3–7]. Waste associated with prescribed medicines cost the National Health Service (NHS) in England an estimated £300 million a year in 2009, £110 million of which related to medicines returned to community pharmacies for disposal [6]. However, the financial cost is only one part of the medication waste burden. The negative impact on the environment is also significant with one reason for finding pharmaceuticals in the water environment [7] being the improper disposal of medication waste [8,9]. The presence of medication waste in the environment can modify the physiological function of living creatures and has been linked to the possible emergence of antibiotic-resistant bacteria such as vancomycin-resistant enterococci and beta-lactam-hydrolysing Enterobacteriaceae [10], as well as the feminising effects of endocrine deactivating compounds such as ethinyl estradiol [11]. The risk to human health is not limited to pollution and contamination of the drinking water, as there is also a risk when others in the home consume unused medicines that have been stockpiled but ought to have been dealt with safely. For example, patients might self-medicate for a new illness with medication previously prescribed for a different illness, causing harm through misdiagnosis or mistreatment [12]; there might be accidental poisoning if children use stockpiled medicines; and medicine abuse might occur where the medicines are controlled or have addictive properties [13].

The causes of medication waste are divided into preventable (e.g., patient stockpiles medicines, overprescribing, or repeat dispensing of unwanted medicines), non-preventable (e.g., death of a patient, or a change in the prescription meaning the previous medicines are no longer required) and non-adherence behaviours [1,6,14]. Therefore, prevention is one way to reduce medication waste. Preventing waste is in fact the top option according to the Waste Hierarchy, which is a grading framework that ranks waste management options according to what is best for the environment, with "prepare for reuse", "recycle", "other recovery", and "disposal" following "prevention" in decreasing preference order [15]. Many interventions have been attempted to prevent medication waste, but these have not always been effective, as the most common causes of medication waste are actually non-preventable [14]. Medicines reuse—the idea of re-dispensing returned medicines to others following quality control—is an underexplored concept in the UK but could help reduce medication waste regardless of the cause. What is more, qualitative studies have previously analysed intentions and actions towards the reusing of medication waste, reporting a possible future for the idea [16–19]. Numerous factors influence the practicalities of such an idea, including the prior storage conditions, as well as the therapeutic classes and the dosages forms of medicines considered to be waste but which might then be reused. Knowing information about the different therapeutic classes and dosage forms of medication waste creates some understanding of which medicines might potentially be up for reuse. For example, it is helpful to know if medicines being returned are mostly solid-dosage forms (thus having the potential to be reused), or liquids, injectables, etc., and whether these medicines are over the counter (cheaper/not critical to NHS costs) or other therapeutic classes that could be more relevant in terms of environmental sustainability or cost-effectiveness.

Despite a thorough literature review on the causes of medication waste [6,14,20–23], the financial [4,6,20,24–28] and environmental impact of medication waste [7,10,11], medicine disposal practices [8,9,22,24,28–34], and management strategies of medication waste [6,14], only some studies have reported the type and therapeutic classes and dosage forms of unused or returned medication waste, and none have brought the information together in a focused review [6,23,28]. This study aimed to narratively review and report findings from the literature about the different therapeutic classes and the dosage forms of medication waste that are returned by patients to community pharmacies, hospitals, general practitioners' clinics, or collected through waste campaigns in different countries around the world. Results from studies based on surveys (without the physical return of medicines) were also included to take account of relevant data collected via this alternative method.

2. Materials and Methods

A search of electronic databases was carried out over one month in 2017 and updated in 2020 ending on 5 November 2020 to identify reports and studies published in English detailing therapeutic classes and dosage forms of medication waste. Electronic databases searched comprised PubMed/Medline, Cochrane library, Grey literature (open grey and British library), National Audit Office (NAO), and National Institute for Health and Care Excellence (NICE) evidence. The bibliographies of retrieved references were also searched.

The search activity used combinations of a list of terms that included the following: types of unused medicines OR classes of unused medicines OR dosage forms of unused medicines OR types of medicine waste OR classes of medicine waste OR dosage forms of medicine waste OR types of unused drugs OR classes of unused drugs OR dosage forms of unused drugs OR types of drug waste OR classes of drug waste OR dosage forms of drug waste.

The inclusion criteria aimed to select studies published in English that reported the therapeutic classes and dosage forms of returned medication waste, either dispensed following a prescription or purchased over the counter (OTC), or a medicine sample that had expired (or had no clear expiry date) or was never fully consumed (or not used at all). Studies describing medical waste, medical device waste, and/or clinical tissue waste were excluded.

Study selection was completed by two researchers (H.A. and N.P.) using a Preferred Reporting Items for Systematic Reviews and Meta-Analyses (PRISMA) flow of identification, screening, eligibility, and inclusion [35] (Figure 1). At first, 3390 candidate studies were identified; then, 18 duplicates were removed. All study titles and abstracts of the remaining 3372 studies were screened, with 3311 studies removed, resulting in 61 potentially eligible studies. After a thorough full-text review of the 61 studies to assess for eligibility, 45 studies published between 2002 and 2020 were included in this narrative review. Data obtained from the retrieved studies described demographic information of the participants, the types and dosage forms of medication waste, study settings and sample size, and the time/duration of the collection of the returned medicines (varying from 4 weeks up to 12 months).

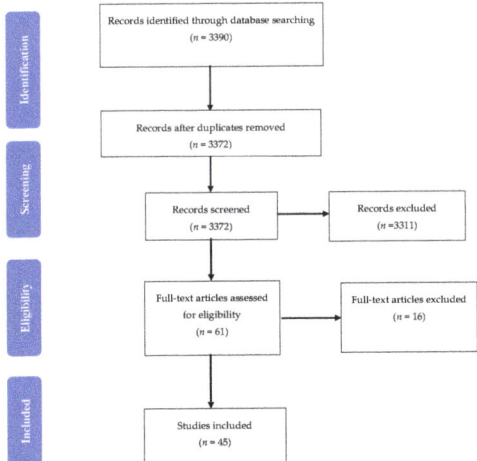

Figure 1. Literature search scope using the PRISMA flow chart adapted from the PRISMA Group, 2009 [35].

3. Results

The search yielded 3390 candidate studies. A total of forty-five studies published between 2002 and 2020 and comprising data from 26 different countries from around the world (Australia, Austria, Egypt, Ghana, India, Jordan, Kuwait, Malaysia, Mexico, New Zealand, Oman, Qatar, Saudi Arabia, Spain, Taiwan, Tanzania, Thailand, United Arab Emirates, United Kingdom, United States of America, China, Malta, Indonesia, Iraq, Nigeria, and Ethiopia) were included and reviewed. In some of these studies, medication waste was returned by patients to community pharmacies, general practitioners' clinics, hospitals or sometimes collected via medicine take-back and medicine waste campaigns. However, twenty nine (the majority) studies used a survey to collect information about the therapeutic classes and dosage forms of medication waste by asking participants for information without physically collecting the waste: six studies from Ethiopia [36–41], three from India [42–44], two from Malaysia [24,45], two from the USA [34,46], two from Jordan [47,48], two from Egypt [26,49], two from Thailand [20,50], one from Qatar [51], one from China [52], one from Iraq [53], one from Indonesia [54], one from Nigeria [55], one from Spain [56], one from Saudi Arabia [27], one from Tanzania [57], one from Malta [58], and one from Ghana [59]. The methodologies used and the targeted populations are summarised in Appendix A Table A1.

3.1. Studies' Samples

The studies' samples were reported in different ways. Most studies reported sample size as the number of medication waste items returned or collected. Other studies reported the sample as per weight (kg), per bag, packs, or containers of the collected returned medication waste. The sample for survey-based studies was reported as the number of completed questionnaires collected or the number of participants surveyed. For more details about the sample of the studies included, please refer to Appendix A Table A1.

3.2. Demographics of the Participants

Gender was not reported in the majority of the studies (Appendix A Table A1). Fifteen studies (36% of the retrieved studies) described the gender of the participants, and it was not apparent that there is a gender difference associated with the presence/reporting of medication waste. For example, more women took part in seven of the studies [20,38,45,52,54,56,57] and more men took part in eight of the studies [36,37,39,40,42,49,55,59]. In the study from Egypt [49], the number of people who returned their medication waste happened to be more male than female and one study from Malaysia [24] recruited female students only.

Age of participants was described in 23 studies out of 45 studies (51%) (Appendix A Table A1). Participants' age profile varied in these studies and was up to 81 years. Twelve studies of the 23 studies (25%) found an apparent relationship between the mean number of returned medicinal items per patient and their age. Here, the majority of medication waste was reported to be from participants with the age ranges of 60–80 years [21,31,32,49,57]. Two studies [43,59] had more data relating to participants in the age range 20–40, but this was an artefact of the study designs, focussing on students who are likely to be in that younger age range. It is not possible to conclude that the age range of 60–80 years was associated with more medication waste as, additionally, age data was absent from half of the studies (49%).

3.3. Dosage Forms of Returned Medication Waste

Dosage forms were investigated in 22 out of the 45 studies (49%) on medication waste (Appendix A Table A2). Dosage forms included a range of oral solid dosage forms (tablets, capsules, granules, powders, and lozenges), liquids (syrups, injections, eye drops, suspensions, emulsions, and lotions), semisolids (ointments, creams, gel, paste and suppositories), and other items such as inhalers, sprays, patches, strips, and chewing gum. Oral dosage forms were the most commonly reported formulation in fourteen studies out of 22 (64%) with percentages ranging from 40.6% to 95.6% of all medication waste. Moreover, tablets were reported to be the most common of the oral dosage forms.

One study from Oman (60) reported that during handling of the dosage forms, most of them appeared in a suitable condition for reuse and were still in their original container. However, some had changed in colour, consistency, and odour and therefore were deemed not to be suitable for reuse. Results from a UK study [36] were consistent with the Oman study [60] in which many of the returned medication waste items were reported to be in a condition suitable for reuse as assessed by a pharmacist. These were the only two studies that directly commented on whether the medication waste returned was potentially suitable for reuse.

3.4. Therapeutic Category of the Returned Medication Waste

Except for two studies [31,57] in which only prescribed medicines were included in the authors' analysis, the majority of the studies include both prescribed and OTC medicines. Moreover, only three studies [25,26,61] included medicinal samples in addition to prescribed and OTC medicines.

The majority of the studies (42 out of the total 45) reported the therapeutic category of the medication waste, and these were included in the current analysis (Appendix A Table A2). The remaining three studies reported the medication waste individually by generic or brand name and were therefore excluded from the current analysis.

The therapeutic categorisation systems used for reporting the findings were not the same in all studies. Seven studies used the British National Formulary (BNF) categories [6,26,49,60,62–64]. Seven studies used the Anatomical Therapeutic Chemical Coding (ATC) of the WHO [33,36,48,56,58,65,66]. Other ways of therapeutic categorisation included national codings such as the Saudi National Formulary (SNF) [27], Chinese Pharmacopoeia [52], and the Monthly Index of Medical Specialities online (MIMS) [20]. The remaining studies used disease and class of medicine classification such as diabetes/anti-diabetic. A breadth of therapeutic categories reported included cardiovascular system (CVS), central nervous system (CNS), alimentary tract/gastrointestinal tract (GIT), respiratory system, musculoskeletal system and joint disease, analgesics and antipyretics, non-steroidal anti-inflammatory drugs (NSAIDs), endocrine system, malignant disease and anticancer medicines, nutrition and blood, vitamins and minerals, gynaecology and medicines for urinary tract infection (UTI), antibiotics, medicines for ear, nose, and oropharynx, and skin medicines.

Eight studies out of the 42 (19%) reported that CVS medicines were the most common therapeutic category of medication waste [6,32,49,60,62–64,66]. Similarly, eight studies out of 42 (19%) reported that anti-infective medicines were the most common therapeutic category of medication waste [26,36–41,57]. CNS medicines were reported in five studies out of the 42 (12%) as the most common therapeutic category of medication waste [21,31,47,51,65].

The different therapeutic categorisation systems used in reporting medication waste (sometimes in studies completed in the same country) make the interpretation of results difficult. For example, two studies, one from India [42], and one from the USA [25], combined analgesics with nonsteroidal anti-inflammatory drugs (NSAIDs) into one therapeutic category, while five studies from India [43], the USA [34,46], Mexico [61], and Thailand [50] described analgesics and antipyretics as one category and musculoskeletal and joint disease medicines as another category. In addition, the number of studies that investigated medication waste by therapeutic categorisation was more likely to be from a small number of countries. For example, seventeen studies out of forty-two (40%) were from four countries: the UK [6,13,62,64], Ethiopia [36–41], New Zealand [21,31,65,67], and the USA [25,34,46]. This makes reporting of the results by the number of studies less representative of the international literature.

Therefore, in order to synthesise the results for this narrative review, all the different therapeutic categories were re-classified according to the BNF categorisation system and then represented by country (Figure 2). For example, NSAIDs were re-classified under musculoskeletal system medicines (BNF Chapter 10), analgesic and antipyretics were re-classified under CNS medicines (BNF Chapter

4), and alimentary tract system medicines were re-classified under gastrointestinal system medicines (BNF Chapter 1). In addition, in countries where more than one report was found, such as the Ethiopia, UK, New Zealand, Jordan, and Egypt, the sum of all returns of medication waste was calculated and reported by country.

Figure 2 shows the results of the common therapeutic categories of medication waste reported by country and after re-classification according to the BNF categorisation system. In the UK, CVS medicines were the most common therapeutic class of medication waste, with CNS medicines being the second most common therapeutic class. Other therapeutic categories of medication waste, such as gastrointestinal and respiratory medicines, were also reported but less commonly in the UK. Similar results to the UK were reported from countries such as Australia, Austria, Mexico, and Oman where CVS medicines were the most common therapeutic class of medication waste. Moreover, in Mexico, Australia, and Austria, musculoskeletal system medicines were also common and the second most reported category.

In New Zealand, CNS medicines were the most common therapeutic class of medication waste. Other therapeutic categories such as gastrointestinal, cardiovascular, and musculoskeletal system medicines (with diclofenac sodium and ibuprofen reported to be commonly returned as waste) were also reported in studies from New Zealand but less than CNS medicines. In Jordan and Qatar, results were similar to New Zealand, where CNS medicines were the most common therapeutic class of medication waste. In Jordan and Qatar, paracetamol was the most common individual tablet considered as waste. In addition, in Jordan, gastrointestinal medicines were reported as the second most common therapeutic class of medication waste followed by anti-infective medicines. In Qatar, anti-infective medicines were reported as the second most common therapeutic class of medication waste. Other therapeutic categories of medication waste such as musculoskeletal system medicines were reported in Jordan and Qatar but less commonly.

In Spain, both the gastrointestinal system and CNS medicines were the most common therapeutic classes of medication waste. In Taiwan, gastrointestinal system and CVS were the most common therapeutic classes of medication waste. While in Saudi Arabia, both the respiratory system and CNS medicines were the most common therapeutic classes of medication waste.

In Ethiopia, Egypt, and Tanzania, anti-infective medicines were the most common therapeutic class of medication waste. The CNS medicines (in Ethiopia), and CVS medicines (in Egypt and Tanzania) were reported as the second most common therapeutic class of medication waste. Other therapeutic categories of medication waste such as musculoskeletal and gastrointestinal system medicines were reported in Ethiopia, Egypt, and Tanzania, but less so.

Studies from the USA, Thailand, India, and Indonesia showed that musculoskeletal system medicines were the most common therapeutic class of medication waste in these countries. Finally, in Malaysia, vitamins and minerals were the most common therapeutic category of medication waste.

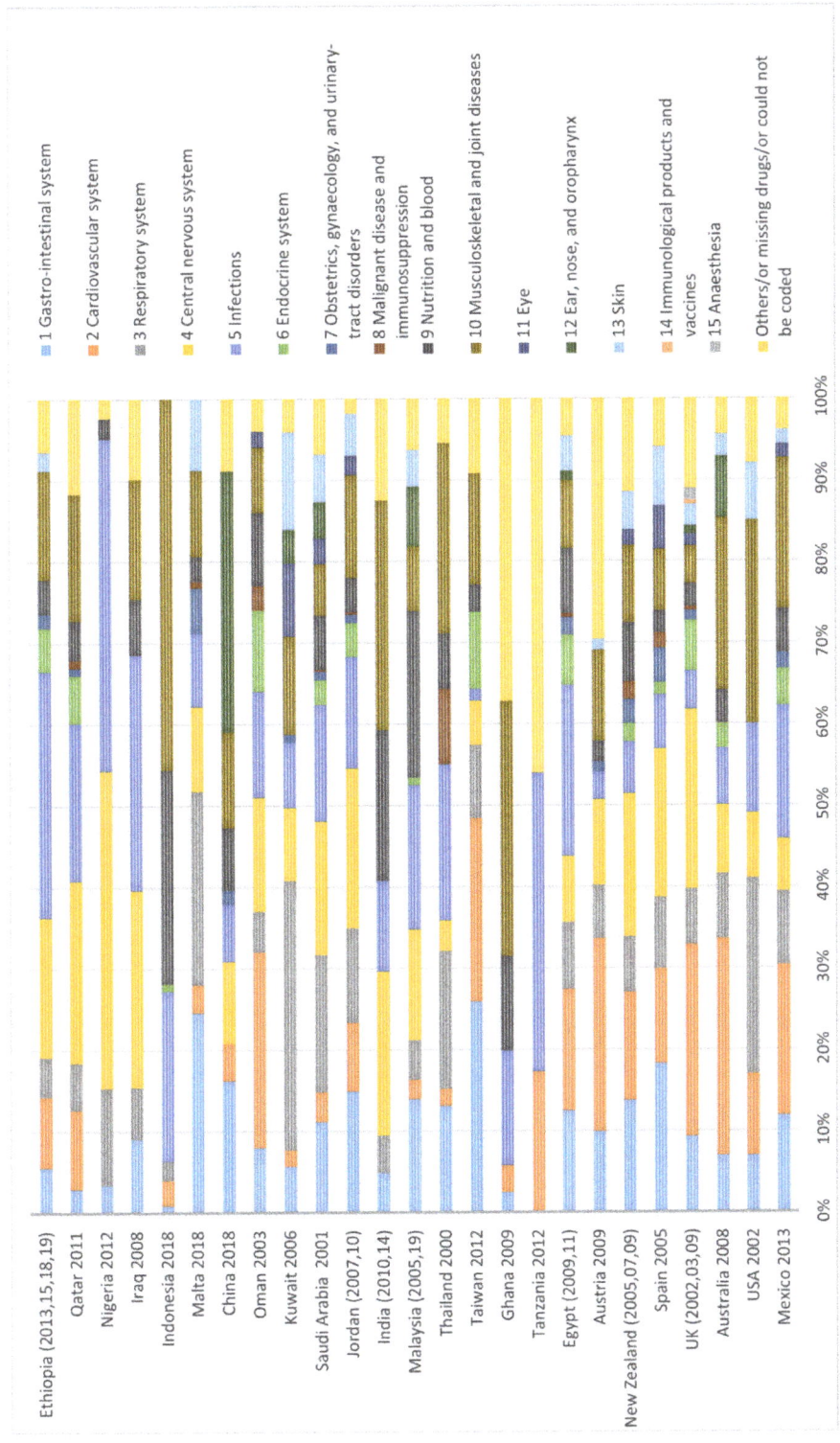

Figure 2. The common therapeutic categories of medicine waste reported from different countries in the world by year of data collection, re-classified according to the British National Formulary (BNF) categorisation system.

4. Discussion

Despite the extensive literature on medication waste, no literature review to date had explicitly focused on the therapeutic classes and the dosage forms of medication waste items. This narrative review addresses that gap. The principal finding is that CVS (certainly in the UK) and anti-infective (certainly in some African countries) medicines are reported as some of the most commonly returned/accumulated medication waste category. Arguably, knowing the therapeutic category of medication waste is as crucial as the quantity of the returned medication waste in terms of environmental and financial potential for medicines reuse. This is because medicines in certain therapeutic categories cost more. For example, one UK study [63] reported the volume of waste relating to respiratory system medicines to be about half (8%) that reported for CNS medicines (19%), but the cost of the medicines in the respiratory group was about the same as those in the CNS category. Thus, knowing the therapeutic categorization of medication waste makes it easier to judge where medicines reuse might be financially logical. It is of course essential to quality assure the safety of any returned medicines using criteria related to the storage conditions (such as heat and humidity), physical shape (such as being sealed, unopened, unused, and within blister packs), and tampering. Two studies conducted in Oman [60] and the UK [63] directly commented on whether the medication waste returned was potentially suitable for reuse. These studies reported that during handling of the dosage forms, most of the returned medicines appeared in a suitable condition for reuse and were still in their original container, with only a few having changed in colour, consistency, and odour; thus, these were deemed unsuitable for reuse. Findings of these studies are also important considering that unused medicines from the so-called developed world are sometimes sent for reuse to so-called developing countries.

In the UK, CVS medicines were the most common therapeutic class of medication waste. A possible explanation is that CVS medicines are one of the commonly prescribed medicines in the UK, comprising approximately 20% of all the medicines prescribed because of the prevalence of cardiovascular disease. Moreover, CVS medicines are one of the commonly amended classes of medicines because of frequent changes in doses and drugs necessitated by guidelines [62]. In Ethiopia, Egypt, and Tanzania, anti-infective medicines were the most common therapeutic class of medication waste. This is possibly because antibiotics have been available without a prescription in these countries, where also it is common for people not to complete their course of antibiotic treatment when their symptoms resolve. In New Zealand and Jordan, CNS medicines were the most common therapeutic class of medication waste with paracetamol as the most common individual tablet returned as waste. The potential explanation here is that analgesics (with paracetamol reported to be the most common) are frequently used for the self-medication of headaches, which is a commonplace discomfort. Similarly, in the USA, Thailand, and India, the musculoskeletal system medicines were the most common therapeutic class of medication waste with NSAIDs being the most common group reported in these countries, again reflecting their common usage. In the study from Malaysia, vitamins and minerals were reported as the most common therapeutic category of medication waste, but this is likely an artefact of the methods, which only sampled female students.

This narrative review synthesised information about the most commonly found medication waste products from different countries around the world. However, the results should be interpreted carefully. First, the findings apply to medication waste that was returned by patients only or reported in surveys and does not take into account the substantial amount of medication waste likely to be disposed of into household garbage or via the sink or simply kept stockpiled unreported at home [65]. Second, the small sample size and the small number of returns of medication waste in the majority of the studies made these studies less likely to be representative of a global picture. Third, the CNS classification of paracetamol as the most commonly reported item as waste raised the percentages of waste from the CNS therapeutic class compared to other therapeutic classes such as musculoskeletal, alimentary tract, and respiratory systems. Paracetamol is considered cheap, and one may argue that it is not worthwhile to set up a medicines reuse system if this is the largest category of returned medicines in any one country. Fourth, the quality of the studies included in this narrative review was not checked because of the disparity of methods and a lack of specific criteria, which could affect the results reported (as none of the papers found were excluded) and could be seen as another limitation of this study. Finally, the results of this narrative review cannot be generalised. For example, results from Ethiopia, Egypt, and Tanzania of having antibiotics as the most common therapeutic category of medication waste cannot be generalised (although reported to be the commonest along with CVS medicines) to other countries where antibiotics are only available with a prescription such as in the UK or the USA. In addition, results from the two Malaysian studies, which reported that vitamins and minerals were the most common therapeutic category of medication waste, is impossible to generalise to the larger population, as one study was only completed with female Malaysian students (no males). The other Malaysian study was also completed by more females than males.

This narrative review has other limitations that should also be acknowledged. First, it included results from reports, theses, audits, and the grey literature, but there is always a risk that some studies were not included as a result of not performing a thorough enough systematic search. Second, the search strategy was restricted to studies that were published in the English language only and so could have missed other valuable research. Third, the reasons behind the accumulation of the returned medication waste from each therapeutic category were not clearly evidenced in all the studies. Some studies provided possible explanations that may apply only to the country from which data were obtained, and therefore, it may not be appropriate to generalise these explanations. Finally, information about what motivates people to return their medication waste and if they returned a certain type of medication waste over others were not investigated and remain unknown.

This review is the first to provide narrative information about the different therapeutic categories and dosages forms of returned medication waste from different countries around the world. Pooling information about the different therapeutic classes and dosage forms of medication waste can help increase knowledge about medicines that are returned unused and or otherwise classed as wasted medicines, so that extrapolations can be made about the costs of waste and whether it is worthwhile to reuse these medicines. For example, paracetamol is considered cheap, and one may argue that it is not worthwhile to set up a medicines reuse system if this is the largest category of returned medicines in any one country. In addition, oral solid dosage forms are more likely to be suitable candidates for reuse compared to other dosage forms such as liquids or injectables; therefore, it is useful to know where this is the most commonly returned formulation. However, a pharmacist's hand inspection of such medicines would not be sufficient to address concerns about the quality and the safety of returned medicines. For example, there would also need to be additional checks in place for storage conditions (e.g., under excessive heat and humidity), and physical characteristics (such as being sealed, unopened, unused, and being in a blister) which could indicate (non-)tampering, degradation or contamination, in addition to the visual indicators. These concerns would need to be addressed before medicines reuse becomes a reality [23,68], and one way to do this would be through the application of technology [69,70].

This narrative review identified a large number of studies from the literature that investigated the different therapeutic classes and the dosage forms of medication waste returned by patients to healthcare settings, and through waste campaigns, as well as information obtained from survey responses. Although there was variability among the levels of medication waste reported in different countries, findings from some countries such as the UK and Ethiopia were relatively consistent and appeared to reflect the local usage of these medicines. This suggests that medication waste categories might be proportional to the prevalence of medicines in each specific country, which remains to be tested in future studies. Future studies that focus on assessing the quality and the safety of retuned medicines, and exploring public and healthcare providers' perception about medicines reuse should also be performed before medicines reuse becomes a reality. For example, contained sites such as long-term care facilities or hospice care settings where the medications are presumably stored correctly might be more capable of reusing medicines and could be a realistic site for trialling medicines reuse in the future.

5. Conclusions

Findings from this narrative review provide insight about the different dosages forms and the therapeutic classes of medication waste, which can be used to support future medicines reuse-related research and explorations. It appears that the therapeutic categories of medication waste are reflecting prevalence of usage, inviting policy makers in each country to reflect on whether medicines reuse could be cost-effective in their own settings. Any medicines reuse scheme would still need to consider quality and safety checking of returned medicines over and above the pharmacists' visual checks.

Author Contributions: P.D.: Conceptualisation, Supervision, Project administration, Validation, Visualisation, Writing—Reviewing and Editing, Resources. N.P.: Conceptualisation, Supervision, Project administration, Validation, Visualisation, Writing—Reviewing and Editing, Resources. H.A.: Conceptualisation, Methodology, Investigation, Data Curation, Formal analysis, Validation, Visualisation, Writing—Original draft preparation. All authors have read and agreed to the published version of the manuscript.

Funding: This research was part of a PhD project sponsored and funded by Al-Zarqa University (under the regulation of the Jordanian Ministry of Higher Education).

Acknowledgments: We thank Zarqa University for the funding of the PhD project.

Conflicts of Interest: The authors declare that they have no conflict of interest to disclose.

Appendix A

Table A1. Summary of the research instrument, sample, and demographics of the included studies.

Year of Study	Author(s)	Country/Settings	Research Instrument	Wasted Medicines Information (e.g., Take Back Campaigns vs. Survey)	Sample	Demographics
2015	Gracia-Vásquez et al. [61]	Mexico; nine cities of Monterrey	Unused/expired medications were collected from households in a special container placed in a visible and accessible location in 85 collection centres in community pharmacies located in nine cities in the Monterrey metropolitan area over 12 months from March 2012 to February 2013	Take back program.	Random sample of 22,140 items, 30% of total drugs collected over 12 months), as 70% were unable to be classified.	Not studied.
2008	Braund et al. [21]	New Zealand	Over a five-week period medications were returned to two collection point pharmacies and questionnaires were completed by returners.	Take back program. In addition, a questionnaire was completed to determine the reasons that the medications were not used.	163 returns, comprising of 1399 items, with only 126 returned questionnaires.	The majority of those returning medications fall within the age range of 61–80 years.
2007	Braund et al. [67]	New Zealand; Otago Pharmacies	Medications returned unsolicited to Otago pharmacies over a 9-month period, from 1 April to 31 December 2005.	Take back program.	A random sample (159 kg, 12%) of the 1294 kg of medications returned for destruction over a nine-month period from the Otago region were identified.	Not studied.
2009	Braund et al. [31]	New Zealand; Hutt Valley District Health Board	A Disposal of Unwanted Medication Properly (DUMP) campaign was conducted for 4 weeks in November 2007 in 31 community pharmacies. Questionnaires were completed by the returners.	Take back program. 'Disposal of Unwanted Medication Properly (DUMP)' campaign.	Of the total 1605 bags returned over 4 weeks for disposal, only 329 bags (20%), containing a total of 1253 items were fully analysed. Only 653 questionnaires were completed (41%).	The age distribution of the patients with unused medications was <20 (8%), 21–40 (13%), 41–60 (28%), 61–80 (40%) and >81 years (11%).
2010	Caroline et al. [29]	New Zealand; Nelson Bays region	A Disposal of Unwanted Medication Properly (DUMP) campaign was conducted for 5 weeks in November and December 2009 and for 3 weeks afterwards. Surveys were completed in 379 bags.	Take back program. 'Disposal of Unwanted Medication Properly (DUMP)' campaign.	Of the 6500 DUMP bags distributed across the Nelson Bays region, 1244 bags were returned (response rate 19%), with an average of 7 items per bag (number of items returned 8609).	Not studied.

Table A1. Cont.

Year of Study	Author(s)	Country/Settings	Research Instrument	Wasted Medicines Information (e.g., Take Back Campaigns vs. Survey)	Sample	Demographics
2009	James et al. [65]	New Zealand: Taranaki region (around 37,000 households)	Unused medications returned for disposal to the 24 community Pharmacies in the Taranaki region (≈37,000 households) of New Zealand over 6 weeks.	Take back program.	716 individuals returned 3777 items of unused medications. Of the 3777, information for the amount issued and returned was complete for 2704. The majority (51%) of returns contained 75–100% of the original dispensed amount of medication.	Not studied.
2005	Langley et al. [62]	United Kingdom; East Birmingham	Unused medications returned to 8 community pharmacies and 5 general practices (G.P.) surgeries over 4 weeks each (4 weeks during August 2001, 4 weeks during March 2002, respectively).	No return campaign was conducted and no attempt was made to encourage patients or carers into returning medicines. Medicines returned to 8 community pharmacies and 5 general practices (G.P.) surgeries over 4 weeks were assessed.	A total of 114 returns; 24 (21.1%) to G.P. surgeries and 90 (78.9%) to community pharmacies. The total returns comprised 340 items, of which 42 (12.4%) were returned to G.P.s and 298 (87.6%) to community pharmacies.	Older patients (60 years and over) returned 61.4% of items with 24.6% of returns coming from patients aged 30–59 years and 5.3% of returns originating from patients under 30. Ages were not recorded for 8.7% of returns.
2007	Mackridge et al. [63]	United Kingdom; Eastern Birmingham Primary Care Trust (P.C.T.)	Unused medications returned to pharmacies and G.P. surgeries were collected over 8 weeks in May and June 2003 in Eastern Birmingham Primary Care Trust (P.C.T.). Three-quarters of the P.C.T. sites participated, 51/60 (85%) pharmacies and 42/61 (70.5%) G.P. surgeries.	Unused medicines were returned and data were collected in Eastern Birmingham Primary Care Trust (PCT), a predominantly urban PCT with an ethnic minority population of 20%.	934 return events were made from 910 patients (190 GP surgeries, 744 pharmacies), comprising 3765 items (431 GP surgeries, 3334 pharmacies) and totalling 4934 individual packs.	The mean age of 63.5 ± 0.78 years (10 months to 99 years) and there was no detectable correlation between the mean number of items returned per patient and their age.
2008	Bradley [64]	United Kingdom; Cumbria	A medicine waste audit in community pharmacies of Cumbria where each pharmacy asked to analyse 20 returns of unused medicines. Further qualitative data were collected by interviewing the patients and their representatives.	Unused medicine were returned to community pharmacies in Cumbria where each pharmacy was asked to analyse 20 returns of unused medicines.	A total 4563 items was received from 87 community pharmacies across Cumbria.	Not studied.
2010	Trueman et al. [6]	United Kingdom	Unused medications returned to 114 pharmacies (51 from London/urban, 32 from North-West/rural and urban, 24 from Yorkshire and Humber/rural and urban, 7 from West-Midlands/rural) from 5 primary care trusts.	Unused medicine were returned to 114 pharmacies in 5 primary care trusts.	In total, 8626 items were reported as returned with 7500 of the returned items identified and coded for analysis.	Not studied.

Table A1. *Cont.*

Year of Study	Author(s)	Country/Settings	Research Instrument	Wasted Medicines Information (e.g., Take Back Campaigns vs. Survey)	Sample	Demographics
2008	Coma et al. [56]	Spain; Barcelona	Unused medications returned to random sample of 118 community pharmacies in Barcelona invited to participate. 38 (32%) agreed to participate. Data were collected from February to April 2005. Questionnaires were completed by the returners.	Unused medications were collected from 38 community pharmacies over a period of 7 consecutive working days (excluding Sundays). A questionnaire was designed to evaluate each returned medicine.	In total, 1176 packages were returned by 227 patients. The majority were medicines (96.6%), and the rest were medical supplies or devices (0.5%) or other products sold in the community pharmacy (2.9%; e.g., personal care, nutrition). Most medicines returned were drugs for human use (99.8%) and only 0.2% were for veterinary use.	54.6% women, 64 ± 20 years old.
2015	Law et al. [46]	U.S.A.; Southern California	Cross-sectional, observational two phases study was conducted using a convenience sample in Southern California. In Phase I, a web-based survey was conducted at one health sciences institution; and in Phase II, a paper-based survey at drug take back events.	Web and paper-based survey.	Phase I: A total of 539 prescription medications were reported, with an average of 4 per household. Approximately 7% of the unused medications were expired, and 30% were brand name. Phase II: Of the 776 unused medications returned for disposal, 311 (40%) medications were brand name. Nearly two-thirds (66.2%) were expired, discontinued by the physician (25%), or became unused after the patient indicated feeling better (17.6%).	Phase I: Average household age was 36.4 years, but not described in Phase II which the drug take back program.
2004	Garey et al. [25]	U.S.A.; Houston, Texas	Unused medications returned to community pharmacy during "Medicine Cabinet Clean up Campaign" over 6 months between April and September 2002 (pilot study).	"Medicine Cabinet Clean up Campaign"	In total, 1315 medication containers were returned to the community pharmacy. 63% of returned medications were dispensed between 2000 and 2002, 31% from 1995 to 1999, and 6% before 1995.	Not studied.
2015	Maeng et al. [34]	U.S.A.; Regional health plan in Central Pennsylvania	Telephone survey conducted by a survey research centre.	Telephone survey.	Not studied.	Not studied.

Table A1. Cont.

Year of Study	Author(s)	Country/Settings	Research Instrument	Wasted Medicines Information (e.g., Take Back Campaigns vs. Survey)	Sample	Demographics
2014	Vogler et al. [66]	Austria; Vienna	Unused medications collected from household garbage in all districts of Vienna between 12 October and 24 November 2009.	Unused medicines ending up in household garbage were analysed in all districts of Vienna.	In total, 152 packs were identified from manually investigated sample from household garbage in Vienna.	Not studied.
2013	Chien et al. [71]	Taiwan; Shuang-Ho university teaching hospital	Discarded drugs were collected from the Drug Discarding Bin at the Shuang-Ho Hospital over 4 weeks.	Discarded drugs from the Drug Discarding Bin at the Shuang-Ho Hospital in Taiwan were collected and analysed. A paper-based questionnaire was utilised to study the attitudes and perspectives of the out-patients and/or patients' family members about discarding unused medications that were prescribed and covered by the National Health Insurance policy.	A total of 98 kg (51,972) discarded medications collected from the hospital Drug Discarding Bin.	Not studied.
2013	Abushanab et al. [48]	Jordan; Amman	Cross sectional survey using a pre-piloted questionnaire was used in the interview of 219 households in 9 areas of Amman to about the types of drugs stored at home conducted between November 2009 and April 2010.	Survey study.	From the 2393 drug products presented in surveyed households, 24.99% was considered as drug waste (drug wastage, calculated as the sum of drug products that had expired 10.91%, had no clear expiration date 1.84%, or which had never been used since dispensing 15.04%).	Age of the interviewee (years) 42.15 ± 14.67.
2012	Al-Azzam et al. [47]	Jordan; North of Jordan particularly Irbid	Validated questionnaire was administered to 435 households selected randomly from different areas in the north of Jordan (particularly in Irbid governorate) in the period from April 2007 and until August 2007.	Survey study.	Of the total of 2835 medication items found in the 435 selected houses, 65.3% were in use, and 34.7% were not in use.	Age of the interviewee (years) 36.4 (±11.9).

Table A1. Cont.

Year of Study	Author(s)	Country/Settings	Research Instrument	Wasted Medicines Information (e.g., Take Back Campaigns vs. Survey)	Sample	Demographics
2002	Abou-Auda [27]	5 regions in Saudi Arabia and other Gulf countries (Kuwait, U.A.E., Qatar, and Oman)	A questionnaire was administered to a total of 1641 households participated in the study (1554 in Saudi Arabia; 87 in other countries).	Survey study.	A total of 12,463 drug products were found in 1554 households in Saudi Arabia. Among the 87 households surveyed in the 4 other Gulf countries, 616 drug products were found.	Not studied.
2011	Kheir et al. [51]	Qatar	This was a cross-sectional, exploratory, descriptive study. Households included in the study were identified using a list of home telephone numbers was selected randomly from the telephone directory maintained by Qtel®, Qatar's national telephone company.	Survey study.	Four hundred and thirty-two phone calls were made to invite respondents to take part in the study. Eighty-one household representatives initially expressed interest in being part of the research during the first call, of whom 49 participants (18% of the targeted sample size) answered all survey questions.	Not reported.
2007	Al-Siyabi et al. [60]	Oman; Sultan Qaboos University Hospital (SQUH)	Observational study of returned unused medicines to the pharmacy at SQUH between February and June 2003.	Returned medicines received by pharmacy staff were analysed in the study.	A total of 1171 items (medications) were returned to the pharmacy at SQUH; among these, 99 drugs were excluded. Medicines were included only if they had SQUH patients' labels, and any items without SQUH patient' labels were excluded from study.	Not studied.
2004	Wongpoowarak et al. [20]	Thailand; Songkhla	A cross-sectional survey of unused medicines of a random sample of 931 households in the Songkhla. Of the 931 households surveyed and interviewed by using a structured questionnaire, there were 453 (48.7%) where at least one person reported having unused medications.	Survey study.	A total of 1004 unused medication (items) were identified from 523 respondents who had unused medications in 453 households. Nine items could not be identified because their physical appearance did not match that of any known medication. Thus, 995 items were included.	Gender: Male: 224 (42.8%). Female: 299 (57.2%). Age: 0–9 years: 167 (31.9%). 10–19 years: 52 (10.0%). 20–29 years: 66 (12.6%). 30–39 years: 76 (14.5%). 40–49 years: 64 (12.2%). 50–59 years: 40 (7.7%). ≥60 years: 58 (11.1%).

Table A1. Cont.

Year of Study	Author(s)	Country/Settings	Research Instrument	Wasted Medicines Information (e.g., Take Back Campaigns vs. Survey)	Sample	Demographics
2013	Sooksriwong et al. [50]	Thailand; 4 regions of Thailand: Bangkok, Chiang Mai, Khon Kaen, Mahasarakham and Songkla	Structured questionnaire developed to survey 357 households which were interviewed and during January and March 2011: 46% in Bangkok and 54% in upcountry.	Survey study.	2208 drug items were found in 357 households. 952 items (43%) of these drug items were dispensed by public hospitals, 750 items (34%) were from drug stores, 163 items (8%) were from private hospitals and 210 items (10%) were from others.	Not studied.
2011	El-Hamamsy [26]	Egypt; Cairo	Pilot study where all drugs returned unused to 20 community pharmacies in Cairo over period of one month (April 2009).	All drugs returned unused to 20 community pharmacies located in Cairo, Egypt were documented during April 2009. A total of 316 patients completed a survey about medication disposal practices.	A total of 541 drugs were returned and collected over one month.	Not studied.
2012	Ibrahim et al. [49]	Egypt; Alexandria	A cross-sectional descriptive study where all drugs returned unused to randomly selected 60 pharmacies in Alexandria over a period of one month during March 2011.	Survey study.	A total of 657 drugs were returned from 600 patients to the 60 pharmacies over one month.	Males constituted the higher percentage of the participants 56.7%. Elderly having 60 years or above constituted the highest proportion of the sample (28.3%), while the lowest percentage (4.0%) was within the age group (10 to less than 20).
2010	Guirguis et al. [32]	Australia; St Vincent's Hospital, Melbourne	Retrospective audit looked at all expired medications or those no longer needed were collected at St Vincent's Hospital, Melbourne over 2 months (July and August 2008).	Retrospective audit looked at all the items collected over a period of 2 months: July and August 2008.	A total of 293 items were collected from 40 patients recruited over 2 months.	Older than 65 years of age.

Table A1. Cont.

Year of Study	Author(s)	Country/Settings	Research Instrument	Wasted Medicines Information (e.g., Take Back Campaigns vs. Survey)	Sample	Demographics
2014	Kagashe et al. [57]	Tanzania; tertiary hospital in Dar ES-Salaam city	Cross-sectional study carried out at a tertiary hospital in Dar es Salaam city Tanzania where patient files were analysed for last admission treatment information for the year 2012.	Survey study.	About 56.3% of medicines prescribed were dispensed to patients. Out of the total 1418 dispensed drugs, 730 medicines were wasted.	The mean age of the study population was 44 years, with minimum age of 11 years and maximum of 88 years. Medicines wastage was reported from female more than in male (404 (55.7%) vs. 326 (47.1%), respectively).
2007	Abahussain et al. [33]	Kuwait; Kuwait city	Municipal collection program of unwanted medicines from households in Kuwait City.	Take back collection program.	Sample of 200 households in Kuwait received an educational letter and special plastic bags in which to place unwanted medicines to be collected by the municipality. A second convenience sample of an additional 14 households in Kuwait received the same educational letter together with a face-to-face interview and assistance in collecting unwanted medicines.	Not studied.
2013	Aditya [43]	India; dental hospital in North India	Descriptive cross-sectional survey of dental students based on a structured questionnaire format) was carried out in a teaching dental hospital in North India.	Survey study.	244 students, with 8 students were excluded due to incomplete forms only 236 were included.	Age of participants from 20 to 40 years.
2011	Gupta et al. [42]	India; Greater Noida City	A simple randomised prospective survey study that was carried out for a period of six months in selected areas of Greater Noida City. Randomly selected 102 houses were visited to educate and assess the people about Home Medicine Cabinet.	Survey study.	A total of 392 people were surveyed in 92 houses with the exception of 10 houses.	Of the total 392 people surveyed: The male vs. female for those with age >12 years is 144 (36.73%) vs.133 (33.93%), respectively. The male vs. female for those with age <12 years is 69 (17.6%) vs. 46 (11.74%), respectively.

Table A1. Cont.

Year of Study	Author(s)	Country/Settings	Research Instrument	Wasted Medicines Information (e.g., Take Back Campaigns vs. Survey)	Sample	Demographics
2014	Mirza and Ganguly [44]	Anand district of Gujarat, India	A cross-sectional study was conducted during 2012–2014. Data were collected from 800 houses, 400 each from urban and rural areas and then analysed for the details of medicines available in the house.	Survey study.	A total of 800 houses, 400 each from urban and rural areas, were included for the study, which was based on the prevalence of self-medication as per a previous study done in India.	The participants above the age of 18 years, capable of giving information of medicine use within the family (the heads of the households or their spouses or any adult capable of delivering required information) were interviewed for the study. The presence of any healthcare professional amongst the family members in a visited house was excluded in order to avoid biased answers.
2009	Ali et al. [24]	Malaysia; Universiti Sains	A prospective descriptive, cross-sectional survey was conducted from February to June 2005 in the Universiti Sains, Malaysia.	Survey study.	A total of 481 single female respondents were targeted for a questionnaire-based survey on randomly sampled students. A total of 1724 different types of medicines were found with an average number of 4 medicines found per student.	Respondent were only females ages varied from 19 to 54 years old. 89.2% ($n = 429$) of the students were categorised in the 19–24 years age category, while 8.7% ($n = 42$) were aged between 25 and 30 years old. The remaining 2.1% ($n = 10$) were aged between 31 and 54 years.
2020	Hassali and Shakeel [45]	Selangor, Malaysia	The quantitative, cross-sectional study was conducted by face-to-face interviews using a pre-validated structured survey form in Selangor, Malaysia from September to December 2019.	Survey study.	Among the approached 600 individuals, 426 showed their willingness to participate in the study. Hence, the response rate of the present study was 71%.	A large proportion of the respondents (269; 63.1%) were females. Most of the respondents were Malay (378; 88.7%), followed by Chinese (32; 7.5%). The study population included students, private and public sector employees, and housewives, who were over 18 years of age. More than half of the respondents were bachelor's degree holders (220; 51.6%).

Table A1. *Cont.*

Year of Study	Author(s)	Country/Settings	Research Instrument	Wasted Medicines Information (e.g., Take Back Campaigns vs. Survey)	Sample	Demographics
2014	Aboagye et al. [59]	Ghana	The study was conducted over selected areas in Ghana with a questionnaire were randomly issued out from 13 to 20 December 2009.	Survey study.	Out of the 200 questionnaires sent out, 180 were retrieved and analysed.	The majority of the respondents 62.8% (113/180) were between the ages of 21 and 40 years, and the minority 5.6% (10/180) were above 61 years. A total of 99 (55%) of the respondents were males corresponding to 81 (45%) females.
2019	Huang et al. [52]	China, six provinces in North, Central, and Southern regions of China	A cross-sectional survey of 625 households survey was carried out between March and April 2018 in China.	Survey study.	We randomly sampled 1000 households from the communities according to community population information registration forms. At the end of the period, after removal of incomplete responses, a total of 625 completed and usable questionnaires were received, equating to a response rate of 62.5% (625/1000).	The majority of respondents, 61.9% (387/625) in the households visited were females. A high proportion 60.6% (379/625) of the respondents were employees from different companies. In terms of age groups, 78.4% (490/625) of respondents were less than 30 years old, and 12.0% (75/625) of the respondents were aged between 31 and 45.
2019	Vella and West [58]	Malta, Maltese village	The study was conducted from 1 April to 31 December 2018 within a community pharmacy in a small Maltese village with 3500 inhabitants.	Survey study.	A total of 411 medications were collected, amounting to a total cost of approximately €2600.	Not reported.

Table A1. *Cont.*

Year of Study	Author(s)	Country/Settings	Research Instrument	Wasted Medicines Information (e.g., Take Back Campaigns vs. Survey)	Sample	Demographics
2020	Insani et al. [54]	Bandung, Indonesia	A descriptive cross-sectional study was conducted in Bandung, Indonesia, from November 2017–January 2018.	Survey study.	A total of 497 respondents completed the questionnaire.	A total of 497 respondents completed the questionnaire of which many were female (n = 366, 73.6%) and aged between 18 and 30 years (n = 424, 85.3%). More than half of them completed secondary education (n = 326, 65.6%) and about one-third (n = 167, 33.6%) were university graduates. A large proportion of respondents were students/university students (n = 342, 69.0%).
2010	Jassim [53]	Basrah, Iraq	This is a descriptive study involving a questionnaire survey to determine the extent of drug storage and self-medication in 300 household units Basrah, Iraq between 2007 and 2008.	Survey study.	A total of 300 household units in Basrah, Iraq included in this study. A survey was conducted in 300 households in Basrah, southern Iraq to determine the availability, source, and storage conditions of medicinal drugs and the prevalence of self-medication with antimicrobials.	Not reported.
2012	Auta et al. [55]	Nigeria	A cross-sectional survey of a random sample of 240 undergraduate pharmacy students of the University of Jos, Jos, Nigeria, was carried out.	Survey study.	A total of 240 students were chosen randomly with at least 50 from each professional level/year to participate in the study. A pre-tested, self-administered questionnaire was distributed among participants after explaining the purpose of the study and obtaining oral informed consent.	A total of 188 of the 240 (representing 78.3%) questionnaires administered were completely filled and returned by respondents. The respondents consisted of 55.3% males and 44.7% females with the majority of the respondents between the ages of 21 and 25 years.

Table A1. Cont.

Year of Study	Author(s)	Country/Settings	Research Instrument	Wasted Medicines Information (e.g., Take Back Campaigns vs. Survey)	Sample	Demographics
2015	Wondimu et al. [41]	Tigray Region, Northern Ethiopia	A community-based cross-sectional study was conducted in April 2013 in Tigray Region, Ethiopia.	Survey study.	A total of 1034 participants were enrolled in the study. A multi-stage sampling method was employed to select households.	Overall, 1000 (97%) households responded to the interview, among them 504 urban and 496 were rural. The median family size of the households was 5; just above half (52%) of the households had at least five family members. Only 7% of the surveyed households had a health professional as a family member.
2017	Teni et al. [36]	Gondar town, northwestern Ethiopia	A cross-sectional household survey was conducted from 5 April to 6 May 2015. In the study, 809 households were surveyed from four sub-cities selected through multi-stage sampling with 771 included in the final analysis.	Survey study.	In the study, 809 households were surveyed from four sub-cities selected through multi-stage sampling with 771 included in the final analysis.	Of the participants of the study that represented their respective households, upwards of three quarters (76.3%) and two-fifths (40.9%) were female and those in the age group of 18 to 29 years, respectively. Nearly three-fourths (73.3%) followed Orthodox Christianity, and almost all (90.3) were Amhara in their ethnic identity.

Table A1. Cont.

Year of Study	Author(s)	Country/Settings	Research Instrument	Wasted Medicines Information (e.g., Take Back Campaigns vs. Survey)	Sample	Demographics
2019	Ebrahim et al. [37]	Awi zone, Amhara regional state, Ethiopia	A facility-based cross-sectional study design supplemented by a qualitative approach was conducted from 23 April to 22 May 2018.	Survey study.	A total of 4 health facilities were included in the study. During the 1 month of the study period, 56 types of medications were found unused at the health facilities.	Three of the heads were male and one was a female. All of them were BSc nurses with a work experience of a minimum of 4.6 and a maximum of 8 years. All the pharmacy heads were male and degree holders with a minimum experience of 4 years and maximum experience of 8 years. A total of 3 store women and 1 store man were interviewed. All the store men/women were diploma holders with a work experience of a minimum of 4 years and a maximum of 8 years.
2020	Gudeta and Assefa [39]	Jimma city, Ethiopia	A facility-based descriptive cross-sectional study was conducted among private practitioners in retail outlets of Jimma city from 20 November to 19 December 2018.	Survey study.	All drug shops, 35 (62.5%) and pharmacies, 21 (37.5%) in Jimma city, were visited, 3 of which were used for pre-testing. A total of 106 questionnaires were distributed to practitioners in 53 retail outlets, of which 87 returned the completed questionnaires, making a response rate of 82.1%.	The majority of the practitioners, 44 (50.6%) were within the age range of 25 to 31 years. More than half, 56 (64.4%) of them were males. Regarding their profession, the majority of them were pharmacy professionals, 73 (83.9%).

Table A1. Cont.

Year of Study	Author(s)	Country/Settings	Research Instrument	Wasted Medicines Information (e.g., Take Back Campaigns vs. Survey)	Sample	Demographics
2020	Kahsay et al. [40]	Adigrat city, Ethiopia	A cross-sectional study was conducted using semistructured questionnaires, which focussed on knowledge, attitudes, and disposal practices for unused and expired medications were used to collect data from respondents.	Survey study.	The study was conducted among 359 respondents from the residents of Adigrat city, Ethiopia. All of the 359 returned questionnaires were valid for data entry and analysis.	All the approached 359 individuals agreed to participate in the study. Of the 359 respondents, 207 (57.7%) were males. The majority (137; 38.2%) of the respondents were 32 years old and above. Concerning their educational level, one hundred and twelve (31.2%) respondents completed secondary education, 178 (49.6%) had a college/university degree and above, and 31 (8.6%) were illiterate.
2020	Yimenu et al. [38]	Awi zone, Amhara regional state, Northwestern Ethiopia	A community-based cross-sectional study was conducted through interviews with representatives of households.	Survey study.	A total of 23 kebeles (the smallest an administrative unit in Ethiopia) (2 urban and 21 rural kebeles) from four woredas were selected using a multi-stage sampling technique. A total of 507 households were included in the study.	The majority of the study participants, 368 (72.6%), were female. The mean age of the study participants was 40 years, and the majority were between the ages of 30 and 65 (67.9%)
2020	Yimenu et al. [38]	Awi zone, Amhara regional state, Northwestern Ethiopia	A community-based cross-sectional study was conducted through interviews with representatives of households.	Survey study.	A total of 23 kebeles (the smallest an administrative unit in Ethiopia) (2 urban and 21 rural kebeles) from four woredas were selected using a multi-stage sampling technique. A total of 507 households were included in the study.	The majority of the study participants, 368 (72.6%), were female. The mean age of the study participants was 40 years, and the majority were between the ages of 30 and 65 (67.9%)

Table A2. Summary of the therapeutic classes, dosage forms, and limitations of the included studies.

Year of Study	Author(s)	Settings/Country	Therapeutic Category of the Unused, Wasted Medicine	Dosage Form	Study Limitation
2015	Gracia-Vásquez et al. [61]	Mexico; nine cities of Monterrey	The most commonly returned medications were of nonsteroidal anti-inflammatory followed by cardiovascular drugs. Nonsteroidal anti-inflammatory drugs: 16.11%. Cardiovascular drugs: 14.21% (Anti-hypertensive 55%). Gastrointestinal drugs 11.43%. Antibacterial drugs: 10.05%. Respiratory system drugs: 8.75%. Neurological drugs: 6.13% (anti-depressant: 34%). Dietary supplement: 5.23%. Anti-diabetic drugs: 4.34%. Miscellaneous drugs: 3.79%. Hypolipemic drugs: 3.67%. Anti-parasitic drugs: 2.48%. Hormonal drugs: 1.89%. Anti-micotic drugs: 1.84%. Steroidal anti-inflammatory drugs: 1.72%. Dermatological drugs: 1.71%. Ophthalmic drugs: 1.64%. Anti-viral drugs: 1.53%.	The majority of unused/expired medications collected (73%) was in solid dosage form (tablets, capsules, granules, powders, and lozenges). 20% were liquid pharmaceutical forms (syrups, injections, eye drops, suspensions, emulsions, and lotions). 6% were semisolid (ointments, creams, gel, paste, and suppositories). 1% were other forms, such as metered dose inhalers, sprays, patches, strips, and chewing gums.	Unable to describe respondent demographic information.
2008	Braund et al. [21]	New Zealand	The most commonly returned medications were of the nervous system drugs, followed by alimentary tract and metabolism. Nervous system drugs: 17%. Alimentary tract and metabolism system drugs: 14%. Cardiovascular system drugs: 12%. Respiratory system and allergies: 11%. Musculoskeletal system drugs: 11%. Infections—agents for systemic use: 9%. Blood and blood-forming organs: 8%. Oncology agents and immunosuppressants: 6%. Genitourinary system: 5%. Dermatologicals: 3%. Sensory organs: 2%. Hormone preparations—systemic: 2%.	Only oral dosage form reported.	Small number of returned unused medication.
2007	Braund et al. [67]	New Zealand; Otago Pharmacies	The returned medications were not classified by therapeutic group, but by generic name. The most commonly returned tablet was paracetamol (9% of all tablets returned). The most commonly returned capsule was omeprazole 20 mg (8% of capsules); additionally, omeprazole 40 mg accounted for a further 5% of all capsules.	There were 65,907 tablets returned and 7599 capsules returned. Others include injections, inhalers, eye drops, creams, gels, ointment, test strips, liquids, and suppositories.	Unable to describe respondent demographic information. Unable to report unused medicines as therapeutic group.
2009	Braund et al. [31]	New Zealand; Hutt Valley District Health Board	The predominant therapeutic group was drugs affecting the nervous system, but individually, diclofenac sodium and ibuprofen were the most returned medications, respectively. Nervous system drugs: 19%. Alimentary tract and metabolism: 13%. Cardiovascular system: 12%. Musculoskeletal system: 11%. Respiratory system and allergies, and miscellaneous: 8%. Blood and blood-forming organs: 7%. Dermatological and anti-infective: 7%. Genitourinary: 3%. Hormones: 3%.	Oral solid forms (tablets and capsules) were counted. Liquid medications were quantified by the amount left in the original container, semisolid preparations were estimated as a proportion of original container. Inhalers were recorded as either full, half-full, or empty. Anything almost empty was excluded from the analysis.	The chosen sample of the total returned unused medicine was around 20%, which maybe not representative of the whole sample.

Table A2. *Cont.*

Year of Study	Author(s)	Settings/Country	Therapeutic Category of the Unused, Wasted Medicine	Dosage Form	Study Limitation
2010	Caroline et al. [29]	New Zealand; Nelson Bays region	The most common returned (top 20) by quantities (individual unit) were (n = 435,397): Salazopyrin: 94,271 tablets. Paracetamol: 23,251 tablets. Lactulose: 11,324 mL. Aspirin: 10,047 tablets. Simvastatin: 7380 tablets. Diclofenac: 7014 (mixed preparation). Prednisolone: 7004 tablets. Metoprolol: 6627 tablets. Warfarin: 6590 tablets. Furosemide: 6117 tablets. Lemnis fatty cream: 6095g. Cilazapril: 5687 tablets. (Paracetamol and codeine) preparation: 5003 tablets. Ibuprofen: 4873 tablets. Codeine: 4794 tablets. Laxsol: 4267 tablets. Morphine: 4107 (mixed preparations). Emulsifying ointment 4030 g. Quinapril: 3890 tablets.	Oral solid forms (tablets and capsules) with tablets as the most common returned dosage form. Oral liquid forms. Cream and ointment.	Unable to describe respondent demographic information.
2009	James et al. [65]	New Zealand: Taranaki region (around 37,000 households)	The predominant therapeutic group was drugs affecting the nervous system, but individually, paracetamol (acetaminophen) was the most returned medication respectively. Nervous system drugs (n = 658, 24.3%). Cardiovascular system (n = 559, 20.7%). Alimentary tract and metabolism (n = 529, 19.6%). Blood and blood-forming organs (n = 283, 10.5%). Respiratory system and allergies (n = 190, 7.1%).	Not studied.	Unable to describe respondent demographic information. In addition, due the different policies for collection and disposal of medicines, the majority of unused medicines were disposed into landfills and water system, which may mean that the returned amount may be underestimate of the extent of unused medicines.
2005	Langley et al. [62]	United Kingdom: East Birmingham	The predominant therapeutic group was drugs affecting cardiovascular system. Cardiovascular system drugs: 28.5%. Central nervous system drugs: 18.8%. Respiratory system drugs: 14.7%. Gastrointestinal drugs: 10.6%. Endocrine system drugs: 5.6%. Musculoskeletal and joint disease drugs: 5%. Anti-infective Drugs: 4.7%. Eye Drugs: 3.5%. Nutrition and blood drugs: 2.1%. Skin drugs: 1.8%. Obstetrics, gynaecology, and urinary tract disorders: 1.5%. Nutrition and blood and unknown: 1.2%. Malignant disease and immunosuppression: 0.9%.	Tablet or capsule, oral liquid, cream or ointment, and inhalers.	Sample size and the number of returns are small, which makes it difficult to extrapolate the result to the whole United Kingdom.

Table A2. Cont.

Year of Study	Author(s)	Settings/Country	Therapeutic Category of the Unused, Wasted Medicine	Dosage Form	Study Limitation
2007	Mackridge et al. [63]	United Kingdom; Eastern Birmingham Primary Care Trust (P.C.T.)	The predominant therapeutic groups were drugs affecting cardiovascular system and drugs acting on the central nervous system, respectively. The most commonly returned drugs were aspirin (102 items), co-codamol (98 items), salbutamol (96 items), furosemide (90 items), and glyceryl trinitrate (78 items). Drugs affecting cardiovascular system (1003 items, 26.6%). Drugs acting on the central nervous system (884 items, 23.5%). Drugs affecting respiratory system (358 items, 9.5%) and gastrointestinal system (358 items, 9.5%). Drugs affecting endocrine system (257 items, 6.8%). Drugs treating musculoskeletal and joint diseases (235 items, 6.2%). Anti-infective drugs (165 items, 4.4%). Drugs for skin (124 items, 3.3%). Drugs for nutrition and blood (116 items, 3.1%). Drugs for eye (65 items, 1.7%). Obstetrics, gynaecology, and urinary tract disorders (59 items, 1.6%). Drugs for ear, nose, and oropharynx (58 items, 1.5%) and others (58 items, 1.5%). Drugs for malignant disease and immunosuppression 20 items, 0.5%). Drugs for anaesthesia (5 items, 0.1%).	Tablet or capsule, oral liquid, cream or ointment, and inhalers.	The author reported that this study did not attempt to estimate the quantities of unused medicines at patient's home; as a result, it is more likely that the unused medicines from primary care was underestimated.
2008	Bradley [64]	United Kingdom; Cumbria	The greatest value of returned of medicines was from cardiovascular and central nervous system categories (BNF), total number of returns (n = 4562): Cardiovascular (n = 1232), Central nervous system (n = 1149). Gastrointestinal system (n = 468) Endocrine (n = 334). Respiratory (n = 307). Anti-infective (n = 250). Musculoskeletal and joint (n = 228). Nutrition and blood (n = 141). Skin (n = 134). Others (n = 319)	Not studied.	It is an audit report with a result from Cumbria/northwest of England, which may not representative of the whole United Kingdom and may underestimate the extent of unused medicines.
2010	Trueman et al. [6]	United Kingdom	Coding was based on guidance provided by the Royal Pharmaceutical Society of Great Britain/BNF. The most common retuned medication was for the cardiovascular and central nervous system. Cardiovascular system drugs (1950 items, 22.6%). Central nervous system drugs (1907 items, 22.11%). Gastrointestinal system drugs (828 items, 9.6%). Respiratory system drugs (528 items, 6.12%). Endocrine system drugs (518 items, 6.01%). Anti-infective drugs (444 items, 5.15%). Musculoskeletal, joint disease drugs (364 items, 4.22%). Nutrition and blood drugs (249 items, 2.89%). Skin drugs (192 items, 2.23%). Eye drugs (129 items, 1.5%). Ear, nose, oropharynx drugs (68 items, 0.79%). Malignant disease and immunosuppression drugs (53 items, 0.61%). Wound management drugs (34 items, 0.39%). Borderline substances (25 items, 0.29%). Drugs for Anaesthesia (9 items, 0.10%).	Not studied.	Unable to describe respondent demographic information.

48

Table A2. Cont.

Year of Study	Author(s)	Settings/Country	Therapeutic Category of the Unused, Wasted Medicine	Dosage Form	Study Limitation
2008	Coma et al. [56]	Spain; Barcelona	The predominant therapeutic groups were drugs affecting the alimentary tract and metabolism, nervous system, and cardiovascular system, respectively. All drugs were categorised according to Anatomical Therapeutic Chemical (A.T.C.) system/code of the World Health Organisation (WHO). Alimentary tract and metabolism drugs (215 items, 18.3%). Nervous system drugs (214 items, 18.2%). Cardiovascular drugs (137 items, 11.6%). Respiratory system drugs (103 items, 8.8%). Musculoskeletal system drugs (88 items, 7.5%). Dermatological drugs (85 items, 7.2%). Anti-infective drugs (77 items, 6.5%). Missing drugs (could not be coded according to the A.T.C. system), (66 items, 5.6%). Sensory organs drugs (63 items, 5.4%). Drugs affecting genitourinary system and sex hormones (50 items, 4.3%). Drugs affecting blood and blood-forming organs (32 items, 2.7%). Antineoplastic and immune-modulating drugs (22 items 1.9%). Systemic hormonal preparations excluding sex hormones and insulins, (17 items, 1.4%). Various drugs (5 items, 0.4%). Anti-parasitic products, insecticides, and repellents (2 items, 0.2%).	Not studied.	Unable to describe the respondent demographic information clearly.
2015	Law et al. [46]	U.S.A.; Southern California	Approximately 2 of 3 prescription medications were reported unused. In Phase I, pain medications (23.3%) and antibiotics (18%) were most commonly reported as unused. In Phase II, 17% of medications for chronic conditions (hypertension, diabetes, cholesterol, heart disease) and 8.3% for mental health problems (antidepressants/antipsychotic/anti-convulsant) were commonly reported as unused. 7% painkillers and 4% electrolytes and dietary supplements.	Tablets, pills, capsules, and liquid preparations.	Use of a web-based survey may limit the accessibility of this study to people without computer and Internet access at home, which may to some extent underestimate the extent of unused medicines. Unable to describe respondent demographic information.
2004	Garey et al. [25]	U.S.A.; Houston, Texas	The predominant therapeutic group was nonsteroidal anti-inflammatory drugs/pain 25%. Drugs for cough/cold/allergy 15%. Anti-infective drugs 11%. Cardiovascular drugs 10%. Respiratory drugs 9%. Neurological drugs 8%. Dermatological 7% and gastrointestinal 7%.	Oral medications (capsules or tablets) were most commonly returned (64%), followed by liquid (12%), creams (11%), inhalers (7%), or miscellaneous (6%; e.g., eye glasses, hearing aid batteries, medical equipment). Approximately 17,000 oral pills were collected during the study period.	Unable to describe respondent demographic information.
2016	Maeng et al. [34]	U.S.A.; Regional health plan in Central Pennsylvania	The predominant therapeutic group was pain medication (15%), hypertension (14%), antibiotics (11%), and psychiatric disorders (9%).	Not studied.	Unable to describe respondent demographic information.

Table A2. Cont.

Year of Study	Author(s)	Settings/Country	Therapeutic Category of the Unused, Wasted Medicine	Dosage Form	Study Limitation
2014	Vogler et al. [66]	Austria; Vienna	The predominant therapeutic group was cardiovascular drugs. Cardiovascular drugs (36 packs, 23.7%). Musculoskeletal system drugs (17 packs, 11.2%). Nervous system drugs (16 packs, 10.5%) Alimentary tract and metabolism 15 packs, 9.9%). Anti-infective drugs for systemic use (5 packs, 3.3%). Drugs for blood and blood-forming organs (4 packs, 2.6%). Genitourinary system drugs and sex hormone (2 packs, 1.3%) and Dermatological drugs (2 packs, 1.3%). Other A.T.C. code or not attributable (45 packs, 29.6%).	Oral medications were the most commonly founded 86.8% (usually solid oral), followed by dermal 6.7%, parental 4%, nasal 0.7%, pulmonary 0.7%, eye 0.7%, and dental 0.7%.	Unable to describe respondent demographic information.
2013	Chien et al. [71]	Taiwan; Shuang-Ho university teaching hospital	Among the discarded medications, gastrointestinal drugs were at the top of the list of all discarded medications. The analysis of discarded and unused drugs revealed that Strocain (oxethazine, polymigel) was on top of the list, followed by Glucobay (acarbose), Mopride (mosapride), and Loditon (metformin). Gastrointestinal drugs: 25.93%. Cardiovascular drugs: 22.49%. Anti-inflammatory drugs: 12.15%. Anti-diabetic drugs: 9.49%. Cold medicines: 6.83%. Psychiatric drugs: 5.44%. Respiratory drugs: 2.16%. Rheumatological drugs: 1.52%. Antimicrobial drugs: 1.42%. Others: 9.19%. Health foods: 3.38%.	Tablets, bottles, and tubes.	Unable to describe respondent demographic information.
2013	Abushanab et al. [48]	Jordan; Amman	Alimentary tract and metabolism drugs were the most commonly found in household (both used and unused). Stored drug products were classified by A.T.C. code of WHO. Alimentary tract and metabolism: 519 (20.7%). Nervous system: 370 (17.3%). Musculoskeletal system: 313 (12.9%). Respiratory system: 291 (12%). Cardiovascular system: 256 (10.9%). Anti-infective for systemic use: 252 (10.6%). Dermatological: 149 (5.4%). Blood and blood-forming organs: 109 (4.6%). Genitourinary system and sex hormones: 31 (1.1%). Systemic hormonal preparations, excl. sex hormones and insulin: 18 (1.1%). Anti-parasitic products, insecticides and repellents: 13 (0.7%). Anti-neoplastic and immune-modulating agents 8 (0.3%), sensory organs 63 (2.5%).	Not studied.	Studied the medication stored at home the estimated the unused wasted medicine as the sum of drug products that had expired, had no clear expiration date, or which had never been used since dispensing. So not directly investigate the unused wasted medicine.

Table A2. *Cont.*

Year of Study	Author(s)	Settings/Country	Therapeutic Category of the Unused, Wasted Medicine	Dosage Form	Study Limitation
2012	Al-Azzam et al. [47]	Jordan; North of Jordan particularly Irbid	Central nervous system drugs were found to be the most common, followed by anti-infective agents. The most common individual medications found were amoxicillin, paracetamol, metronidazole, antihistamines, hypoglycaemic medications, and adult cold medications. Central nervous system drugs (713 items, 25.2%). Anti-infective agents (493 items, 17.4%). Musculoskeletal agents (381 items, 13.4%) Respiratory system agents (348 items, 12.3%) Gastrointestinal agents (301 items, 10.6%) Cardiovascular agents (216 items, 7.6%) Endocrine system agents (200 items, 7.0%) Nutrition agents (127 items, 4.5%). Eye, ear, nose and skin agents (56 items, 2.0%).	Tablets (1794 items, 63.3%) Capsules (332 items, 11.7%) Syrups (250 items, 8.8%) Suspensions (201, 7.1%) Suppositories (117 items, 4.1%) Creams/ointments/gels (43 items, 1.5%) All forms of injections (53 items, 1.9%) Drops/nasal or oral puff (45 items, 1.6%).	A sample was selected from northern Jordan, which may not representative of the whole of Jordan.
2002	Abou-Auda [27]	5 regions in Saudi Arabia and other Gulf countries (Kuwait, U.A.E, Qatar, and Oman)	Medications were also categorised according to their pharmacologic or therapeutic class using the classification of drugs adopted in the Saudi National Formulary (SNF). Respiratory system drugs Saudi Arabia: 2095 (16.8%), other gulf countries: 94 (15.3%). Central nervous system drugs Saudi Arabia: 2050 (16.4%), other gulf countries: 84 (13.6%). Antibiotics Saudi Arabia: 1779 (14.3%), other gulf countries: 111 (18.0%). Gastrointestinal drugs Saudi Arabia: 1382 (11.1%), other gulf countries: 60 (9.7%). Miscellaneous Saudi Arabia: 847 (6.8%), other gulf countries: 57 (9.3%). Nutrition and blood drugs Saudi Arabia: 823 (6.6%), other gulf countries: 24 (3.9%). Musculoskeletal/joints drugs Saudi Arabia: 790 (6.3%), other gulf countries: 52 (8.4%). Skin drugs Saudi Arabia: 735 (5.9%), other gulf countries: 33 (5.4%). Ear, nose, and throat drugs Saudi Arabia: 553 (4.4%), other gulf countries: 26 (4.2%). Cardiovascular drugs Saudi Arabia: 465 (3.7%), other gulf countries: 60 (9.7%). Eye drugs Saudi Arabia: 398 (3.2%), other gulf countries: 25 (4.1%). Endocrine drugs Saudi Arabia: 375 (3.0%), other gulf countries: 16 (2.6%). Obstetric/gynaecologic and/or urinary drugs Saudi Arabia: 140 (1.1%), other gulf countries: 12 (1.9%). Cytotoxic drugs Saudi Arabia: 31 (0.2%), other gulf countries: 0 (0.0%). Total drugs Saudi Arabia: 12,463 (100%), other gulf countries: 616 (100%). The mean medication wastage was estimated to be 25.8% Saudi Arabia and 41.3% other gulf countries.	Not studied.	Unable to describe respondent demographic information.

Table A2. Cont.

Year of Study	Authors	Settings/Country	Therapeutic Category of the Unused, Wasted Medicine	Dosage Form	Study Limitation
2011	Kheir et al. [51]	Qatar	The majority of the drugs stored ($n = 58$; 21%) in the participating homes were analgesics. Nonsteroidal anti-inflammatory drugs were the second most commonly stored drugs, representing 16% of all the drugs.	Not reported.	There was potential for selection and social desirability bias as a result of the strategy of using the telephone to conduct an interview. In addition, interviews were conducted during working hours, which could run the risk of excluding highly educated young subjects. Due to the small sample size, the results of this exploratory study should be considered with caution.
2007	Al-Siyabi et al. [60]	Oman; Sultan Qaboos University Hospital (SQUH)	Cardiovascular drugs were the most common pharmacological group of returned drugs. The drugs were classified according to the classification index of the British National Formulary. Cardiovascular drugs: 24%. Central nervous system drugs: 14%. Anti-infective drugs: 13%. Endocrine drugs: 10%. Nutrition: 9%. Gastrointestinal drugs: 8%, and Musculoskeletal system drugs: 8%. Respiratory system drugs: 5%. Immunosuppressant drugs: 3%. Eye/Ear drugs: 2%.	Not studied.	Unable to describe respondent demographic information. As it included only medicines with SQUH labels, others were missed, and this may underestimate the extent of unused medicines.
2004	Wongpoowarak et al. [20]	Thailand; Songkhla	Musculoskeletal system drugs were the most common pharmacological group of returned drugs. The medications were pharmacologically classified using MIMS Thailand, which is a standard reference source. Musculoskeletal system drugs (229 items, 23.3%). Anti-infective drugs (189 items, 19.2%). Respiratory system drugs (166 items, 16.9%). Gastrointestinal system drugs (129 items, 13.1%). Allergy and immune system drugs (91 items, 9.2%). Vitamins and minerals (68 items, 6.9%). Others (54 items, 5.5%). Central nervous system (37 items, 3.8%). Cardiovascular (21 items, 2.1%).	Oral dosage forms compromised 95.6% (951 items). Oral tablets or capsules (636 items, 63.9%). Oral liquids (311 items, 31.3%). Eye drops (23 items, 2.3%). Topical liquids (14 items, 1.4%). Creams (5 items, 0.5%). Oral powders (4 items, 0.4%). Inhalers (2 items, 0.2%).	This study was a snapshot study, as the studied population was one of 14 provinces in southern Thailand.

Table A2. Cont.

Year of Study	Author(s)	Settings/Country	Therapeutic Category of the Unused, Wasted Medicine	Dosage Form	Study Limitation
2013	Sooksriwong et al. [50]	Thailand; 4 regions of Thailand: Bangkok, Chiang Mai, Khon Kaen, Mahasarakham and Songkla	A total of 2208 drug items found in household surveys were classified into 5 groups of the mostly found drugs. These were 343 non-opioid analgesics and antipyretic drugs, 188 antacids, anti-reflux agents and anti-ulcer, 180 nonsteroidal anti-inflammatory drugs (NSAIDs), 127 antihistamine and anti-allergic and 119 anti-diabetic drugs. Top 5 of the most found rarely or unused drugs, classified as leftover medicines, were NSAIDs (49 items), penicillin (38 items), G.I.T. regulators, and antiflatulents (36 items). Of the total of 2208 drug items found in household, 82 items (3.7%) and 45 items (2.0%) of drugs were already expired and deteriorated, respectively.	Not studied.	Unable to describe respondent demographic information.
2011	El-Hamamsy A [26]	Egypt: Cairo	The returned medications were classified according to the British National Formulary (BNF). Antibiotics were the most common pharmacological group of returned medications. Antibiotics (109 items, 20.15%). Gastrointestinal system drugs (88 items, 16.27%). Cardiovascular system drugs (58 items, 10.72%). Respiratory system drugs (44 items, 8.13%). Nervous system drugs (39 items, 7.20%). Analgesics and anti-inflammatory (38 items, 7.02%). Dermatological drugs (35 items, 6.47%). Blood and blood-forming organs (29 items, 5.36%). Systemic hormonal preparations, sex hormones, and insulin's (27 items, 4.99%). Anti-parasitic products, insecticides, and repellents (25 items, 4.62%). Genitourinary system (20 items, 3.69%). Antineoplastic and immune-modulating agents (3 items, 0.55%). Various others (26 items, 4.80%).	Not studied.	Unable to describe respondent demographic information.
2012	Ibrahim et al. [49]	Egypt: Alexandria	Cardiovascular system drugs were the most common pharmacological group of returned medications. The returned medications were classified according to the British National Formulary (BNF). Cardiovascular system (127 items, 19.4%). Anti-infective (126 items, 19.2%). Gastrointestinal system (66 items, 10.9%). Nutrition and blood (69 items, 10.6%). Nonsteroidal anti-inflammatory (64 items, 9.8%). Nervous system (61 items, 9.3%). Respiratory system (58 items, 8.9%). Skin care (19 items, 2.9%). Endocrine System (49 items, 7.5%). Ear, nose, throat (7 items, 1.1%) and genitourinary system (7 items, 1.1%). Musculoskeletal system (2 items, 0.3%).	Not studied.	This study did not estimate the quantities of unused medicines in patient's home. As result, it is likely that it may underestimate the extent of unused medicines in the community.

Table A2. Cont.

Year of Study	Author(s)	Settings/Country	Therapeutic Category of the Unused, Wasted Medicine	Dosage Form	Study Limitation
2010	Guirguis et al. [32]	Australia; St Vincent's Hospital, Melbourne	Cardiovascular system drugs were the most common pharmacological group of returned medications. The smallest group was that of topicals, e.g., creams and ointments. Cardiovascular system drugs (78 items, 26.6%). Analgesics/anti-inflammatories (62 items, 21.2%). Neuropsychiatry drugs (8.5%). Respiratory system drugs (8%). Eye/Ear/Nose drugs (7.5%). Gastrointestinal drugs (7%), and Antimicrobials (7%). Herbals and vitamins (12 items, 4.1%). Diabetes drugs (3%). Topicals, e.g., creams and ointments (8 items, 2.7%). Miscellaneous (4.5%).	They report that they collect topicals, cream, ointment along with other dosage forms (that was not defined).	Sample size and the number of returns are small, which make it difficult to extrapolate the result to the whole of Australia.
2014	Kagashe et al. [57]	Tanzania; tertiary hospital in Dar es Salaam city	Medicines wasted in this study were categorised into three major groups, anti-infective, cardiovascular medications, and others. Anti-infective drugs: 18.9%. Cardiovascular drugs: 8.9%. Other drugs: 23.7%.	Oral solids drugs were the most common wasted dosage form 40.6% followed by injections 9.2%, with very few topicals preparations.	Since only hospital-prescribed medicines was included, others may be missed, which may underestimate the extent of unused medicines.
2007	Abahussain et al. [33]	Kuwait; Kuwait city	No medicines were collected from the 200 households participating in the municipal collection program The second intervention yielded 123 medicines from 14 homes; the most common class of unwanted medicines were drugs for respiratory system. Unwanted medications were classified according to the ATC WHO classification. A third of all unwanted medicines were for the respiratory system (38% of these were cough and cold preparations, 25% nasal preparations). 12% of the medicines were for the musculoskeletal system (53% oral NSAIDs) or were dermatologicals (33% topical antibiotics).	There were 141 items (including duplicates). 508 tablets/capsules, 25 oral liquids, 20 tubes, 21 dropper bottles, and various other dosage forms.	Sample size and the number of returns are small, which make it difficult to extrapolate the result to the whole of Kuwait. Unable to describe respondent demographic information.
2013	Aditya [43]	India; dental hospital in North India	Qualitative analysis of expired medications at home revealed antipyretics (54%), analgesics (64%), followed by antihistamines (35%) to be hoarded in home pharmacies/medicine chests. Other drugs were antibiotics (26%), antacids (23%), topical drugs (39%) and supplements (vitamins) (41%). Excessive buying of over-the counter (O.T.C.) drugs (53%); self-discontinuation (17%), and expiration of drugs (24%) resulted in possession of unused/leftover medications at home.	Not studied.	Small sample size from a specific region in India, which make it difficult to generalise and extrapolate the results to the whole of India.
2011	Gupta et al. [42]	India; Greater Noida City	Most of the expired drugs are in the category of analgesics and NSAIDs (23.93%) followed by nutritional supplements (22.56%), antibiotics (14.94%), expectorants and mucolytics (6.77%), bronchodilators (5.31%), and antacids (6.53%).	Oral tablets were the most common; other dosage forms include syrups, capsules, suspensions, powders, eye drops, gels, churna, cream, and ear wax softener.	Defined medicine wastes as only expired medicines, which may underestimate the extent of unused wasted medicines.

Table A2. Cont.

Year of Study	Author(s)	Settings/Country	Therapeutic Category of the Unused, Wasted Medicine	Dosage Form	Study Limitation
2014	Mirza and Ganguly [44]	Anand district of Gujarat, India	Among the prescribed medicines, the majority of medicines were from cardiovascular disease (19.88%) and from without prescription medicines, nonsteroidal anti-inflammatory drugs (NSAIDs) were the major group available at houses (35.13%).	Not reported.	Since the interviewers were fully aware of the purpose of the project, some information regarding medicines was not shared, which might have led to a skewed result.
2009	Ali et al. [24]	Malaysia; Universiti Sains	The total number of medicines found unused was 1724 drug products with vitamins and minerals as the most common class of unused drugs. Vitamins and minerals: 427 (24.8%). Gastrointestinal drugs: 298 (17.3%). Analgesic and antipyretics: 293 (17.0%). Antibiotics: 174 (10.0%). Ear, nose, and throat drugs: 159 (9.2%). Respiratory drugs: 106 (6.3%). Dermatological products: 97 (5.6%). Anti-rheumatic and anti-inflammatory: 69 (4.0%). Others (C.N.S. drugs, endocrine and metabolic drugs, cardiovascular drugs, genitourinary drugs, and others): 101 (5.8%).	68.5% ($n = 1181$) of the medications were in the form of tablets and pills while capsules constituted 14.6% ($n = 252$) of the overall amount. 5% ($n = 87$) syrups and suspensions while 4.9% ($n = 84$) were creams and ointments. Less than 1.0% ($n = 5$) consisted of inhalers, with 0.2% ($n = 4$) suppositories of the overall total.	Sampling of only female students made it impossible to generalise the results to the whole student population in the campus.
2020	Hassali and Shakeel [45]	Selangor, Malaysia	The major classes of medications that were purchased included antibiotics (207; 48.5%) followed by painkillers/nonsteroidal anti-inflammatory drugs (NSAIDs) (101; 23.7%). In addition, anti-hypertensive 51 (11.9%), anti-diabetic 20 (4.6%), OTC antihistamines 34 (7.9%), and multi-vitamins and other supplements 13 (3.0%).	Not studied.	The sample size of the study was small to depict a clear picture of the entire Selangor population; hence, the findings of the current study are not generalisable to all of Malaysia.
2014	Aboagye et al. [59]	Ghana	Leftover medicines: Paracetamol tablets 27 Amoxicillin capsules 12 Aspirin tablets 4 Metronidazole tablets 5 F-PAC (Paracetamol/Aspirin/Caffeine) 3 Vitamin B complex tablets 7 Multi-vitamins tablets 7 Diclofenac tablets 3 Magnesium trisilicate tablets 3 Ibuprofen tablets 5 Others/Unidentified 45 Do not remember 1.	Not studied.	Sample size and the number of returns are small which make it difficult to extrapolate the result to the whole of Ghana. Leftover medicines were described as individual medicine, not as a group.

Table A2. Cont.

Year of Study	Author(s)	Settings/Country	Therapeutic Category of the Unused, Wasted Medicine	Dosage Form	Study Limitation
2019	Huang et al. [52]	Six provinces in North, Central, and Southern regions of China	Cold medication (86.1%) was the most common category of medicines kept in households. Specifically, the following were the major classes of medicines found in the households: gastrointestinal medicines (27.0%), pain medications (22.9%), vitamins (20.6%), antibiotics (19.0%), external painkillers (16.5%), and external anti-inflammatory antidotes (15.4%).	Not studied.	Not reported.
2019	Vella and West [58]	Maltese village, Malta	The most common class of disposed medications was that pertaining to the alimentary tract (24.6%), closely followed by medicines belonging to the respiratory group (23.8%). 10.5% of the unused disposed medications were from the musculoskeletal group, which includes medications such as nonsteroidal anti-inflammatory drugs (NSAIDs), and supplements, such as glucosamine. The medications with the lowest return rate were anti-neoplastic and immunomodulating agents (0.7%), followed by anti-parasitic medications (0.2%).	Solid dosage forms were counted manually, liquid dosage forms were measured using a calibrated measuring cylinder, dermatological preparations were measured using kitchen weighing scales, and inhalers that had a counter were recorded as per value available on the counter. Unused inhalers without a counter, eye drops, ear drops, nasal drops, and nasal and oral sprays were not quantified as effective entries, as their quantities could not be safely determined.	This study excluded some dosage forms whilst quantifying and costing waste, such as eye drops, inhalers, and nasal sprays. Therefore, the actual cost of waste presented in this study is an underestimate.
2020	Insani et al. [54]	Bandung, Indonesia	NSAIDs were the most common medicines left unused ($n = 372$) followed by vitamins and nutritional supplements ($n = 215$) and antibiotics ($n = 171$).	Not reported.	This study was conducted in one region in Bandung (small sample size); thus, its generalisation for the Indonesian population is limited. In addition, the predictors associated with disposal practice were not identified.
2010	Jassim [53]	Basrah, Iraq	Overall, 4279 items of drugs were analysed. Antibiotics were the leading household stored drugs (26.43%), followed by antipyretic/analgesics (19.58%), and NSAIDs (nonsteroidal anti-inflammatory drugs) (11.45%). These drugs constituted (57%) of the total drugs stored.	Not reported.	This study was conducted in 300 households in Basrah, southern Iraq (i.e., one region in Iraq). Small sample size.

Table A2. *Cont.*

Year of Study	Author(s)	Settings/Country	Therapeutic Category of the Unused, Wasted Medicine	Dosage Form	Study Limitation
2012	Auta et al. [55]	Nigeria	Common classes of medicines reported as leftover medicines were analgesics (36.4%), antibiotics (33.1%), and antihistamines (11.9%).	Respondents reported having about 318 medicines items (representing 2.56 items per student's room) in all, with the tablets (62.3%) being the most common dosage form. Followed by capsules (16.4%), lotions/creams (11.6%), and syrups/suspensions (6.3%).	This study was based on the self-reported presence of medicines in respondents' residence. Therefore, it is possible that the medicines were under-reported or some names of unidentified medicines were wrongly reported. In addition, the sample size was small.
2015	Wondimu et al. [41]	Tigray Region, Northern Ethiopia	The most common classes of drugs found in the households were analgesics (29%) and antibiotics (25%). Generally, more than half (62%) of the medications were used for ongoing treatment.	Most (70%) of the medicines were available in the form of tablets, followed by capsules (13.2%), oral liquid (9.9%), semisolids (2.8%), injections (1.8%), and other dosage forms (2.2%).	One of the study limitations was the cross-sectional design employed, which might be affected by temporal relationship establishment with some variables and could not provide much more substantial evidence of causality, unlike a longitudinal design.
2017	Teni et al. [36]	Gondar town, northwestern Ethiopia	Anti-infectives for systemic use (23.9%), medicines for alimentary tract and metabolism (19.2%) and those for the cardiovascular system (17.7%) ranked top.	Of the total 553 medicines stored, more than three quarters (80.8%) were of solid dosage forms. Liquid dosage forms were (16.6%) and semisolids were (2.5%).	The study did not include the rural parts of Gondar Town. The small sample size makes the findings not representative of the pattern of household medicine storage practice in those areas.
2019	Ebrahim et al. [37]	Awi zone, Amhara regional state, Ethiopia	Anti-infective medications were found to be the most frequently unused medications 63 (36.4%) followed by antipain medications 37 (21.4%) and cardiovascular medications 19 (11%).	Not reported.	Health centres and private health facilities were not included in the study, and thus, the results may have been slightly different if those facilities were included.

Table A2. *Cont.*

Year of Study	Author(s)	Settings/Country	Therapeutic Category of the Unused, Wasted Medicine	Dosage Form	Study Limitation
2020	Gudeta and Assefa [39]	Jimma city, Ethiopia	Antibiotics, 31 (35.6%), and anti-hypertensive, 21 (24.1%) constituted the highest proportion of the waste.	Not reported.	The sample size was small. In addition, the current study was conducted among private practitioners. Thus, prospective researchers may consider both private and public professionals for their comparative study.
2020	Kahsay et al. [40]	Adigrat city, Ethiopia	The common types of medicines kept in households were analgesics (41.5%) and antibiotics (36.7%). In addition, antipain and antibiotic (4.8%), anti-diabetic (5.3%), and anti-hypertensive (8%) medicines were other types of unused medications found in homes.	Not reported.	The small sample size and the cross-sectional nature of the study design prevent us from drawing causal inferences about the relationship between the chosen covariates and outcome variables over a period.
2020	Yimenu et al. [38]	Awi zone, Amhara regional state, northwestern Ethiopia	Anti-infective medicines were found to be the most common unused medicines, 53 (58.9%), followed by antipain medicines, 16 (17.8%).	Not reported.	The small sample size and not including the health centres and private health facilities were limitations to this study. Thus, the results may be slightly different if those facilities were included.

References

1. *Pharmaceutical Waste Reduction in the NHS*. 2015. Available online: https://www.england.nhs.uk/wp-content/uploads/2015/06/pharmaceutical-waste-reduction.pdf (accessed on 30 November 2020).
2. Definition and characterization of health-care waste. In *Safe Management of Wastes from Health-Care Activities*, 2nd ed.; WHO: Geneva, Switzerland, 2014.
3. Opar, A. Rising drug costs prompt new uses for old pills. *Nat. Med.* **2006**, *12*, 1333. [CrossRef] [PubMed]
4. Toh, M.R.; Chew, L. Turning waste medicines to cost savings: A pilot study on the feasibility of medication recycling as a solution to drug wastage. *Palliat. Med.* **2016**, *31*, 35–41. [CrossRef] [PubMed]
5. Bekker, C.L.; Gardarsdottir, H.; Egberts, T.C.; Molenaar, H.A.; Bouvy, M.L.; Bemt, B.V.D.; Hövels, A.M. What does it cost to redispense unused medications in the pharmacy? A micro-costing study. *BMC Health Serv. Res.* **2019**, *19*, 243. [CrossRef] [PubMed]
6. Trueman, P.; Lowson, K.; Blighe, A.; Meszaros, A. Evaluation of the Scale, Causes and Costs of Waste Medicines Evaluation of the Scale, Causes and Costs of Waste Medicines. Available online: https://discovery.ucl.ac.uk/id/eprint/1350234/ (accessed on 30 November 2020).
7. Kümmerer, K. The presence of pharmaceuticals in the environment due to human use—Present knowledge and future challenges. *J. Environ. Manag.* **2009**, *90*, 2354–2366. Available online: https://pubmed.ncbi.nlm.nih.gov/19261375/ (accessed on 14 November 2020). [CrossRef] [PubMed]
8. Bound, J.P.; Voulvoulis, N. Household Disposal of Pharmaceuticals as a Pathway for Aquatic Contamination in the United Kingdom. *Environ. Health Perspect.* **2005**, *113*, 1705–1711. [CrossRef]
9. Radhakrishna, L.; Nagarajan, P.; Vijayanandhan, S.S.; Ponniah, T. Knowledge, attitude and practice (kap) towards disposal of medicines: A qualitative study among health care professionals in south India. *World J. Pharm. Res.* **2014**, *3*, 1955–1963.
10. Schwartz, T.; Kohnen, W.; Jansen, B.; Obst, U. Detection of antibiotic-resistant bacteria and their resistance genes in wastewater, surface water, and drinking water biofilms. *FEMS Microbiol. Ecol.* **2006**, *43*, 325–335. [CrossRef]
11. Länge, R.; Hutchinson, T.H.; Croudace, C.P.; Siegmund, F.; Schweinfurth, H.; Hampe, P.; Panter, G.H.; Sumpter, J.P. Effects of the synthetic estrogen 17α-ethinylestradiol on the life-cycle of the fathead minnow (*Pimephales promelas*). *Environ. Toxicol. Chem.* **2001**, *20*, 1216–1227. [CrossRef]
12. Wu, P.E.; Juurlink, D.N. Unused prescription drugs should not be treated like leftovers. *CMAJ* **2014**, *186*, 815–816. [CrossRef]
13. Medicines Non-Use in Primary Care—Aston Research Explorer. Available online: https://research.aston.ac.uk/en/studentTheses/medicines-non-use-in-primary-care (accessed on 15 November 2020).
14. West, L.M.; Diack, L.; Cordina, M.; Stewart, D. A systematic review of the literature on 'medication wastage': An exploration of causative factors and effect of interventions. *Int. J. Clin. Pharm.* **2014**, *36*, 873–881. [CrossRef]
15. Waste Management Plan for England. 2013. Available online: www.gov.uk/defra (accessed on 15 November 2020).
16. McRae, D.; Allman, M.; James, D. The redistribution of medicines: Could it become a reality? *Int. J. Pharm. Pr.* **2016**, *24*, 411–418. [CrossRef] [PubMed]
17. Bekker, C.L.; Gardarsdóttir, H.; Egberts, T.C.; Bouvy, M.L.; Bemt, B.J.F.V.D. Redispensing of medicines unused by patients: A qualitative study among stakeholders. *Int. J. Clin. Pharm.* **2017**, *39*, 196–204. [CrossRef] [PubMed]
18. Alhamad, H.; Patel, N.; Donyai, P. How do people conceptualise the reuse of medicines? An interview study. *Int. J. Pharm. Pr.* **2018**, *26*, 232–241. [CrossRef] [PubMed]
19. Bekker, C.L.; Bemt, B.V.D.; Egberts, T.C.; Bouvy, M.; Gardarsdottir, H. Willingness of patients to use unused medication returned to the pharmacy by another patient: A cross-sectional survey. *BMJ Open* **2019**, *9*, e024767. [CrossRef] [PubMed]
20. Wongpoowarak, P.; Wanakamanee, U.; Panpongtham, K.; Trisdikoon, P.; Wongpoowarak, W.; Ngorsuraches, S. Unused medications at home—Reasons and costs. *Int. J. Pharm. Pr.* **2004**, *12*, 141–148. [CrossRef]
21. Braund, R.; Chuah, F.; Gilbert, R.; Gn, G.; Soh, A.; Tan, L.Y.; Yuen, Y.-C. Identification of the reasons for medication returns. *NZFP* **2008**, *35*, 248–252.
22. Makki, M.; Hassali, M.A.; Awaisu, A.; Hashmi, F.K. The Prevalence of Unused Medications in Homes. *Pharmacy* **2019**, *7*, 61. [CrossRef] [PubMed]

23. Bekker, C.L.; Bemt, B.J.F.V.D.; Egberts, A.C.G.; Bouvy, M.L.; Gardarsdottir, H. Patient and medication factors associated with preventable medication waste and possibilities for redispensing. *Int. J. Clin. Pharm.* **2018**, *40*, 704–711. [CrossRef] [PubMed]
24. Ali, S.; Ibrahim, M. Extent of Medication Wastage and Cost among Female Students in a University Setting. *Mahidol Univ. J. Pharm. Sci.* **2009**, *36*, 34–43.
25. Garey, K.W.; Johle, M.L.; Behrman, K.; Neuhauser, M.M. Economic Consequences of Unused Medications in Houston, Texas. *Ann. Pharmacother.* **2004**, *38*, 1165–1168. [CrossRef] [PubMed]
26. El-Hamamsy, M.; Manal El-Hamamsy, A. Unused medications: How cost and how disposal of in Cairo, Egypt. *Int. J. Pharm. Stud. Res.* **2011**, *2*, 21–27.
27. Abou-Auda, H.S. An economic assessment of the extent of medication use and wastage among families in Saudi Arabia and Arabian Gulf countries. *Clin. Ther.* **2003**, *25*, 1276–1292. [CrossRef]
28. Jafarzadeh, A.; Mahboub-Ahari, A.; Naja, M.; Youse, M. Medicine Storage, Wastage and Associated Determinants among Urban Households: A Systematic Review of Household Surveys. Available online: https://doi.org/10.21203/rs.3.rs-71586/v1 (accessed on 18 November 2020).
29. DUMP—Bewell.org.nz—Nelson Bays Primary Health. Available online: https://www.yumpu.com/en/document/view/18584754/dump-bewellorgnz-nelson-bays-primary-health (accessed on 15 November 2020).
30. Tong, A.Y.C.; Peake, B.M.; Braund, R. Disposal practices for unused medications around the world. *Environ. Int.* **2011**, *37*, 292–298. [CrossRef] [PubMed]
31. Braund, R.; Peake, B.M.; Shieffelbien, L. Disposal practices for unused medications in New Zealand. *Environ. Int.* **2009**, *35*, 952–955. [CrossRef]
32. Guirguis, K. Medications collected for disposal by outreach pharmacists in Australia. *Pharm. World Sci.* **2009**, *32*, 52–58. [CrossRef]
33. Abahussain, E.A.; Ball, D.E.; Matowe, W.C. Practice and Opinion towards Disposal of Unused Medication in Kuwait. *Med. Princ. Pr.* **2006**, *15*, 352–357. [CrossRef]
34. Maeng, D.D.; Snyder, R.C.; Medico, C.J.; Mold, W.M.; Maneval, J.E. Unused medications and disposal patterns at home: Findings from a Medicare patient survey and claims data. *J. Am. Pharm. Assoc.* **2016**, *56*, 41–46.e6. [CrossRef]
35. Moher, D.; Liberati, A.; Tetzlaff, J.; Altman, D.G. Preferred reporting items for systematic reviews and meta-analyses: The PRISMA statement. *PLoS Med.* **2009**, *6*, e1000097. [CrossRef]
36. Teni, F.S.; Surur, A.S.; Asrie, A.B.; Wondimsigegn, D.; Gelayee, D.A.; Shewamene, Z.; Legesse, B.; Birru, E.M. A household survey of medicine storage practices in Gondar town, northwestern Ethiopia. *BMC Public Heal.* **2017**, *17*, 238. [CrossRef]
37. Ebrahim, A.J.; Teni, F.S.; Yimenu, D.K. Unused and Expired Medications: Are They a Threat? A Facility-Based Cross-Sectional Study. *J. Prim. Care Community Health* **2019**, *10*. [CrossRef]
38. Yimenu, D.K.; Teni, F.S.; Ebrahim, A.J. Prevalence and Predictors of Storage of Unused Medicines among Households in Northwestern Ethiopia. *J. Environ. Public Health* **2020**, *2020*, 8703208-10. [CrossRef] [PubMed]
39. Gudeta, T.; Assefa, D. Assessment of Pharmaceuticals Waste Practices Among Private Drug Retail Outlets in Ethiopia. *J. Prim. Care Community Health* **2020**, *11*. [CrossRef] [PubMed]
40. Kahsay, H.; Ahmedin, M.; Kebede, B.; Gebrezihar, K.; Araaya, H.; Tesfay, D. Assessment of Knowledge, Attitude, and Disposal Practice of Unused and Expired Pharmaceuticals in Community of Adigrat City, Northern Ethiopia. *J. Environ. Public Health* **2020**, *2020*, 1–11. [CrossRef] [PubMed]
41. Wondimu, A.; Molla, F.; Demeke, B.; Eticha, T.; Assen, A.; Abrha, S.; Melkam, W. Household storage of medicines and associated factors in Tigray Region, Northern Ethiopia. *PLoS ONE* **2015**, *10*, e0135650. [CrossRef]
42. Gupta, J.; Alam, N.; Bhardwaj, A.; Amin, F.; Alam, M.N. Prospective survey study on assessment and education of home medicine cabinet in general population of community. *IJPSR* **2011**, *2*, 1237–1243.
43. Aditya, S. Safe medication disposal: Need to sensitize undergraduate students. *Int. J. Pharm. Life Sci.* **2013**, *4*, 2476–2480.
44. Mirza, N.; Ganguly, B. Utilization of Medicines Available at Home by General Population of Rural and Urban Set Up of Western India. *J. Clin. Diagn. Res.* **2016**, *10*, FC05–FC09. [CrossRef]
45. Hassali, M.A.; Shakeel, S. Unused and Expired Medications Disposal Practices among the General Public in Selangor, Malaysia. *Pharmacy* **2020**, *8*, 196. [CrossRef]

46. Law, A.V.; Sakharkar, P.; Zargarzadeh, A.; Tai, B.W.B.; Hess, K.; Hata, M.; Mireles, R.; Ha, C.; Park, T.J. Taking stock of medication wastage: Unused medications in US households. *Res. Soc. Adm. Pharm.* **2015**, *11*, 571–578. [CrossRef]
47. Al-Azzam, S.I.; Al-Husein, B.A.; Alzoubi, F.; Masadeh, M.M.B. Self-Medication with Antibiotics in Jordanian Population. *Int. J. Occup. Med. Environ. Health* **2007**, *20*, 373–380. [CrossRef]
48. Abushanab, A.S.; Sweileh, W.M.; Wazaify, M. Storage and wastage of drug products in Jordanian households: A cross-sectional survey. *Int. J. Pharm. Pract.* **2013**, *21*, 185–191. [CrossRef] [PubMed]
49. Ibrahim, S.; Mamdouh, H.; El-Haddad, I.Z. Analysis of medications returned to community pharmacies in Alexandria, Egypt. *Life Sci. J.* **2012**, *9*, 746–751.
50. Sooksriwong, C.; Jarupas, C.; Chinawong, D.; Supakul, S.; Ploylermsang, C.; Sornlumlertwanich, K.; Janto, S. Values of leftover drugs in households: Preliminary study in 5 major Thai cities. *J. Asian Assoc. Sch. Pharm.* **2013**, *2*, 235–242.
51. Kheir, N.M.; El Hajj, M.; Kaissi, R.; Wilbur, K.; Yousif, A. An exploratory study on medications in Qatar homes. *Drug Health Patient Saf.* **2011**, *3*, 99–106. [CrossRef] [PubMed]
52. Huang, Y.; Wang, L.; Zhong, C.; Huang, S. Factors influencing the attention to home storage of medicines in China. *BMC Public Health* **2019**, *19*, 1–10. [CrossRef] [PubMed]
53. Jassim, A.-M. In-home Drug Storage and Self-medication with Antimicrobial Drugs in Basrah, Iraq. *Oman Med. J.* **2010**, *25*, 79–87. [CrossRef] [PubMed]
54. Insani, W.N.; Qonita, N.A.; Jannah, S.S.; Nuraliyah, N.M.; Supadmi, W.; Gatera, V.A.; Alfian, S.D.; Abdulah, R. Improper disposal practice of unused and expired pharmaceutical products in Indonesian households. *Heliyon* **2020**, *6*, e04551. [CrossRef]
55. Auta, A.; Banwat, S.B.; Sariem, C.N.; Shalkur, D.; Nasara, B.; Atuluku, M.O. Medicines in pharmacy students' residence and self-medication practices. *J. Young Pharm.* **2012**, *4*, 119–123. [CrossRef]
56. Coma, A.; Modamio, P.; Lastra, C.F.; Bouvy, M.L.; Mariño, E.L. Returned medicines in community pharmacies of Barcelona, Spain. *Pharm. World Sci.* **2007**, *30*, 272–277. [CrossRef]
57. Kagashe, G.A.; Makenya, F.B.; Buma, D. Medicines Wastage at a Tertiary Hospital in Dar Es Salaam Tanzania. *J. Appl. Pharm. Sci.* **2014**, *4*, 98–102.
58. Vella, V.; West, L.M. Analysis of Disposed Unused Medications at a Village Community Pharmacy. *Pharmacy* **2019**, *7*, 45. [CrossRef] [PubMed]
59. Aboagye, V.S.; Kyei, K.A. Disposal of Leftover Drugs in Ghana. *Pharm. Res.* **2014**, *4*, 84–91.
60. Al-Siyabi, K.; Al-Riyami, K. Value and Types of Medicines Returned by Patients to Sultan Qaboos University Hospital Pharmacy, Oman. *Sultan Qaboos Univ. Med. J. [SQUMJ]* **2007**, *7*, 109–115. [PubMed]
61. Gracia-Vásquez, S.L.; Ramírez-Lara, E.; Camacho-Mora, I.A.; Cantú-Cárdenas, L.G.; Gracia-Vásquez, Y.A.; Esquivel-Ferriño, P.C.; Ramírez-Cabrera, M.A.; Gonzalez-Barranco, P. An analysis of unused and expired medications in Mexican households. *Int. J. Clin. Pharm.* **2015**, *37*, 121–126. [CrossRef]
62. Langley, C.; Marriott, J.; Mackridge, A.; Daniszewski, R. An analysis of returned medicines in primary care. *Pharm World Sci.* **2005**, *27*, 296–299. [CrossRef]
63. Mackridge, A.J.; Marriott, J.F. Returned medicines: Waste or a wasted opportunity? *J. Public. Health* **2007**, *29*, 258–262. [CrossRef]
64. Bradley, M. *Waste Medication: Community Pharmacy Audit Report 2008/09*; NHS Cumbria: Cumbria, UK, 2009.
65. James, T.H.; Helms, M.L.; Braund, R. Analysis of Medications Returned to Community Pharmacies. *Ann. Pharmacother.* **2009**, *43*, 1631–1635. [CrossRef]
66. Vogler, S.; Leopold, C.; Zuidberg, C.; Habl, C. Medicines discarded in household garbage: Analysis of a pharmaceutical waste sample in Vienna. *J. Pharm. Policy Pr.* **2014**, *7*, 6. [CrossRef]
67. Braund, R.; Yuen, Y.C.; Jung, J. Identification and quantification of medication returned to Otago pharmacies. *NZFP* **2007**, *34*, 258–262.
68. Alhamad, H.; Donyai, P. Intentions to "Reuse" Medication in the Future Modelled and Measured Using the Theory of Planned Behavior. *Pharmacy* **2020**, *8*, 213. [CrossRef]
69. Hui, T.K.; Donyai, P.; McCrindle, R.; Sherratt, R.S. Enabling Medicine Reuse Using a Digital Time Temperature Humidity Sensor in an Internet of Pharmaceutical Things Concept. *Sensors* **2020**, *20*, 3080. [CrossRef] [PubMed]

70. Hui, T.K.L.; Mohammed, B.; Donyai, P.; McCrindle, R.; Sherratt, R.S. Enhancing Pharmaceutical Packaging through a Technology Ecosystem to Facilitate the Reuse of Medicines and Reduce Medicinal Waste. *Pharmacy* **2020**, *8*, 58. [CrossRef] [PubMed]
71. Chien, H.-Y.; Ko, J.-J.; Chen, Y.-C.; Weng, S.-H.; Yang, W.-C.; Chang, Y.-C.; Liu, H.-P. Study of Medication Waste in Taiwan. *J. Exp. Clin. Med.* **2013**, *5*, 69–72. [CrossRef]

Publisher's Note: MDPI stays neutral with regard to jurisdictional claims in published maps and institutional affiliations.

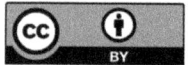 © 2020 by the authors. Licensee MDPI, Basel, Switzerland. This article is an open access article distributed under the terms and conditions of the Creative Commons Attribution (CC BY) license (http://creativecommons.org/licenses/by/4.0/).

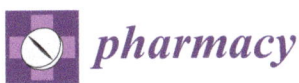

Article

Medication Use and Storage, and Their Potential Risks in US Households

SuHak Lee * and Jon C. Schommer

College of Pharmacy, University of Minnesota, 308 Harvard Street, S.E., Minneapolis, MN 55455, USA; schom010@umn.edu
* Correspondence: leex6829@umn.edu

Abstract: Background: Medications stored in US households may pose risks to vulnerable populations and the environment, potentially increasing societal costs. Research regarding these aspects is scant, and interventions like medication reuse may alleviate negative consequences. The purpose of this study was to describe medications stored in US households, gauge their potential risk to minors (under 18 years of age), pets, and the environment, and estimate potential costs of unused medications. Methods: A survey of 220 US Qualtrics panel members was completed regarding medications stored at home. Published literature guided data coding for risks to minors, pets, and the environment and for estimating potential costs of unused medications. Results: Of the 192 households who provided usable and complete data, 154 (80%) reported storing a medication at home. Most medications were taken daily for chronic diseases. The majority of households with residents or guests who are minors and those with pets reported storing medications with a high risk of poisoning in easily accessible areas such as counters. Regarding risk to the aquatic environment, 46% of the medications had published data regarding this risk. For those with published data, 42% presented a level of significant risk to the aquatic environment. Unused medications stored at home had an estimated potential cost of $98 million at a national level. Implications/Conclusions: Medications stored at home may pose risks to vulnerable populations and the environment. More research regarding medications stored in households and their risks is required to develop innovative interventions such as medication reuse to prevent any potential harm.

Keywords: medication; storage; risk; reuse; household; inventory

1. Introduction

With the increasing use of prescription and over-the-counter (OTC) medications, more drug products are being accumulated in US households [1–14]. Larger medication inventories at home, and subsequent waste can endanger patient safety, reduce quality of care, and harm the environment. To develop interventions that efficiently mitigate unintended, negative consequences, there is a need to study medication use, storage, and disposal in households more in-depth and comprehensively. For instance, medication reuse pertains to redispensing of medications that were once acquired by an individual or healthcare facility. Redistributing unused medications can reduce healthcare waste and costs, and enhance access to care [15–22]. Patients are recognized as the primary consumers of reused medications and as one of the potential primary sources of medications to be reused [23–27]. Therefore, understanding the interplay between patients and their medications will clarify the types of risk that medication reuse can minimize, guide its efficient implementation, and illuminate its benefit. However, comprehensive research regarding the use, storage and disposal of their medications especially in the US is scant.

Accumulating medication inventories at home can harm patients and their families by increasing the risk of medication poisoning. Sorensen et al., found that the higher number of medications stored at home may increase the risk of taking someone else's medications

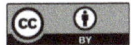

within the same household [28]. According to the 2019 report of the American Association of Poison Control Center's National Poison Data System (NPDS), out of over two million reported exposure cases, 92.1% occurred in residence either of their own or someone else's. The poisoning of patients younger than 20 years of age comprised 57.5% of the reported exposure cases, so they seem to be particularly at higher risk than other age groups [29]. The NPDS reports from the previous years showed similar trends [30–33]. In addition to the high rate of occurrence, poisoning accidents of minors can cause injuries leading to emergency department visits and at times be fatal, but they are preventable and should be critically discussed [29–36].

Selective serotonin reuptake inhibitors (SSRIs), nonsteroidal inflammatory drugs (NSAIDs), acetaminophen (APAP), histamine-1 receptor antagonists (H1RAs), and sedatives/hypnotics/antipsychotics (SHAs) have been identified as medications commonly involved in child poisoning in the NPDS reports [12–14,28,29]. Opioids have also been identified as harmful and high-risk medications for poisoning of minors [35–45]. Regardless of the types of medications, the ease of access seems to play a significant role in pediatric exposure. For example, one survey that analyzed children who were poisoned by their grandparents' medications found medications stored in easily accessible locations such as shelves lower than three feet from the floor were significantly more involved in poisoning than those stored in high shelves [34]. Storing in closed spaces like drawers and closets would also provide additional physical barriers and keep medications away from children more effectively. Nevertheless, for opioids which are extremely habit forming, two studies found that 26% and 36% of the participants stored them in open spaces at home, respectively, noting unsafe storage of the high-risk medication [37,38].

The NPDS report also showed that 98.6% of all non-human exposures involved dogs or cats, implying that these household pets may be at risk of poisoning [29]. The NPDS reports did not specify the substances involved in these cases, but Cortinovis et al. comprehensively reviewed the drugs intended for human use that were frequently involved in poisoning of dogs and cats. Most medications of concern in the review were the same as the high-risk medications for humans, while some, such as vitamin D, iron salts, and β2-agonists seem to be high-risk more specifically for dogs and cats [46].

In addition to poisoning, accumulation of unused, unwanted, and expired (UUE) medications at home in the US has been frequently reported in the literature [13,14,37,39–43]. The accumulation of UUE medications may represent inefficient medication utilization and a potential source of financial waste in healthcare. The economical loss may not seem so apparent, as no significant difference in total prescription costs between those who had any unused medications and who did not was found [14]. However, these medications are stored without fulfilling their intended consumption goals. They can continuously require storage costs and hamper adequate access to medications for other potential purchasers that could have benefited from their use [47,48].

It is concerning when UUE medications are discarded in the end, especially because the most common locations of medication disposal were identified as garbage, toilet and sink in the literature [11,38,39,42]. These disposal methods are also recommended by the Food and Drug Administration (FDA) [49]. However, with these methods, pharmaceuticals still can be introduced into the water system and eventually into the groundwater, lakes, and streams, harming the environment and potentially humans [12,22,27,50–52]. Considering the negative implications, assessment of the potential environmental effects of medications stored at home is imperative. Such an assessment would reaffirm the significance of the environmental issues associated with these medications and help develop better disposal practices to minimize environmental harm.

The 2014–15 Environmentally Classified Pharmaceuticals report by the Stockholm County Council provides the most comprehensive assessment of various medications' environmental effects [53]. However, the evidence provided by the report was based on the Swedish water system and their standard medication doses, and may not be fully applicable in the US. Despite the shortcomings, no study has critically explored the potential environmental risk of medications stored in US households. The Stockholm report can serve as a foundational reference for exploration and basic assessment of the potential risk.

Besides the different types of risk discussed above, the higher number of medications stored at home has been associated with deeper underlying issues with patients such as high severity of illness, therapeutic duplication, confusion between generic and trade names, low medication adherence and lack of medication administration routine [28]. Possessing unused medications also has been associated with a greater number of comorbidities, more frequent visits to emergency departments, primary care physicians, or specialists, and higher total medical cost of care [14]. Similar to these factors, polypharmacy, commonly defined as concurrent use of five or more medications, seems to be strongly associated with greater and unnecessary medication use [54]. The older population especially has a higher chance of comorbidity and is more likely to experience polypharmacy. Maneuvering through multiple, intricate medication therapies can be burdensome for many [54–58]. For this reason, when older patients manage their medications on their own, polypharmacy can arguably contribute to low medication adherence [59–61], potentially creating an unnecessary reservoir of medications stored at home.

Research assessing the aforementioned risks and economic implications of medications stored in the US households is scant. To fill the gaps in the literature, the first objective of the study was to describe medications stored in U.S. households including the number, indications, frequency of use, and storage locations. The second objective was to evaluate unintended consequences of these medications regarding (a) risk for poisoning of minors, (b) risk for poisoning of pets, and (c) risk to the environment. The third objective was to estimate the potential economic cost of the unused medications stored at home.

2. Materials and Methods

The 2018 National Household Medication Inventory Survey was the data source for this cross-sectional study. The survey was deemed to be non-human research and exempt from full review by the University of Minnesota Institutional Review Board. A total of 220 Qualtrics panel members in the U.S. were surveyed from May–June 2018. The Qualtrics Panel members who volunteered to participate in the survey received an invitation from Qualtrics, and the survey was self-administered. Upon completing the survey, each panel member earned credits which were reimbursed monetarily later. The overview of the data analysis is shown in Figure 1.

General Assessment of Households and Stored Medications	
Household Analysis o Number of Medications stored in each o Residents younger than 18 years old o Monthly guests younger than 18 years old o Residents older than 65 years old o Pets	*Medication Analysis* o Categorizations of Medications (Rx [a], OTC [b], controlled, and indications) o Frequency of use o Storage location
Potential Risk Assessment	
Pediatric and Adolescent (Minor) Poisoning Risk Assessment o SSRIs [c], NSAIDs [d], APAP [e], H1Ras [f], SHAs [g], Opioids o Counter (open space) storage status	*Environmental Risk Assessment* o Environmental risk level assignment o PBT [h] score assignment
Pet Poisoning Risk Assessment o NSAIDs, APAP, H1RAs and hydroxyzine, CCBs [i], Baclofen, Sedatives, Vitamin D, β-2 agonists o Counter (open space) storage status	*Cost Analysis* o Potential cost of medications reported to be "not taken" in study households o Extrapolation for the entire US households

Figure 1. Study Overview ([a]: prescription only, [b]: over-the-counter, [c]: serotonin reuptake inhibitors, [d]: nonsteroidal inflammatory drugs, [e]: acetaminophen, [f]: histamine-1 receptor antagonists, [g]: sedative/hypnotics/antipsychotics, [h]: persistence (P), bioaccumulation (B), and toxicity (T), [i]: calcium channel blockers).

2.1. General Assessment of Households and Stored Medications

2.1.1. Household Analysis

In the survey, the participants were asked to choose from "0 medication," "1–4 medication(s)," "5–10 medications," or "more than 10 medications" for the number of medications stored by each household. The participants who reported storing no medication were asked to stop at the beginning of the survey without answering any subsequent questions about the household members.

The survey also assessed whether a household had a resident under 18 years old, a monthly guest under 18 years old, a resident older than 65 years old, and a pet. The Fisher's exact test was utilized to compare the number of medications stored by the households with at least one resident older than 65 years and those without.

2.1.2. Medication Analysis

(a) Categorization of medications

The names of medications the participants stored in their households were reviewed and categorized by their prescription status (prescription, controlled substance, or OTC) and common indications. The controlled substance status was determined based on the Controlled Substances Act, following the federal classification. Medications like aspirin and omeprazole which can be available both as prescription and OTC, were categorized as OTC.

The typical indications of the reported medications were determined by the principal investigator (S.L.) who practices as a pharmacist in Minnesota, USA. The categorization of indications intended to be as inclusive as possible without having much overlap among the indications. A detailed description of the process of assigning medication indications is provided in Appendix A. A response with a typo that hindered interpretation of the exact name of the medication was categorized as "invalid." When the same medication was reported more than once by the same household, any responses reported subsequently to the first response were categorized as "duplicate."

(b) Medication frequency of use and storage locations

For the frequency of use of each medication, the participants were asked to choose from "taken daily," "taken as needed," "not taken, saving for future," "not taken, would like to discard," and "other." The participants were not given an option to specify "other." For the storage location of each medication, they were asked to choose from "bathroom counter," "bathroom cabinet," "garage," "kitchen counter," "kitchen cabinet or drawer," "utility room," "hallway closet," "bedroom counter," "bedroom cabinet," "bedroom closet," and "other." The participants were not asked to specify "other" in the survey.

2.2. Potential Risk of Poisoning Analysis

The risk analysis assessed whether high-risk medications for poisoning of minors and pets were stored on the counter by the households with a resident or monthly guest younger than 18 years old and a pet. Based on the literature, high-risk medications were determined as those more commonly involved in poisoning or associated with serious poisoning with harmful outcomes for minors and pets, particularly dogs and cats. The types of pets owned by the households were not asked in the survey, and it was assumed that the households owned either dogs or cats for simplicity and to adapt the findings of Cortinovis et al. [46].

The high-risk medications for minors included selective serotonin reuptake inhibitors (SSRIs), nonsteroidal inflammatory drugs (NSAIDs), acetaminophen (APAP), histamine-1 receptor antagonists (H1RAs), sedative/hypnotics/antipsychotics (SHAs), and opioids [29–33]. In the National Poison Data System (NPDS) reports, the SHA medications are comprised of barbiturates, atypical antipsychotics, benzodiazepines, buspirone, chloral hydrate, ethchlorvynol, meprobamate, methaqualone, phenothiazines, and histamine-related OTC sleep aids excluding diphenhydramine [29–33]. The high-risk medications for dogs and cats included analgesics (NSAIDs and acetaminophen), antihistamines (diphenhydramine, doxylamine, hydroxyzine, loratadine), calcium channel blockers (CCBs), SSRIs, baclofen, sedative-hypnotic drugs such as benzodiazepines, and non-benzodiazepine hypnotic sedatives, loperamide, vitamin D, and β2-adrenergic receptor agonists [46].

2.3. Potential Environmental Risk Analysis

Based on the 2014–15 Environmentally Classified Pharmaceuticals published by the Stockholm County Council, each reported medication was assigned with a risk of toxicity to the aquatic environment and Persistence, Bioaccumulation, Toxicity (PBT) score. The persistence (P), bioaccumulation (B), and toxicity (T) of the PBT scores represent the ability to resist degradation in the aquatic environment, accumulation in adipose tissues of aquatic organisms, and the potential to poison aquatic organisms, respectively. Each characteristic is assigned a score ranging from 0–3, with a higher value indicating a higher risk. The sums of the scores of the three characteristics of medications have been reported as the PBD Index and utilized for the analysis in the current study [53].

The risk levels were classified as "insignificant," "low," "moderate," and "high." Medications that had undetermined risk levels due to insufficient evidence or were not mentioned in the report were categorized as "insufficient data." Vitamins, electrolytes, amino acids, peptides, proteins, carbohydrates, lipids, vaccines, and herbal medicine were not considered to pose a risk to the environment in the Stockholm report and were given the "exempt" status [53].

For combination medications whose active ingredients could be identified with the given response, the highest known risk level and highest known PBT score of the comprising ingredients were assigned. For example, when the comprising ingredients had both "insufficient data" and "insignificant" risk levels, the "insignificant" ingredient was determined to have more conclusive evidence for the risk and deemed the higher known risk level.

2.4. Cost Analysis

The potential cost of the medications that were reported to be either "not taken, saving for future" or "not taken, would like to discard" was assessed. The survey did not specify the units for quantities and strengths of medications to be reported for the participants. Without standardized units, the responses for quantities and strengths did not show a particular trend and could not be used for cost analysis. In order to estimate the potential cost, the sum of the lowest package Average Wholesale Price (AWP) on Red Book® for each medication regardless of the dosage form, strength, and package size was utilized [62]. The sum was then extrapolated to a national level, based on the US census data [63]. Utilizing the lowest unit AWP was considered, but it was suspected that the chance of storing multiple units of a medication would be higher than storing just one unit. Therefore, the next lowest cost estimate available which was the lowest package AWP at the time of the analysis in 2021 was utilized for the analysis.

Once the total potential cost of "not taken" medications was determined, the ratio of the number of US households based on the US census data (120,756,048 households) [63] and the number of households storing those medications was used to extrapolate the cost nationally.

The survey results were analyzed with Microsoft Excel 2016, SPSS (v. 27.0), and R (v.4.1.0).

3. Results

3.1. General Assessment of Households and Stored Medications

3.1.1. Household Analysis

A total of 192 households (87.3%) out of the 220 households who volunteered to participate completed the survey. The zip codes of the participating households matched the geographic distribution of the US census data, indicating that the collected data were nationally representative [63]. The number of medications stored in the households is shown in Table 1. Note that 154 households (80.2%) reported storing at least one medication at home.

Table 1. Number of medications stored by households with at least one resident older than 65 years vs. without a resident older than 65 years.

Number of Medications Stored in Households	Number of Households Storing at Least One Medication ($n = 154$)		p-Value [a]
	With at Least One Resident Older than 65 Years ($n = 46$)	Without a Resident Older than 65 Years ($n = 108$)	
1–4 medication(s)	102 (66.2%)		
	27 (58.7%)	75 (69.4%)	
5–10 medications	42 (27.3%)		0.10
	13 (28.3%)	29 (26.9%)	
>10 medications	10 (6.5%)		
	6 (13%)	4 (3.7%)	

[a] Fisher's exact test.

Forty-six households (24%) had at least one resident older than 65 years old (Table 1). The Fisher's exact test determined no significant difference in the number of medications reported by the households with a resident older than 65 years and the number reported by those without ($p = 0.10$).

3.1.2. Medication Analysis

(a) Categorization of medications

A total of 457 medications stored at home were reported. After excluding eight "invalid" and 45 "duplicate" responses, a total of 404 valid responses were included in the analysis. Of the valid responses, 261 medications (64.6%) were prescription-only and 143 medications (35.4%) were OTC. Among the prescription-only medications, 25 medications (9.6%) were controlled substances. Table 2 has the breakdown of the indications of the reported prescription, controlled, and OTC medications. The three most commonly reported indications for prescription-only medications were cardiovascular therapy (33.5%), mental health therapy (18.6%), and endocrine therapy (16.5%). Mental health conditions (60%) such as attention deficit hyperactivity disorder (ADHD), and anxiety were the most commonly reported indications for controlled substances. The three most commonly reported indications for OTC medications were pain (37.1%), supplements (18.2%), and gastrointestinal therapy (13.3%) (Table 2). Among the households storing at least one medication at home, 72 households (46.7%) had at least one OTC medication stored at home. The crude responses for medication names are categorized by indications in Appendices B and E.

(b) Medication frequency of use and storage locations

Some of the responses for medication names categorized as "invalid" had their valid frequencies and locations reported. Also, a majority of the medications categorized as "duplicate" had different storage locations. For comprehensiveness, the frequency and location responses corresponding to "duplicate" or "invalid" in the medication indication analysis were included in the current analysis. The inclusion of these responses in the analysis yielded a total number of samples higher than the number of medications reported in the categorization.

A total of 465 responses for the frequency of use was collected. Table 3 shows most of the reported medications were being used: "taken daily," and "taken as needed" (93.8%).

Table 2. Indications of the medications stored in the households ($n = 404$ [a]).

Prescription Medications				OTC Medications	
Non-Controlled		Controlled Substances			
Indications	$n = 236$	Indications	$n = 25$	Indications	$n = 143$
Cardiovascular therapy	79 (33.5%)	Mental health [c]	15 (60%)	Pain	53 (37.1%)
Mental health	44 (18.6%)	Pain [d]	9 (36%)	Supplements	26 (18.2%)
Endocrine therapy	39 (16.5%)	Weight loss	1 (4%)	Gastrointestinal therapy	19 (13.3%)
Antibiotics	9 (3.8%)			Cardiovascular therapy and pain	11 (7.7%)
Others [b]	57 (24.1%)			Others [e]	34 (23.8%)

[a] "Invalid" and "duplicate" responses were excluded from the current analysis, [b] Includes indications with counts of 8 or fewer (complete counts provided in Appendix F), [c] Notably includes 9 benzodiazepines and 1 non-benzodiazepine hypnotic sedative, [d] Notably includes 4 opioids and 1 neuropathic pain, [e] Includes indications with counts of 8 or fewer (complete counts provided in Appendix F).

Table 3. Medication frequency of use.

Frequency of Use ($n = 465$)	
Taken daily	306 (65.8%)
Taken as needed	130 (28%)
Not taken, saving for future	12 (2.6%)
Not taken, would like to discard	7 (1.5%)
Other	10 (2.2%)

For storage locations, a total of 464 responses was collected. Most medications were stored in kitchens (31.9%), bathrooms (28.9%), and bedrooms (21.3%). A total of 147 medications (31.7%) were stored on open counters in bathrooms, kitchens, or bedrooms, which would be more accessible than those stored in drawers, closets, or cabinets (Figure 2). Two households submitted different numbers of responses for the frequencies and locations for their medications, and yielded different sample sizes ($n = 465$ vs. $n = 464$).

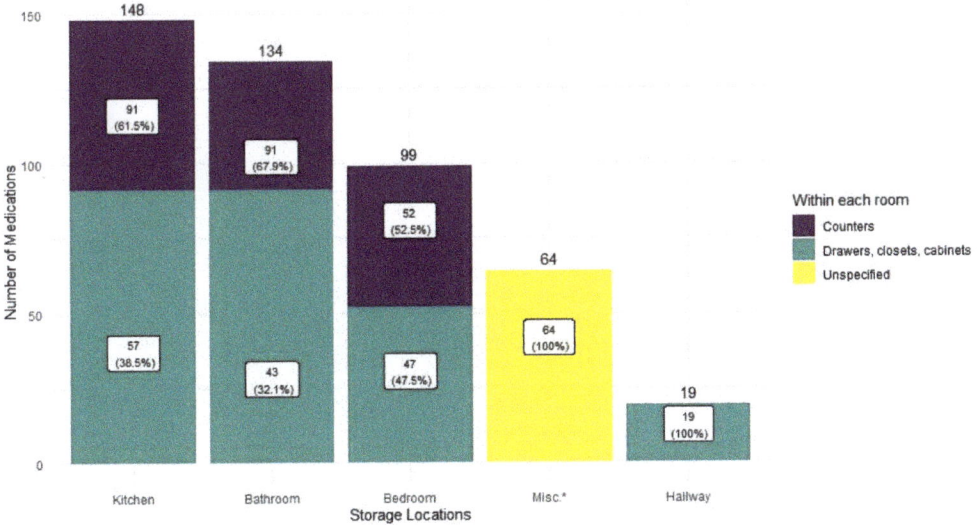

Figure 2. Medication storage locations ($n = 464$) * Misc. in the x-axis includes 14 "utility room," 8 "garage," and 42 "other." The participants were not asked to specify "other" in the survey.

3.2. Potential Risk of Poisoning Analysis

Among households storing at least one medication ($n = 154$), 75 (39.1%) had at least one resident younger than 18 years old, 55 (28.6%) had at least one monthly guest younger than 18 years old, and 112 (58.3%) had at least one pet.

A total of five out of the six (83%) high-risk medications (all except opioids) was being stored on the counter by at least one household with one or more resident(s) younger than 18 years old. At least one household with one or more monthly guest(s) younger than 18 years old stored four out of the six (67%) high-risk medications (all except selective serotonin reuptake inhibitors (SSRIs) and opioids) on the counter. Of the nine high-risk medications, seven (78%) (all except vitamin D and baclofen) were being stored on the counter by at least one household with one or more pet(s). In fact, baclofen storage was not reported by any households with one or more pets.

3.3. Potential Environmental Risk Analysis

After excluding "duplicate" and "invalid" responses, a total of 404 valid medications reported in the survey were included in the environmental analysis and reviewed. Of the valid responses, six OTC medications had only their brand names reported, and were excluded from the current analyses. These brand medications are available in different variations of active ingredients, but the specific types were not reported in the survey. A total of 27 medications were "exempt" from the risk analysis per the 2014–15 Environmentally Classified Pharmaceuticals by the Stockholm County Council [53].

A majority of the medications, 53.9% and 60.1% of the medications did not have sufficient data to determine their risk of toxicity to the aquatic environment and their Persistence (P), Bioaccumulation (B), Toxicity (T) scores respectively (Figures 3 and 4). Among those with data, medications with insignificant-risk level (26.7%) were most prevalent (Figure 3). On the other hand, medications with PBT scores of 4 or higher (35%) were far more frequently identified compared to those with PBT scores lower than 4 (4.9%) (Figure 4).

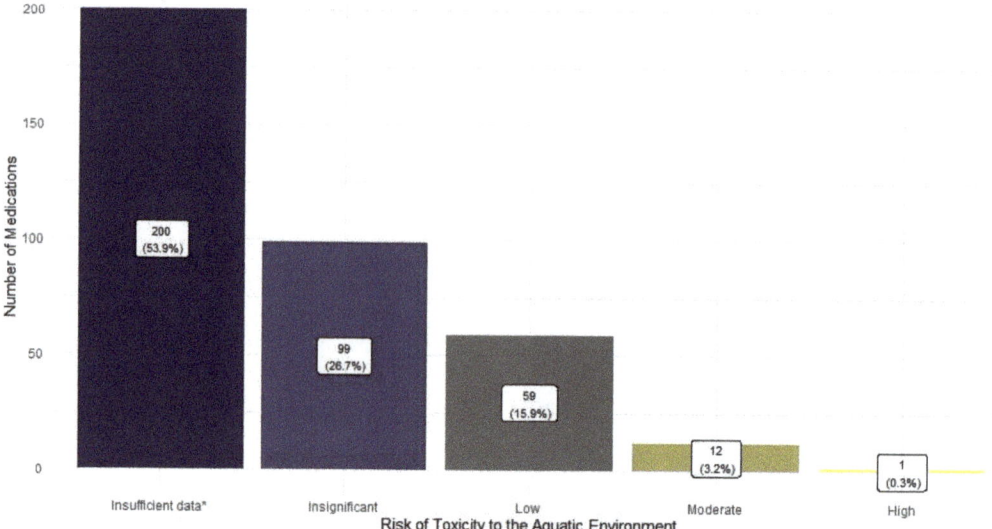

Figure 3. Toxic risk levels assigned to the aquatic environment of the reported medications based on the 2014–15 Environmentally Classified Pharmaceuticals by the Stockholm County Council [53] ($n = 371$) * "Insufficient data" includes medications with undetermined risk levels due to insufficient evidence or those that were not mentioned in the Stockholm report.

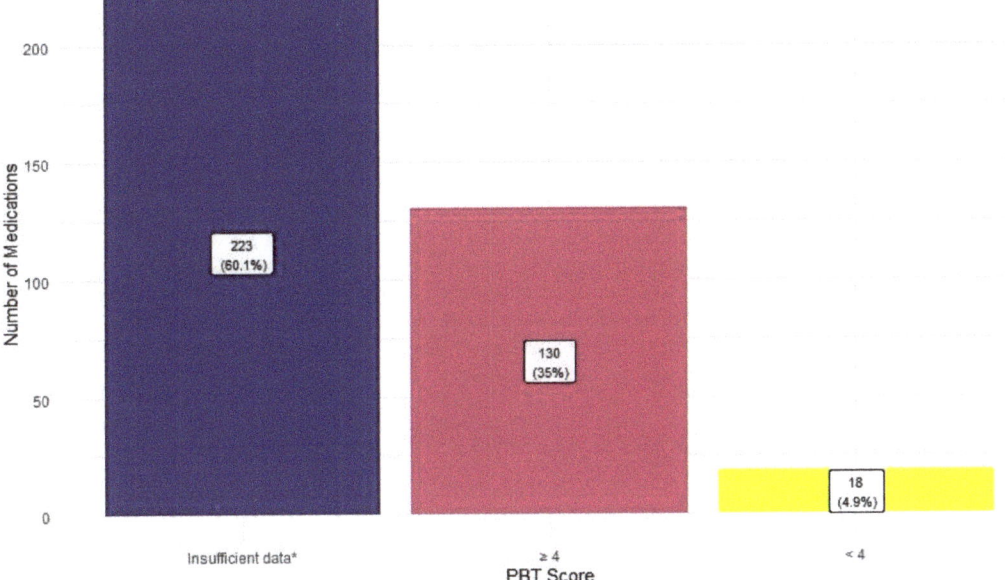

Figure 4. Persistence (P), Bioaccumulation (B), and Toxicity (T) scores of the reported medications. The PBT score is a sum of the P, B, and T score, each ranging from 0–3, assigned to a particular medication reported in the 2014–15 Environmentally Classified Pharmaceuticals by the Stockholm County Council. The higher the score, the higher the risk [53] (n = 371) * Medications without a PBT score in the Stockholm report were categorized as "insufficient data.".

3.4. Cost Analysis

Out of the 19 "not taken, saving for future" or "not taken, would like to discard" responses, 14 had appropriately reported medication names. Based on the lowest package AWP, the 14 medications were worth $156.54. Extrapolating this result to a national level, $98,453,915.39 of medications were potentially stored at home without being used and potentially being wasted.

4. Discussion

4.1. Objective #1: To Assess the US Household Members and the Number, Indications, Frequency of Use and Storage Locations of Their Medications Stored at Home

Approximately 20% of the participating households did not store any medications at home. On the other hand, a household survey conducted in IL found all participating households storing at least one prescription or OTC medication at home [11]. No other US household surveys that could be used as a reference were identified during the literature review. Other similar studies assessed medication possession by individuals, not households.

The bivariate comparison of the number of medications between the households with and without any residents older than 65 found no statistical difference. However, the current survey did not collect the number of medications specifically stored by the individual residents older than 65, and the statistical analysis was explorative at best. The self-administered and online nature of the survey may have also heightened the barrier for the elderly to actively participate in the household survey.

The three most prevalent indications of the reported prescription medications were cardiovascular therapy, mental health, and endocrine therapy including diabetes. The Centers for Disease Control and Prevention (CDC) reported that 6 in 10 US adults suffer from chronic diseases including but not limited to the three identified in the current study. The most common indication of the reported OTC medications was "pain." This result may correspond to arthritis, another prevalent chronic disease reported by the CDC and often managed with analgesics. The prevalence of chronic diseases was also reflected in the most common medication frequency of use being "taken daily" [64–67].

Approximately a half of the households reported storing at least one OTC medication at home, consistent with the high prevalence of OTC medication use published in the literature. 8 of 10 US patients do not seek help from a healthcare professional initially for their minor illnesses and resort to OTC medications [9]. Considering the high barrier to healthcare access in the US, OTC treatment can be a convenient option for many patients.

Most medications reported in the study were stored in bedrooms, kitchen, and bathrooms. The alarming trend was a high number of medications being stored in bathrooms, which is inappropriate for medication storage. Funk et al. did a separate analysis for the appropriateness for each reported medication and their storage space, utilizing the published humidity and temperature ranges of various household locations and specific medication storage recommendations [68].

4.2. Objective #2: To Evaluate the Potential Risk for Poisoning of Minors and Pets and for the Environment Posed by the Medications Stored in the Study Households

4.2.1. Poisoning Risk

A considerable amount (37.1%) of the reported medications were being stored on open counters in kitchens, bathrooms, and bedrooms. In addition, most of the high-risk medications for pediatric and adolescent poisoning were stored on counters by at least one household with a minor or pet. Counters are easily accessible and are not appropriate for medication storage, especially for households with vulnerable populations. In order to prevent and minimize harm by pediatric medication poisoning at home, the CDC recommends storing medications up and away and out of sight in a cabinet where a child cannot reach, never leaving medications unattended when a child is around, and having the Poison Help number readily available in the household [69]. It is uncertain whether patients living with minors or frequently having minor guests are educated about the importance of storage locations and how appropriately they store medications to prevent poisoning. As for pets, although only a small number of calcium channel blockers were reported, they have a small margin of safety, and ingestion of a small amount can be fatal for dogs and cats [46,70], and the pet owners should be appropriately educated.

Opioids were another type of high-risk medications reported in the literature. All the reported opioids in the study were not stored on a counter, suggesting that the study households were able to alleviate the risk of opioid poisoning and diversion to some degree. Locked spaces would be the optimal storage locations for opioids, but the survey did not assess whether the reported opioids were stored in locked spaces. Unlike the previous surveys with at least 30% of their samples having leftover opioids [37–43,71], the current study only had a small number of opioids reported. The discrepancy could also have been caused by inaccurate reporting or social desirability bias of the sample. The study sample might not have included a reasonable number of households with opioids and UUE medications in general.

4.2.2. Environmental Risk

Almost a half of the reported medications had a Persistence, Bioaccumulation, Toxicity (PBT) score of 4 or higher, where a higher score indicated a higher environmental risk. In contrast, those with insignificant or low toxic risk to the aquatic environment combined took up a similar proportion. This finding highlights that medications without direct toxic effects on the aquatic environment can harm the environment via other mechanisms such as high persistence (P) and bioaccumulation (B). Despite the various ways of pharmaceuticals harming the environment, the literature found that up to 80% of the US patients are not educated about proper disposal methods of medications [11,37–39,42]. Additionally, the current disposal mechanisms and systems in the US have apparent limitations. The Resource Conservation and Recovery Act (RCRA) governs the framework for the generation, transportation, treatment, storage, and disposal of hazardous waste, but it recognizes only a small fraction of OTC medications as hazardous waste [52]. A new rule passed under RCRA in 2018 also set the threshold for pharmaceutical waste from healthcare facilities [72]. However, the rule seems to request the stakeholders to accomplish the set outcomes without providing sufficient support for achieving those goals. More efficient support can only be provided after more thoughtful consideration of the sources of pharmaceutical waste.

In addition to addressing the sources of the waste, the environmental effects of pharmaceutical substances need to be more extensively researched. In the current study, more than a half of the reported medications did not have any or enough environmental information available to determine their toxic risk to aquatic organisms or PBT score. The Stockholm report is the most comprehensive resource for the environmental effects of medications to this date, but it lacks considerable evidence and cannot be generalized to countries other than Sweden. PharmEcovigilance is a dimension of pharmacovigilance that governs the environmental effects of pharmaceuticals. The concept of pharmEcovigilance should be more actively promoted for accurate assessment of potential environmental risk and development of interventions protecting the environment from the potential harm [22]. Under this agenda, more pharmaceutical manufacturers should also be encouraged to research the environmental effects of their medications and share the findings with the public.

4.3. Objective #3: To Calculate the Potential Cost of the Unused Medications or Medications Reported to Be "Not Taken" and Stored in the US Households

The cost of the unused medications estimated based on the nationally representative sample was extrapolated to a national level, and the result was unremarkable. The national estimate reported by Law et al., was much higher than the estimate from the current study, ranging from $2.4B to $5.4B [13]. Their calculation may have overestimated the cost, as their data from the convenience samples were collected at drug-take-back events. At the same time, their estimate may be more accurate than the estimate of the current study, as they were able to tally the number of units and exact strengths of unused, unwanted and expired (UUE) medications collected from the sample. In spite of the deviation from the published estimate, the basic cost analysis of the current study would promote discussions about potential costs of UUE medications in the US.

Besides the apparent costs of the UUE pharmaceutical products, their invisible costs are equally concerning. When medications are stored at home, the transfer of medication inventories from suppliers to consumers incurs costs for acquisition and storage [47,48]. The limited access to healthcare in the US adds an additional cost to acquisition for most prescription medications. As for the storage costs, solid dosage medications may not take up a huge volume or require significant storage costs. However, liquid formulations such as insulin or biologics may require delicate storage conditions and additional storage costs. The storage costs can be further increased indirectly, considering the risk of harm via intentional or accidental poisoning or drug diversion, and its potential contribution to the total healthcare costs.

4.4. Potential Solutions for Risk Mitigation

Most existing interventions such as drug-take-back programs intend to minimize the environmental and poisoning risks by removing the unnecessary stocks stored at home. Their benefits have been studied mostly from an environmental perspective. Although any consolidated data regarding disposal methods of pharmaceutical waste in the US could not be identified during the literature review, most of the collected medications are suspected to be incinerated and contribute to more pollution [73]. On the other hand, medication reuse or drug repository programs may be a more environmentally friendly and economical alternative. As of 2018, 38 states and Guan in the US have enacted laws for medication donation and reuse, but about a third of them still do not have operational programs. In order for medications to be donated, they have to meet multiple criteria including but not limited to being unexpired and unopened in their original, sealed, tamper-evident packaging, and having no signs of adulteration or misbranding. With the stringent provisions, the types of donors and medications are limited to certain oral medications [74,75]. These provisions are necessary as aligned with the general public concerns and perception about medication reuse [23,24,26,76], but innovative approaches such as packaging for pharmaceuticals, enhancing the quality and safety of medications and enabling their reuse are needed [77,78].

Despite the challenges, the medication reuse programs in the US have shown prospects for growth and benefit. Iowa and Wyoming reported their success in redistributing $17.7 million and $12.5 million worth of medications in one fiscal year, respectively [74]. The American Society of Clinical Oncology also publicly expressed its commitment to supporting drug repository programs in 2020. Although their support is only for redistribution of oral medications maintained in a controlled and supervised healthcare environment, this may indicate that more sectors within healthcare are recognizing the need for such programs [75]. In addition, better success and expansion of the repository programs can be realized with services or technologies that streamline donation, and inspection of donated medications. For instance, SIRUM, a non-profit organization in California, which provides streamlined donation packaging and shipping services, has now expanded into Colorado, Oregon, and Ohio [79,80].

Ruhoy et al., however, have determined that these "downstream" approaches may incur high costs and have inefficiently captured all medications accumulated as waste historically [12]. Instead, "upstream" approaches targeting the sources of pharmaceutical waste that can reduce the overall healthcare costs and burden of proper medication disposal should also be considered. Some of the recommended upstream approaches are unit packaging, providing trial scripts for new medications, low-quantity packaging of OTC medications, free samples, and drug repository programs that accept donations from patients [12]. Sweden has developed "Kloka Listan" or the Wise List that provides healthcare clinicians with a list of medications for common diseases recommended based on cost-effectiveness and environmental effects [53]. This type of comprehensive database would greatly help US health providers make more economical and environmentally appropriate decisions when prescribing.

4.5. Limitations

The findings suggested certain areas of improvement in healthcare and aspects for which patients and their household members should be better educated. As a household survey, however, the analysis did not reflect the medication use and storage by individuals. Some of the variables could have been more accurately and precisely collected. Both frequencies of use and storage locations did not specify the response collected as "other." The unit for quantities and strengths of medications, and the type of pets owned by the households were not specified as well. Sampling bias, recall bias and social desirability bias may have led to under-reporting of certain medications. Without collecting actual poisoning incidences and disposal methods, the results of the risk analyses could not be determinative. The Stockholm report that was utilized as the reference for the environmental risk analysis did not have conclusive evidence for various medications. Their Sweden-based data also may not be completely applicable in the US.

In-person and on-site assessment would be the most accurate method for evaluating medications stored at home and overcome the limitations that the current study had. The study by Sorenson et al. that found the association between the number of medications stored at home and the risk factors and health outcomes was done through in-person home visits in Australia [28]. Similar direct observations of the medication use, storage, and disposal by investigators in US homes may help tailor patient education and systemic interventions to minimize waste and maximize the efficiency of care and medication use.

5. Conclusions

Various areas of medications stored at home including, the use, storage, and poisoning and environmental risk, have been discussed in this paper. The study especially highlighted the negative implications of medications stored in US households. Notably, a significant portion of the medications stored in the participating households could put the vulnerable populations at risk of accidental exposure and harm the environment. Without studying more about these risks and their intricate associations with patients and household members, the society may keep suffering from the negative consequences. Thus, the findings attest to the dire need for more extensive research in this field to complements the limitations of the study. Those limitations include, but are not limited to, a small sample size and the explorative nature of the study that could not measure direct risks. Such research will guide efficient development and implementation of innovative interventions like medication reuse to prevent any potential harm.

Author Contributions: Conceptualization, S.L. and J.C.S.; methodology, S.L. and J.C.S.; software, S.L. and J.C.S.; validation, S.L. and J.C.S.; formal analysis, S.L.; investigation, S.L. and J.C.S.; resources, S.L. and J.C.S.; data curation, S.L. and J.C.S.; writing—original draft preparation, S.L.; writing—review and editing, S.L. and J.C.S.; visualization, S.L. and J.C.S.; supervision, J.C.S.; project administration, J.C.S.; funding acquisition, J.C.S. All authors have read and agreed to the published version of the manuscript.

Funding: The University of Minnesota provided funding for data collection and for software support (Qualtrics^{XM}; IBM SPSS Statistics 27; R v.4.1.0; and Microsoft Excel 2016).

Institutional Review Board Statement: University of Minnesota, Institutional Review Board Exempt from Full Review Number: HRP-503.

Informed Consent Statement: Your participation is voluntary and your response is confidential. Only aggregate responses will be reported. By completing the survey form, you are providing your consent to participate in the project.

Data Availability Statement: Data files are stored in encrypted format at University of Minnesota. Requests for access to the files may sent to the corresponding author at schom010@umn.edu.

Acknowledgments: Expert advice regarding research referenced in this paper from Ya-Feng Wen, Anthony W. Olson, Donald L. Uden, and Ronald S. Hadsall is greatly appreciated.

Conflicts of Interest: The authors declare no conflict of interest.

Appendix A. Process of Assigning Medication Indications

The categorization of indications intended to be as inclusive as possible without having much overlap among the indications. For instance, "cardiovascular therapy medications" included antihypertensive, anticholesteremic, antithrombotic, antianginal, and heartrate control medications. For medications with multiple active ingredients, their most likely common indication was assigned. For instance, the common indication of a combination of acetaminophen, dextromethorphan, and doxylamine was "cold," rather than a more specific indication for each ingredient. If the multiple active ingredients, however, did not have a common indication, all of their typical indications were assigned. For example, the indication of Yosprala containing aspirin and omeprazole was categorized as "cardiovascular therapy/gastrointestinal therapy." If a medication had multiple indications, the more commonly used indication was reported. For example, gabapentin was initially developed to treat seizures, but in current practice, it is predominantly used for neuropathic pain. Hence, for this study, its indication was categorized as "neuropathic pain." If one medication had multiple competing indications equally common in practice, then all of the indications were reported. For example, hydroxyzine was categorized as "mental health therapy" for its use for both anxiety and "allergies." For medications with various indications and without any distinct, predominantly common indications, their medication class was used for categorization. For instance, methotrexate which can be used for various autoimmune diseases was categorized as "immunosuppressants." For responses classified as "duplicate," when a participant reported a medication in its brand name first and generic name afterward, for instance, Advil and ibuprofen, only the first response was assigned with an indication, and the rest was deemed "duplicate."

Appendix B. Crude Responses (Prescription-only Non-Controlled Medications)

Indications	Entries
Cardiovascular therapy	lipitor, lipitor, Simvastatin, provastatin, AMLODIPINE, lisinopril, atenolol, lisinopril, lisinopril, linsinopril, Simvistatin, simvastatin, Benazapril, elanapril, Benezipril, lisinopril, rosuvastatin calcium, carvedilol, hydrocholotyide, lisinopril, Olmesartan Medoxomil, Lisinoprill, Diltiazem, Verapamil, Pravastatin, amlodipine, Spironolactone, metoprolol tarrate, metoprolol l tartrate, amlodopin, atorvastatin, losartan, diltiazem, lisinopril, Nifedipine, simvastatin, Lisinopril, atenolol, pravostatin, carvedilol, fenofibrate, Propranolol, Trilipix, warfarin, eliquis, hydrochlothazide, Losartan Potassium, simvastatin, Lovastatin, finofibrate, lisinopril, Simvastatin, Isosorbide Mononitrate, ATORVASTATIN, Atorvastatin, Brillintal, losartan, lisinopril, pravastatin, propranolol, clopidogrel, LOSARTAN, Diltiazem, lisinopril, Astrovastatin, Losartan, sotalol, Metoprolol Tartrate, Metoprolol Tartrate, metoprolol, spironalactone, clopidogrel, pravastatin, isosorbide mononitrate, niacin, metoprolol succ er, metoprolol, lovastatin, lisinopril
Mental health	CYMBALTA, Zoloft, Duloxetine, Paxel, lexapor, zoloft, lexapro, Fluoxetine, abilify, paroxetine, Paxil, Prozac, Paxil, ESCITALOPRAM, Sertraline, Paxil, celexa, Risperidone, Geodone, citaopram, paxil, Prozac, duloxetine, Lithium, Risperidone, Lamotrigine, Zoloft, Wellbutrin, Wellbutrin, cymbalta, aripiprazole, Buspirone, cymbolta, effexor, prozac, duloxetine, Atomoxetine HCL, duloxetine, escitalopram oxalate, venaflaxine, Buspirone, buspar, QUETIAPINE, Buspirone
Endocrine therapy	metformin, Metformin, Levothyroxin, levothyroxine, MEDFORMIN, Fosamax, Glimepride, levoxyl, Levoxylthrine, metformin, Starlix, levothyroxine sodium, allopernol, levothyroxine, Levothyroxine, Alendronate, Tradjenta, synthroid, Metformin, Finesteride, metformin, Calcitriol, levthyroine, Glimepiride, Onglyza, metformin, glimeperide, glipizide, glipizide, prednisone, Lantus, lantus, humalog, apidra, Victoza, Estrofem, vivelle dot patch, estarylla, Microgestin
Antibiotics	Amoxicillin, zythromician, amoxicillin, CLINDAMYCIN, ciprofloxacin, metronidazole, Peniclin, penacillian, doxycycline
Muscle spasm	tizanadine, tizanidine, cyclobednzaprine, cyclobenzaprine hcl, cyclobenzaprine, Tizanidine, cyclobenzapran, tizanidine
Insomnia	trazadone, Trazadone, Mirtazapine, Mirtazapine, trazodone, remeron, mirtazapine
Inhalers (COPD, Asthma)	Ventolin inhaler, flovent 220, proair inhaler, ventolin, proair albuterol, advair
Neuropathic pain	gabapentin, gabapentin, Gabapentin, gabapentin, gabapentin, GABAPENTIN
Specialty injections	humira, humira, Remicade, humira, humira, enbrel
Anticonvulsant	dilantin, zonegran, zonisamide, CARBAMAZEPINE, carbamazepine
Gastrointestinal therapy	bentyl, librax, dexilant, dicyclomine
Fluid retention	furosemide, furosemide, furosamide
Pain	meloxicam, meloxicam, Meloxicam
Asthma (oral)	singular, singular
Cardiovascular therapy and mental health	Clonidine HCl, Clonidine
Incontinence	Vesicare, oxybutynin
Immunosuppressants	methotrexate, ARAVIA
Mental health and allergies	hydroyoxyzine

Indications	Entries
Anticonvulsant and antiglaucoma	acetazolamide
Cough	BENZONATATE
Cardiovascular therapy and gastrointestinal therapy	yosorala
Hair loss (topical)	vaniqa
Antiviral (HIV)	atripla
Migraine	immetrex
Steroid (topical)	Triamcinalone
Electrolyte supplementation	klor con

Appendix C. Crude Responses (Controlled Substances)

Indications	Entries
Mental health	Phenobarbiyol, Concerta, ritalin, Adderall, Focalin *Benzodiazepines* clonazepam, Xanax, ativan, Xanax, Klonopin, Xanax, xnax, lorazepam, alprazolam *benzodiazepine-like non-benzodiazepines* Ambean
Pain/controlled	tramadol, Tramadol, Tramadol, tramadol hcl *Opioids* oxycodone, vicodin, Norco, Norco *Neuropathic pain* lyrica
Weight loss/controlled	phentermine

Appendix D. Crude Responses (OTC Medications)

Indications	Entries
Pain	Tylenol, alieve, advil, tylenol, advil, ibuprofen, advil, ADVIL, aleeve, Acetametophin, advil, Ibuprofen, advil, Acetaminophen, advil, aleve, Advil, ibprofen, Advil, ibupfrofen, Tylenol, tylenol, advil, tylenol, tylenol, aleve, acetaminophen, tynol, motrin, tylanol, tylenol, Ibrfrophen, advil, Tylenol, advil, Tylenol, ibuprofen, IBUPROFEN, tylenol, Ibiprogen, ibuprofen, advil, Ibuprofen, NAPROXEN, tylenol, Extra Strength Tylenol, IBUPROFEN, TYLENOL, acetaminophen, Ibruprofen pm, Naproxen, ibuprofen, ibuprofen
Supplements	pnv, vitamins, multivitamins, b12, Flintstone Vitamins, folic acid, oneaday, cinnamon, iron, cholecalciferol vd3, calcium with D, Vitamin C, Biotin, vitamin d, multi-vitamin, b12, B12, cinnamon, ONE DAY WOME;S MULTIVITAMINS, vitamin d, IRON, coq10, vitamin d3, glucosamine, magnesium, hydrangea root
Gastrointestinal therapy	omezaprole, omeprezole, omeprosole, SENNA-LAX, Zantac, Omeprazole, Equate antacid, omeprazole, meta-mucil, omeprazol, Omeprazole, OMEPRAZOLE, nexium, omeprazole, Pepto Bismal, Omeprazole, senexon, polyethylene glycol, simethicone
Cardiovascular therapy and pain	aspirin, ASPHRAN, aspirin, aspirin, ASPIRIN, Aspirin, aspirin, aspirin, aspirin, aspirin, aspirine
Allergies	zyrtec, Loratadin, claritin, Fexofenadine, allegra, wal-zyr, loratadine, Xyzal
Cold	NyQuil, Advil PM, dimatep, Tylenol PM, nyquil, acetaminophen phenylephrine dextromethorphan, dextromethorphan doxylamine succinate
Nasal sprays (decongestants)	nasacort, Flonase, flonase, flonase, flournase, luticasone

Indications	Entries
Allergies and insomnia	Benadryl, Simply Sleep, benadryl
Cardiovascular therapy	fish oil, fish oil
Migraine	excedrin, Excedrin
Pain (topical)	arnicare, Therapain
Eye drops	Refresh
Insomnia	Melatonin
Sore throat (topical)	Chloraseptic
Antiseptic (topical)	hydrogen peroxide

Appendix E. "Duplicate" and "Invalid" Responses

Duplicate	advil, ibuprophen, levoxyl, advil, atorvastatin, advil, Lipitor, VITAMINS
Invalid	good, ahn, one, yes, one, one, Nore, hgygu, borg, medizel, Fevers, gius, metrolmsop, gtreth, one, as, sustain, unknown, dol, idk, CAPSULES, Jetson, BANDAGE, Fevers, oxy, metrokoloious, Unsure, Muscle Relax, birth control, trats, Nite Time, ear drops, Sleep Aid, Exelium, Bayer, tyroid, after sun lotion, Avien, callous liquid, mucus relief, Anti Allergy, birth control, Sinus Relief, hydrochloride, allergy relief

Appendix F. Complete Counts of Indications of Medications Stored in the Households ($N = 404$)

Prescription Medications				OTC Medications	
Non-Controlled		Controlled Substances			
Indications	$N = 236$	Indications	$N = 25$	Indications	$N = 143$
Cardiovascular therapy	79 (33.5%)	Mental health	15 (60%)	Pain	53 (37.1%)
Mental health	44 (18.6%)	Pain	9 (36%)	Supplements	26 (18.2%)
Endocrine therapy	39 (16.5%)	Weight loss	1 (4%)	Gastrointestinal therapy	19 (13.3%)
Antibiotics	9 (3.8%)			Cardiovascular therapy and pain	11 (7.7%)
Muscle spasm	8 (3.4%)			Allergies	8 (5.6%)
Insomnia	7 (3.0%)			Cold	7 (4.9%)
Inhalers (COPD, Asthma)	6 (2.5%)			Nasal sprays (decongestants)	6 (4.2%)
Neuropathic pain	6 (2.5%)			Allergies and insomnia	3 (2.1%)
Specialty injections	6 (2.5%)			Cardiovascular therapy	2 (1.4%)
Anticonvulsant	5 (2.1%)			Migraine	2 (1.4%)
Gastrointestinal therapy	4 (1.7%)			Pain (topical)	2 (1.4%)
Muscle spasm	8 (3.4%)			Eye drops	1 (0.7%)
Insomnia	7 (3.0%)			Insomnia	1 (0.7%)
Inhalers (COPD, Asthma)	6 (2.5%)			Sore throat (topical)	1 (0.7%)
Neuropathic pain	6 (2.5%)			Antiseptic (topical)	1 (0.7%)
Specialty injections	6 (2.5%)				
Anticonvulsant	5 (2.1%)				
Gastrointestinal therapy	4 (1.7%)				

Prescription Medications				OTC Medications	
Non-Controlled		Controlled Substances			
Indications	N = 236	Indications	N = 25	Indications	N = 143
Fluid retention	3 (1.3%)				
Pain	3 (1.3%)				
Asthma (oral)	2 (0.9%)				
Cardiovascular therapy and mental health	2 (0.9%)				
Incontinence	2 (0.9%)				
Immunosuppressants	2 (0.9%)				
Mental health and allergies	1 (0.4%)				
Anticonvulsant and antiglaucoma	1 (0.4%)				
Cough	1 (0.4%)				
Cardiovascular therapy and gastrointestinal therapy	1 (0.4%)				
Hair loss (topical)	1 (0.4%)				
Antiviral (HIV)	1 (0.4%)				
Migraine	1 (0.4%)				
Steroid (topical)	1 (0.4%)				
Electrolyte supplementation	1 (0.4%)				

References

1. Mikulic, M. Drug Prescription Volume U.S. Available online: https://www.statista.com/statistics/238702/us-total-medical-prescriptions-issued/ (accessed on 10 June 2021).
2. Schumock, G.T.; Li, E.C.; Suda, K.J.; Matusiak, L.M.; Hunkler, R.J.; Vermeulen, L.C.; Hoffman, J.M. National Trends in Prescription Drug Expenditures and Projections for 2014. *Am. J. Health Syst. Pharm.* **2014**, *71*, 482–499. [CrossRef] [PubMed]
3. Schumock, G.T.; Li, E.C.; Suda, K.J.; Wiest, M.D.; Stubbings, J.; Matusiak, L.M.; Hunkler, R.J.; Vermeulen, L.C. National Trends in Prescription Drug Expenditures and Projections for 2015. *Am. J. Health Syst. Pharm.* **2015**, *72*, 717–736. [CrossRef] [PubMed]
4. Schumock, G.T.; Li, E.C.; Suda, K.J.; Wiest, M.D.; Stubbings, J.; Matusiak, L.M.; Hunkler, R.J.; Vermeulen, L.C. National Trends in Prescription Drug Expenditures and Projections for 2016. *Am. J. Health Syst. Pharm.* **2016**, *73*, 1058–1075. [CrossRef] [PubMed]
5. Schumock, G.T.; Li, E.C.; Wiest, M.D.; Suda, K.J.; Stubbings, J.; Matusiak, L.M.; Hunkler, R.J.; Vermeulen, L.C. National Trends in Prescription Drug Expenditures and Projections for 2017. *Am. J. Health Syst. Pharm.* **2017**, *74*, 1158–1173. [CrossRef]
6. Schumock, G.T.; Stubbings, J.; Wiest, M.D.; Li, E.C.; Suda, K.J.; Matusiak, L.M.; Hunkler, R.J.; Vermeulen, L.C. National Trends in Prescription Drug Expenditures and Projections for 2018. *Am. J. Health Syst. Pharm.* **2018**, *75*, 1023–1038. [CrossRef]
7. Schumock, G.T.; Stubbings, J.; Hoffman, J.M.; Wiest, M.D.; Suda, K.J.; Rim, M.H.; Tadrous, M.; Tichy, E.M.; Cuellar, S.; Clark, J.S.; et al. National Trends in Prescription Drug Expenditures and Projections for 2019. *Am. J. Health Syst. Pharm.* **2019**, *76*, 1105–1121. [CrossRef]
8. Tichy, E.M.; Schumock, G.T.; Hoffman, J.M.; Suda, K.J.; Rim, M.H.; Tadrous, M.; Stubbings, J.; Cuellar, S.; Clark, J.S.; Wiest, M.D.; et al. National Trends in Prescription Drug Expenditures and Projections for 2020. *Am. J. Health Syst. Pharm.* **2020**, *77*, 1213–1230. [CrossRef]
9. OTC Use Statistics—Consumer Healthcare Products Association. Available online: https://www.chpa.org/about-consumer-healthcare/research-data/otc-use-statistics (accessed on 10 June 2021).
10. Mikulic, M. Prescription Drug Spending in U.S. 1960–2020. Available online: https://www.statista.com/statistics/184914/prescription-drug-expenditures-in-the-us-since-1960/ (accessed on 10 June 2021).
11. Wieczorkiewicz, S.M.; Kassamali, Z.; Danziger, L.H. Behind Closed Doors: Medication Storage and Disposal in the Home. *Ann. Pharmacother.* **2013**, *47*, 482–489. [CrossRef]
12. Ruhoy, I.S.; Daughton, C.G. Beyond the Medicine Cabinet: An Analysis of Where and Why Medications Accumulate. *Environ. Int.* **2008**, *34*, 1157–1169. [CrossRef]
13. Law, A.V.; Sakharkar, P.; Zargarzadeh, A.; Tai, B.W.B.; Hess, K.; Hata, M.; Mireles, R.; Ha, C.; Park, T.J. Taking Stock of Medication Wastage: Unused Medications in US Households. *Res. Soc. Adm. Pharm.* **2015**, *11*, 571–578. [CrossRef]
14. Maeng, D.D.; Tom, L.A.; Wright, E.A. Patient Characteristics and Healthcare Utilization Patterns Associated with Unused Medications among Medicare Patients. *Res. Soc. Adm. Pharm.* **2017**, *13*, 1090–1094. [CrossRef] [PubMed]

15. Bekker, C.L.; Gardarsdottir, H.; Egberts, A.C.G.; Molenaar, H.A.; Bouvy, M.L.; van den Bemt, B.J.F.; Hövels, A.M. What Does It Cost to Redispense Unused Medications in the Pharmacy? A Micro-Costing Study. *BMC Health Serv. Res.* **2019**, *19*, 243. [CrossRef] [PubMed]
16. Toh, M.R.; Chew, L. Turning Waste Medicines to Cost Savings: A Pilot Study on the Feasibility of Medication Recycling as a Solution to Drug Wastage. *Palliat. Med.* **2017**, *31*, 35–41. [CrossRef] [PubMed]
17. Patrick, P.A.; Jibilian, A.; Herasme, O.; Valencia, J.; Hernandez, E.C.; Jurado, S.; Aguais, J. The Efficacy of a US-Based Medicine Recycling Program Delivering Antiretroviral Drugs Worldwide. *J. Int. Assoc. Physicians AIDS Care* **2009**, *8*, 25–29. [CrossRef] [PubMed]
18. Briones, N. Current State of Drug Recycling Programs in the United States. Available online: https://chicagounbound.uchicago.edu/cgi/viewcontent.cgi?article=1121&context=international_immersion_program_papers (accessed on 25 January 2022).
19. HIV Medicine Recycling Program. Available online: https://aidforaids.org/hiv-recycling-program/ (accessed on 25 January 2022).
20. About RAMP—RAMP—Recycled AIDS Medicine Program. Available online: http://rampusa.org/about-ramp/ (accessed on 25 January 2022).
21. Nicoli, F.; Paudel, D.; Bresciani, G.; Rodi, D.; Siniscalchi, A. Donation Programme of Returned Medicines: Role of Donors and Point of View of Beneficiaries. *Int. Health* **2018**, *10*, 133–136. [CrossRef]
22. Daughton, C.G.; Ruhoy, I.S. PharmEcovigilance: Aligning Pharmacovigilance with Environmental Protection. In *An Introduction to Environmental Pharmacology*; Rahman, S.Z., Shahid, M., Gupta, V., Eds.; Ibn Sina Academy: Aligarh, India, 2008; pp. 21–34.
23. Bekker, C.; van den Bemt, B.; Egberts, T.C.; Bouvy, M.; Gardarsdottir, H. Willingness of Patients to Use Unused Medication Returned to the Pharmacy by Another Patient: A Cross-Sectional Survey. *BMJ Open* **2019**, *9*, e024767. [CrossRef]
24. Bekker, C.L.; Gardarsdottir, H.; Egberts, T.C.G.; Bouvy, M.L.; van den Bemt, B.J.F. Redispensing of Medicines Unused by Patients: A Qualitative Study among Stakeholders. *Int. J. Clin. Pharm.* **2017**, *39*, 196–204. [CrossRef]
25. Alshemari, A.; Breen, L.; Quinn, G.; Sivarajah, U. Can We Create a Circular Pharmaceutical Supply Chain (CPSC) to Reduce Medicines Waste? *Pharmacy* **2020**, *8*, 221. [CrossRef]
26. Donyai, P.; McCrindle, R.; Hui, T.K.L.; Sherratt, R.S. Stakeholder Views on the Idea of Medicines Reuse in the UK. *Pharmacy* **2021**, *9*, 85. [CrossRef]
27. Ruhoy, I.S.; Daughton, C.G. Types and Quantities of Leftover Drugs Entering the Environment via Disposal to Sewage—Revealed by Coroner Records. *Sci. Total Environ.* **2007**, *388*, 137–148. [CrossRef]
28. Sorensen, L.; Stokes, J.A.; Purdie, D.M.; Woodward, M.; Roberts, M.S. Medication Management at Home: Medication-Related Risk Factors Associated with Poor Health Outcomes. *Age Ageing* **2005**, *34*, 626–632. [CrossRef] [PubMed]
29. Gummin, D.D.; Mowry, J.B.; Beuhler, M.C.; Spyker, D.A.; Brooks, D.E.; Dibert, K.W.; Rivers, L.J.; Pham, N.P.T.; Ryan, M.L. 2019 Annual Report of the American Association of Poison Control Centers' National Poison Data System (NPDS): 37th Annual Report. *Clin. Toxicol.* **2020**, *58*, 1360–1541. [CrossRef] [PubMed]
30. Gummin, D.D.; Mowry, J.B.; Spyker, D.A.; Brooks, D.E.; Beuhler, M.C.; Rivers, L.J.; Hashem, H.A.; Ryan, M.L. 2018 Annual Report of the American Association of Poison Control Centers' National Poison Data System (NPDS): 36th Annual Report. *Clin. Toxicol.* **2019**, *57*, 1220–1413. [CrossRef] [PubMed]
31. Gummin, D.D.; Mowry, J.B.; Spyker, D.A.; Brooks, D.E.; Osterthaler, K.M.; Banner, W. 2017 Annual Report of the American Association of Poison Control Centers' National Poison Data System (NPDS): 35th Annual Report. *Clin. Toxicol.* **2018**, *56*, 1213–1415. [CrossRef]
32. Gummin, D.D.; Mowry, J.B.; Spyker, D.A.; Brooks, D.E.; Fraser, M.O.; Banner, W. 2016 Annual Report of the American Association of Poison Control Centers' National Poison Data System (NPDS): 34th Annual Report. *Clin. Toxicol.* **2017**, *55*, 1072–1254. [CrossRef] [PubMed]
33. Mowry, J.B.; Spyker, D.A.; Brooks, D.E.; Zimmerman, A.; Schauben, J.L. 2015 Annual Report of the American Association of Poison Control Centers' National Poison Data System (NPDS): 33rd Annual Report. *Clin. Toxicol.* **2016**, *54*, 924–1109. [CrossRef] [PubMed]
34. McFee, R.B.; Caraccio, T.R. "Hang Up Your Pocketbook"—An Easy Intervention for the Granny Syndrome: Grandparents as a Risk Factor in Unintentional Pediatric Exposures to Pharmaceuticals. *J. Am. Osteopath Assoc.* **2006**, *106*, 405–411.
35. Bond, G.R.; Woodward, R.W.; Ho, M. The Growing Impact of Pediatric Pharmaceutical Poisoning. *J. Pediatrics* **2012**, *160*, 265270. [CrossRef] [PubMed]
36. Lovegrove, M.C.; Weidle, N.J.; Budnitz, D.S. Trends in Emergency Department Visits for Unsupervised Pediatric Medication Exposures, 2004-2013. *Pediatrics* **2015**, *136*, e821–e829. [CrossRef]
37. Gregorian, R.; Marrett, E.; Sivathanu, V.; Torgal, M.; Shah, S.; Kwong, W.J.; Gudin, J. Safe Opioid Storage and Disposal: A Survey of Patient Beliefs and Practices. *J. Pain Res.* **2020**, *13*, 987–995. [CrossRef]
38. Silvestre, J.; Reddy, A.; de la Cruz, M.; Wu, J.; Liu, D.; Bruera, E.; Todd, K.H. Frequency of Unsafe Storage, Use, and Disposal Practices of Opioids among Cancer Patients Presenting to the Emergency Department. *Palliat. Support Care* **2017**, *15*, 638–643. [CrossRef] [PubMed]
39. Kennedy-Hendricks, A.; Gielen, A.; McDonald, E.; McGinty, E.E.; Shields, W.; Barry, C.L. Medication Sharing, Storage, and Disposal Practices for Opioid Medications Among US Adults. *JAMA Intern. Med.* **2016**, *176*, 1027–1029. [CrossRef] [PubMed]
40. Maughan, B.C.; Hersh, E.V.; Shofer, F.S.; Wanner, K.J.; Archer, E.; Carrasco, L.R.; Rhodes, K.V. Unused Opioid Analgesics and Drug Disposal Following Outpatient Dental Surgery: A Randomized Controlled Trial. *Drug Alcohol Depend.* **2016**, *168*, 328–334. [CrossRef] [PubMed]
41. Neill, L.A.; Kim, H.S.; Cameron, K.A.; Lank, P.M.; Patel, D.A.; Hur, S.I.; Opsasnick, L.A.; Curtis, L.M.; Eifler, M.R.; Courtney, D.M.; et al. Who Is Keeping Their Unused Opioids and Why? *Pain Med.* **2020**, *21*, 84–91. [CrossRef]

42. Reddy, A.; de la Cruz, M.; Rodriguez, E.M.; Thames, J.; Wu, J.; Chisholm, G.; Liu, D.; Frisbee-Hume, S.; Yennurajalingam, S.; Hui, D.; et al. Patterns of Storage, Use, and Disposal of Opioids Among Cancer Outpatients. *Oncologist* **2014**, *19*, 780–785. [CrossRef]
43. McCauley, J.L.; Back, S.E.; Brady, K.T. Pilot of a Brief, Web-Based Educational Intervention Targeting Safe Storage and Disposal of Prescription Opioids. *Addict. Behav.* **2013**, *38*, 2230–2235. [CrossRef]
44. Bailey, J.E.; Campagna, E.; Dart, R.C. RADARS System Poison Center Investigators The Underrecognized Toll of Prescription Opioid Abuse on Young Children. *Ann. Emerg. Med.* **2009**, *53*, 419–424. [CrossRef]
45. Agarwal, M.; Lovegrove, M.C.; Geller, R.J.; Pomerleau, A.C.; Sapiano, M.R.P.; Weidle, N.J.; Morgan, B.W.; Budnitz, D.S. Circumstances Involved in Unsupervised Solid Dose Medication Exposures among Young Children. *J. Pediatr.* **2020**, *219*, 188195.e6. [CrossRef]
46. Cortinovis, C.; Pizzo, F.; Caloni, F. Poisoning of Dogs and Cats by Drugs Intended for Human Use. *Vet. J.* **2015**, *203*, 52–58. [CrossRef]
47. Jensen, D.M.; Granzin, K.L. Consumer Logistics: The Inventory Subsystem. In Proceedings of the 1984 Academy of Marketing Science (AMS) Annual Conference; Lindquist, J.D., Ed.; Springer International Publishing: Cham, Switzerland, 2015; pp. 47–51.
48. Stiff, R.; Johnson, K.; Tourk, K.A. Scarcity and Hoarding: Economic and Social Explanations and Marketing Implications. *ACR N. Am. Adv.* **1975**, *2*, 203–216.
49. Center for Drug Evaluation and Disposal of Unused Medicines: What You Should Know. Available online: https://www.fda.gov/drugs/safe-disposal-medicines/disposal-unused-medicines-what-you-should-know (accessed on 12 June 2021).
50. Batt, A.L.; Bruce, I.B.; Aga, D.S. Evaluating the Vulnerability of Surface Waters to Antibiotic Contamination from Varying Wastewater Treatment Plant Discharges. *Environ. Pollut.* **2006**, *142*, 295–302. [CrossRef] [PubMed]
51. Hirsch, R.; Ternes, T.; Haberer, K.; Kratz, K.-L. Occurrence of Antibiotics in the Aquatic Environment. *Sci. Total Environ.* **1999**, *225*, 109–118. [CrossRef]
52. Glassmeyer, S.T.; Hinchey, E.K.; Boehme, S.E.; Daughton, C.G.; Ruhoy, I.S.; Conerly, O.; Daniels, R.L.; Lauer, L.; McCarthy, M.; Nettesheim, T.G.; et al. Disposal Practices for Unwanted Residential Medications in the United States. *Environ. Int.* **2009**, *35*, 566–572. [CrossRef] [PubMed]
53. Stockholms Lans Landsting 2014–2015 Enviornmentally Classified Pharmaceuticals. Available online: https://noharm-global.org/sites/default/files/documents-files/2633/Environmental%20classified%20pharmaceuticals%202014-2015%20booklet.pdf (accessed on 20 May 2021).
54. Masnoon, N.; Shakib, S.; Kalisch-Ellett, L.; Caughey, G.E. What Is Polypharmacy? A Systematic Review of Definitions. *BMC Geriatr.* **2017**, *17*, 230. [CrossRef]
55. Zia, A.; Kamaruzzaman, S.B.; Tan, M.P. Polypharmacy and Falls in Older People: Balancing Evidence-Based Medicine against Falls Risk. *Postgrad. Med.* **2015**, *127*, 330–337. [CrossRef]
56. Prithviraj, G.K.; Koroukian, S.; Margevicius, S.; Berger, N.A.; Bagai, R.; Owusu, C. Patient Characteristics Associated with Polypharmacy and Inappropriate Prescribing of Medications among Older Adults with Cancer. *J. Geriatr. Oncol.* **2012**, *3*, 228–237. [CrossRef]
57. Turner, J.P.; Shakib, S.; Singhal, N.; Hogan-Doran, J.; Prowse, R.; Johns, S.; Bell, J.S. Prevalence and Factors Associated with Polypharmacy in Older People with Cancer. *Support. Care Cancer* **2014**, *22*, 1727–1734. [CrossRef]
58. Best, O.; Gnjidic, D.; Hilmer, S.N.; Naganathan, V.; McLachlan, A.J. Investigating Polypharmacy and Drug Burden Index in Hospitalised Older People. *Intern. Med. J.* **2013**, *43*, 912–918. [CrossRef]
59. Marcum, Z.A.; Gellad, W.F. Medication Adherence to Multi-Drug Regimens. *Clin. Geriatr. Med.* **2012**, *28*, 287–300. [CrossRef]
60. Saljoughian, M. Polypharmacy and Drug Adherence in Elderly Patients. Available online: https://www.uspharmacist.com/article/polypharmacy-and-drug-adherence-in-elderly-patients (accessed on 25 January 2022).
61. Franchi, C.; Ardoino, I.; Ludergnani, M.; Cukay, G.; Merlino, L.; Nobili, A. Medication Adherence in Community-Dwelling Older People Exposed to Chronic Polypharmacy. *J. Epidemiol. Community Health* **2021**, *75*, 854–859. [CrossRef]
62. RED BOOK Online. IBM Micromedex [Database Online]. Truven Health Analytics/IBM Watson Health. 2021. Available online: https://www.micromedexsolutions.com (accessed on 16 July 2021).
63. US Census Bureau, C.H.S. Statistical Abstracts—History—U.S. Census Bureau. Available online: https://www.census.gov/history/www/reference/publications/statistical_abstracts.html (accessed on 19 July 2021).
64. Chronic Diseases in America | CDC. Available online: https://www.cdc.gov/chronicdisease/resources/infographic/chronic-diseases.htm (accessed on 12 June 2021).
65. Michas, F. Leading Diagnoses for Primary Care Physicians U.S. 2019. Available online: https://www.statista.com/statistics/1029294/leading-diagnoses-for-primary-care-physicians-us/ (accessed on 12 June 2021).
66. Mental Health By the Numbers | NAMI: National Alliance on Mental Illness. Available online: https://www.nami.org/mhstats (accessed on 12 June 2021).
67. National Health Index. Available online: https://www.bcbs.com/the-health-of-america/health-index/national-health-index (accessed on 12 June 2021).
68. Funk, O.G.; Yung, R.; Arrighi, S.; Lee, S. Medication Storage Appropriateness in US Households. *Innov. Pharm.* **2021**, *12*, 16. [CrossRef] [PubMed]
69. Tips to Prevent Poisonings | Home and Recreational Safety | CDC Injury Center. Available online: https://www.cdc.gov/homeandrecreationalsafety/poisoning/preventiontips.htm (accessed on 14 June 2021).
70. Maton, B.L.; Simmonds, E.E.; Lee, J.A.; Alwood, A.J. The Use of High-Dose Insulin Therapy and Intravenous Lipid Emulsion to Treat Severe, Refractory Diltiazem Toxicosis in a Dog. *J. Vet. Emerg. Crit. Care* **2013**, *23*, 321–327. [CrossRef] [PubMed]

71. Lewis, E.T.; Cucciare, M.A.; Trafton, J.A. What Do Patients Do with Unused Opioid Medications? *Clin. J. Pain* **2014**, *30*, 654–662. [CrossRef]
72. Resource Conservation and Recovery Act (RCRA) Overview. Available online: https://www.epa.gov/rcra/resource-conservation-and-recovery-act-rcra-overview (accessed on 14 June 2021).
73. Veolia Medical Waste Disposal, Now and in the Future. Available online: http://blog.veolianorthamerica.com/medical-waste-disposal-now-and-future (accessed on 2 August 2021).
74. National Conference of State Legislatures State Prescription Drug Return, Reuse and Recycling Laws. Available online: https://www.ncsl.org/research/health/state-prescription-drug-return-reuse-and-recycling.aspx (accessed on 1 August 2021).
75. American Society of Clinical Oncology 2020 Drug Repository Position Statement. Available online: https://www.asco.org/sites/new-www.asco.org/files/content-files/advocacy-and-policy/documents/2020-DrugRepositoryPositionStatement.pdf (accessed on 1 August 2021).
76. Alhamad, H.; Patel, N.; Donyai, P. How Do People Conceptualise the Reuse of Medicines? An Interview Study. *Int. J. Pharm. Pract.* **2018**, *26*, 232–241. [CrossRef]
77. Hui, T.K.L.; Donyai, P.; McCrindle, R.; Sherratt, R.S. Enabling Medicine Reuse Using a Digital Time Temperature Humidity Sensor in an Internet of Pharmaceutical Things Concept. *Sensors* **2020**, *20*, 3080. [CrossRef]
78. Hui, T.K.L.; Mohammed, B.; Donyai, P.; McCrindle, R.; Sherratt, R.S. Enhancing Pharmaceutical Packaging through a Technology Ecosystem to Facilitate the Reuse of Medicines and Reduce Medicinal Waste. *Pharmacy* **2020**, *8*, 58. [CrossRef]
79. SIRUM Saving Medicine: Saving Lives. Available online: https://www.sirum.org/ (accessed on 3 October 2021).
80. Kaldy, J. Program Turns Discarded Drugs Into Lifesavers for Needy. *Caring Ages* **2015**, *16*, 9. [CrossRef]

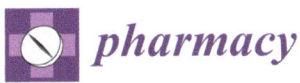

Commentary

Stakeholder Views on the Idea of Medicines Reuse in the UK

Parastou Donyai [1,*], Rachel McCrindle [2], Terence K. L. Hui [2] and R. Simon Sherratt [2]

[1] Reading School of Pharmacy, University of Reading, P.O. Box 226, Whiteknights, Reading RG6 6AP, UK
[2] Department of Biomedical Engineering, School of Biological Sciences, University of Reading, Whiteknights, Reading RG6 6AY, UK; r.j.mccrindle@reading.ac.uk (R.M.); t.hui@reading.ac.uk (T.K.L.H.); r.s.sherratt@reading.ac.uk (R.S.S.)
* Correspondence: p.donyai@reading.ac.uk; Tel.: +44-118-378-4704; Fax: +44-118-378-4703

Abstract: People's views about medicines reuse are being examined in a handful of qualitative studies and this commentary adds to that work by drawing on our own discussions with groups of stakeholders in the UK in the past two years. The reuse of medicines within the community pharmacy setting is not permitted in the UK but our multidisciplinary team anticipates that this position will change in the coming years as medication shortages and worries about environmental waste and financial losses from the destruction of unused medicines are brought to the fore. Indeed, for many stakeholders, the issue of waste is a strong feature of conversations about medicines reuse. In addition to this, stakeholders identify the numerous barriers to medicines reuse in the UK. This includes the current uncertainty about the quality of unused medicines returned to pharmacies, which could otherwise be reused. However, stakeholders have also been very willing to propose solutions to a range of existing barriers. Our commentary draws on stakeholder meetings to elaborate the range of views about medicines reuse within a UK context. The challenge is to move forward from these views to advance the technologies that will facilitate medicines reuse practically as well as legally.

Keywords: medicines; reuse; recycle; medicines reuse; attitudes

Citation: Donyai, P.; McCrindle, R.; Hui, T.K.L.; Sherratt, R.S. Stakeholder Views on the Idea of Medicines Reuse in the UK. *Pharmacy* **2021**, *9*, 85. https://doi.org/10.3390/pharmacy9020085

Academic Editor: Jon Schommer

Received: 7 March 2021
Accepted: 13 April 2021
Published: 16 April 2021

Publisher's Note: MDPI stays neutral with regard to jurisdictional claims in published maps and institutional affiliations.

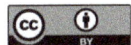

Copyright: © 2021 by the authors. Licensee MDPI, Basel, Switzerland. This article is an open access article distributed under the terms and conditions of the Creative Commons Attribution (CC BY) license (https://creativecommons.org/licenses/by/4.0/).

1. Introduction

A limited number of studies have examined people's views about the concept of 'medicines reuse' [1–4] and the purpose of this commentary is to add to this body of knowledge by reporting on our own discussions about the topic with groups of stakeholders in the UK in the past 24 months.

The concept of 'medicines reuse' itself is open to different interpretations and definitions. For example, some might understand it to relate to reusing a patient's own medicines when they are admitted to a hospital ward [5]; or the concept might be related to the recycling of medicinal components or packaging in future manufacturing processes [6]. The phrase medicines reuse has also been used to refer to the repurposing of old drugs for new conditions. A number of related terminologies also exist, including re-dispense, recycle, redistribute and reverse flow. These ideas and related concepts, although important, are not the focus of the current paper. Here, we use the term 'medicines reuse' to mean the idea that within a community pharmacy context, "medication returned by one patient can be dispensed by a pharmacist to another patient (instead of disposal as waste–which is what currently takes place)". Our paper is focused within a UK context, where pharmacists working within community pharmacies are not permitted to reuse medicines. What prevents medicines reuse in this setting is a combination of the law, professional guidance and past precedence.

In the UK, apparently how a medicine is sourced is not generally relevant as long as a medicine is supplied in accordance with the relevant prescription, for the specific purposes of part 12 of the Human Medicines Regulation 2012 [7]. However, reusing medicines reportedly invalidates the terms and conditions under which medicines are supplied from wholesalers [8]. Additionally, because legislation governing the supply of medicines requires persons trading medicines (other than directly supplying to patients) to hold a wholesale dealer's license [unless supplies are small, take place occasionally, are not-for-profit and not for onward wholesale distribution], this legislation also limits the receipt and redistribution of returned medicines between different units/legal entities along a supply chain (e.g., from one pharmacy to another) [9]. Furthermore, under normal circumstances, medicines reuse is not recommended by the Department of Health because the quality of any medicine that has left the pharmacy cannot be guaranteed [10,11]. In fact, in the UK, none of the regulatory and professional bodies currently support the reuse of medicines within the community pharmacy setting. This includes the Medicines and Healthcare Products Regulatory Agency (MHRA), the Association of British Pharmaceutical Industries (ABPI), the General Pharmaceutical Council (GPhC), the National Health Service (NHS), the British Medical Association (BMA), and the Royal Pharmaceutical Society (RPS). Our research group, however, is investigating the sustainability of this position.

Based on existing knowledge about pharmacy and the technology that might be integrated within pharmaceutical packaging, our multidisciplinary team Reuse of Medicines through Informatics, Networks and Sensors (ReMINDS) (www.reading.ac.uk/ReMINDS, accessed on 14 April 2020) is composed of academics from the pharmacy, computer science and biomedical engineering fields at the University of Reading. 'ReMINDS' communicates our opinion on medicines reuse candidly (we are pro researching medicines-reuse) so our paper is arranged as a commentary rather than a research paper, the aim being to present new viewpoints on an existing problem, while also drawing on original data. Here, we draw on key themes conveyed to our group by a range of stakeholders in meetings organized to discuss medicines reuse, while acknowledging that our paper is imbued with personal opinion, in line with Berterö's definition of a commentary [12].

We draw on our discussions with a range of stakeholders that includes young people, future pharmacists, pharmacists working within the primary-care, community, hospital, and homecare settings, pharmaceutical industry representatives, specialists in medicines supply, patients, and researchers.

2. The Wastage of Medicines

Medicines reuse as a concept stems from the problem of medication waste. After all, if there was zero medication wastage, there would be no medicines *to* reuse. Thus, a range of ideas about medicines reuse are expressed by people, directly in relation to the creation and prevention of medication waste.

A range of practices and settings are thought to contribute to medication waste. For example, using multi-compartment compliance aids (MCCAs) as a practice is thought to be wasteful; in MCCAs, individual doses, having been removed from their packaging, are placed with other medicines within distinct compartments a month or more in advance of actual consumption, rendering the medicines 'expended' as soon as the MCCA is prepared. Then if a patient's medication regimen is changed (e.g., a medication is discontinued), the entire content of their MCCA becomes unusable for that patient—this is because it is too risky to remove individual discontinued tablets from the compartments (risk of error) so the entire contents have to be discarded once the regimen changes. MCCAs are utilized widely within care homes, where there is also a notion by some stakeholders that care-home staff contribute to the wastage of medicines by excessive reordering and the stockpiling of medicines.

Outside of formal care settings, another factor associated with medication waste is medication non-adherence, where patients fail to fully follow the dosage instructions of their medication, for example by not taking their medicines at all or failing to complete the full course. The reasons for non-adherence are complex, multi-factorial and well researched but some noteworthy insights from our patient stakeholders include the need to create conditions that allow patients to disclose their real medication-taking patterns, and to address their fear, disinterest or lack of understanding about medicines, some of which are potentially engendered, it seems, through the physical appearance (design/text) of medicinal packaging.

An additional behaviour recognized and discussed by our stakeholders is the unnecessary/over ordering of medication, for example patients ordering large pack sizes, and stockpiling medication, or over/inappropriate prescribing by doctors. This issue is especially important in the UK since patients are sometimes seen not to be 'accountable' for behaviours such as over-ordering, because many do not directly pay for their medication and bear none of the financial costs. There is arguably then no real barrier to intentional or unintentional medication stockpiling, with some of the people we have spoken to suggesting that notifying patients about the monetary cost (albeit to the NHS) of their medicines (e.g., printing the price on the medicinal packet) might incentivize more responsible re-ordering behaviours—or that in any case alerting patients of their responsibility to reduce the NHS medicines spend is a worthwhile activity.

Doctors, pharmacists and other health professionals are also considered key actors who can reduce medicines waste by 'taking responsibility' for more sustainable practices. For example, by checking, discussing and challenging quantities and medicines being re-ordered, completing medication reviews to ensure rational prescribing, prescribing lower quantities for more expensive medicines or medicines that are new to patients, and ensuring better stock control (including liaising with wholesalers and delivery companies) to avoid accumulating short-dated items (including on hospital wards) or ending up with medicines that are kept at the wrong storage temperature. Related to this is the notion of deprescribing (stopping superfluous medicines), which some patients and doctors avoid out of fear (of therapeutic repercussions). Finally, as patients' own drugs (PODs) can still be used if they are admitted to hospital, another challenge is to ensure patients take their current medicines to hospital, to avoid duplicate dispensing, especially important where people have multiple admissions to hospital within a short period of time. Of course, this is not to deny that some PODs are judged to be of insufficient quality by hospital staff and re-dispensed in any case.

3. Barriers to Medicines Reuse

Similar to that reported elsewhere, our stakeholders had some concerns about medicines reuse. This included questions about the quality and safety of returned medicines and how these might be checked for suitability; and whether patients and consumers really store their medicines correctly at home, especially medicines requiring cold storage—and how people might be educated to do so. Our stakeholders recognized the potential for errors or contamination to occur within the supply chain. Further, they wondered about the cleanliness and potential for contamination of returned medication packs.

One of the concerns about medicines reuse relates to the practicality of operating such a scheme in UK community pharmacies. Community pharmacists have limited time for additional services, meaning that the addition of a medicines reuse scheme would doubtless require effective resourcing and incentivization. It also necessitates additional guidance and standard operating procedures for the receipt, separate storage, quality-assurance, and supply of reusable medicines within relatively small pharmacy spaces. National pharmacy bodies, for example, would be expected to publish consensus guidelines on medicines reuse. Or the NHS might consider taking back returned medication for storage and re-distribution. An additional challenge within community pharmacies relates to the reimbursement of prescription costs and the audit trail needed to prevent duplicate payments to pharmacies, while ensuring pharmacies are paid for the cost of administering medicines reuse.

There is also an expectation for medicines reuse to be financially logical, with implementation costs having to balance against the cost of the original medication. For example, any additional technology that might track the medicine's storage conditions, batch number, manufacturing date/product age, expiry date, etc., to manage resupply, should reasonably be cost-effective. Stakeholders also highlight the potential paradox of having to add to a medicine's carbon footprint in order to reduce its waste—the environmental harm of medicines reuse (e.g., via any additions to the packaging) must thus balance against that created by the medicine's potential wastage if unused.

Two points came up specifically when we spoke to younger people about medicines reuse. Some conceptualized reuse as the process of taking back medicines and re-extracting the constituent elements. For packaged medicines, they thought that these are already routinely sent to other (poorer) countries for their use, but this practice is discouraged by the World Health Organisation which sees it as operating double standards.

Stakeholders pose other relevant questions within the UK context, including whether multiple re-use (re-dispensing) of a medicine might be permitted, and how recall of medicines might affect re-dispensed medicines. Another important issue is how current legislation to hold a wholesale dealer's licence impacts on medicines reuse across different sections of the NHS.

A related matter concerns the falsified medicines directive (FMD), which describes a set of measures introduced in the European Union for the regulation of medicines trade, to prevent the appearance of fake medicines in the legal supply chain. February 2019 saw the implementation of two specific safety features on medicines determined by FMD; a unique identifier (a 2D data matrix code with product code, serial number, batch number, expiry date) on medicinal packaging scannable at fixed points along the supply chain, and tamper evident features (anti-tampering devices) on the pack. Thus, medicines can be verified in their movement through the supply chain, and 'decommissioned' at the final point, on supply to the patient. The stakeholders we engaged with duly ask how medicines then might be placed back within the supply chain in light of FMD, and how the safety features determined by FMD might be harvested to verify medicines for reuse. However, FMD will no longer apply in the UK following its exit from the European Union in 2021, and while this negates the need to 're-commission' a medicine, the absence of safety features that might prevent falsified medicines from entering the supply chain is a less constructive step for medicines reuse.

4. Towards Solutions

Medicines reuse is not currently permitted in the UK but there have been ample questions and ideas from our stakeholders on how to promote engagement with such a scheme in the future. Some questions are, for example, how people might be incentivized to return their unused medicines to pharmacies in the first place, especially within the shelf life of the product. And how they might be educated to store their medication correctly at home to start with. How the stigma around returning medicines to pharmacies might be reduced—after all, these are medicines that would have been ordered/accepted but then left unused. Further, is there a need to take consent before supplying 'reused' medicines? How might we tackle negative perceptions about receiving what some might consider to be 'second-hand medicines', such that medicines reuse becomes socially acceptable, or indeed an obligation in light of eco-friendly movements? Perhaps in the future there might even be a system where people actively 'opt out' of receiving medicines within a reuse scheme.

Suggestions for changing popular opinion and social norms include teaching about the importance of medicines reuse, communicating success stories, and reshaping misconceptions about 're-used' medicines. Stakeholders believe incentivizing uptake, or at least quantifying the overall benefits of medicines reuse could encourage engagement. For example, reusing medicines to prevent medicines shortages is a logical aim. Patients also want clearer information about the current fate of medicines returned to pharmacies. Other suggestions are to learn from existing groups such as 'free cycle', and to train pharmacists and other staff to promote engagement with medicines reuse, and indeed sustainable pharmacy more broadly, and engaging with popular media, celebrity advocates and social media influencers. The use of social media and technology (e.g., smartphones) is seen as plausible, indeed inevitable but patients also express that any developments in this area should be inclusive of older people, who use medicines the most, and poorer patients who might lack access to the newest smartphones.

The support of a range of official bodies too is seen as important for sanctioning medicines reuse in the first place, none of which currently approve medicines reuse within the community pharmacy setting. For example, engaging with medicines reuse might become a part of the community pharmacy contract and embedded within the pharmacy professional standards. Or administering medicines reuse might formally become one of the responsibilities of support staff within a pharmacy. Stakeholders suggest drawing on the experience of similar schemes in Greece [13] and the US [14] to overcome existing barriers to medicines reuse, and aiming to make medicines reuse as acceptable as reusing coffee cups and plastic bags.

Pharmaceutical companies are seen to play a key role and perhaps there could even be tax breaks for companies proactively changing their practices to facilitate reuse; or other incentives in lieu of their social responsibility. For example, pharmaceutical companies are recognized for holding primary raw data relating to the stability of medicines under different storage conditions—gaining access to these data might enable researchers to model and predict the integrity of medication stored in different home environments, to help define medication reuse criteria. Pharmaceutical companies might also explore whether *medication packaging* could be modified to colour-code sensitivity to environmental conditions, increase tolerance to these conditions, accommodate time/temperature indicators or other technology within the surface, or become more sustainable in itself. They might extend the usable shelf life of medicines. They might invest in the development of a secure supply chain for the return of medicines, sustainable technology that monitors medicine integrity during storage and use, or indeed tracks its whereabouts, and provide assurances about the safety, quality and cleanliness of returned medicines. Such technology would need to be secure and ensure the privacy, and even liberty of users. It would also need to be mindful of the primary users of medicines—for example, to prevent creating alarm if a visual quality indicator shows a potentially 'invalidated' medicine during first use.

Hospital pharmacies are recognized for their policies on medicines reuse (for using PODs), and pharmacies in general have risk management tools, which stakeholders expressed would be useful to learn from.

In terms of legislation, our stakeholders recognized the importance of engaging with the various professional and regulatory bodies to enable medicines reuse, recognizing the time and effort that would be required. Activities might include lobbying the MHRA for an exemption that would allow medicines to be reused within the community pharmacy setting; or illustrating potential cost savings to the Department of Health, at least for high-cost items or where drugs are vulnerable to shortages.

5. Discussion

Our stakeholders' ideas about the wastage of medicines can be summarized as relating to practices around MCCAs, especially in care homes, medication non-adherence, over-ordering, over-prescribing, improper stock control and inadequate use of PODs. Their concerns about medicines reuse relate to the quality and safety of returned medicines, pharmacy resources and incentivization to deal with the process, the cost-benefits of such a scheme, and legislative barriers. Finally, their proposed solutions centre on educating and incentivizing the public, removing stigma around returning and reusing medicines, defining consent processes, using technology and social media, engaging with official bodies and the pharmaceutical industry, learning from existing practices in hospitals and lobbying regulators to change the law.

The issues identified as contributing to waste have long been recognized by others and in fact mirror many of the findings of a seminal report on the scale, causes and costs of waste medicines published in 2011 [15]. Indeed, the problem of medication waste is one of the main reasons for debating medicines reuse. This is alongside the high cost of medication, for example expensive cancer drugs in developed countries [16] and the cost of a range of other drugs for chronic and communicable diseases in developing countries such as India [17]. A small pilot in Singapore has also identified the huge potential for medicines reuse to reduce medication wastage and costs [18]. Researchers examining the benefit of long-term donation programmes in Europe, Africa and Latin America, against WHO's formal advice to withhold such donations, also report a decrease in expenditure by both patients and health facilities [19]. The issue of lack of accountability for the over-ordering of medicines identified by our stakeholders associated with free prescriptions has also been debated before, with one suggestion being to charge a nominal £1 fee for prescription items to create a symbolic contract for patients to take their medicines more responsibly [20].

Some of the concerns relating to medicines reuse expressed by our stakeholders, as well as their proposed solutions, also feature in the limited number of studies that have systematically examined medication reuse. For example, Bekker and colleagues who examined views about medicines reuse in The Netherlands in 2014/15 identified two central requirements for the re-dispensing of returned medicines; namely, patient willingness to use and trust re-dispensed medicines and guaranteed product quality of re-dispensed medicines [2]. System requirements in that study were identified as relating to legal feasibility, financial aspects that should be taken into account and the roles stakeholders can fulfil [2]. Interestingly, in 2014 Liou and colleagues devised a quality control programme to ensure the safe recycling of metered dose inhalers within a hospital setting, focusing on microbial decontamination of the partially used devices [21]. When McRae and colleagues interviewed pharmacists in the UK about medicines reuse in 2014, they identified a range of criteria to be met for pharmacists to potentially accept the redistribution of tablet and capsule medication: "protection for pharmacists; guidance from the professional regulator; tamper evident seals; 'as new' packaging; technologies to indicate inappropriate storage and public engagement" [22]. Our own findings from interviews with members of the public in the UK exploring medicines reuse beliefs in 2016 was structured around the theory of planned behaviour [3]. We reported views on the potential economic and environmental benefits of medicines reuse alongside people's worries about medication stability and safety. Our participants then also wondered if pharmacists had the time and storage space to dedicate to medicines reuse. The physical characteristics of reused medicines, and quality assurance and logistics of reuse processes were also seen to enable/obstruct engagement in medicines reuse [3]. Thus, our stakeholders' views outlined here appear to chime with the concerns expressed by others in the past, and appear to be valid and reasonable to address.

While the number of studies in this field are limited, it is also clear that once people are consulted, there is an appetite for exploring how to make medicines reuse safe, and a limited number of ideas on how to do so in practice. One of the ideas that appears to be unique to our own exploration of views here is to engage pharmaceutical companies in sharing their raw stability data to be programmed into a system for monitoring the impact of storage conditions on the continued stability of medication stored in a patient's home. We also found it interesting that when talking to our younger stakeholders, they imagined medicines reuse was already taking place, albeit at least via donations to developing countries. What is important about our work is that is brings together the views of a range of participants and reflects the latest thinking in this area. However, it is also interesting to note that as far back as 2007, Mackridge and Marriott spotted the potential that by using "modern packaging techniques, including tamper-evident seals and 'smart' labels that react to temperature and humidity, it would be possible to identify inappropriately stored medicines" [23].

6. What Next

Alongside stakeholder consultations described here and elsewhere [3], we have been progressing some of the practical ideas relating to medicines reuse within our multidisciplinary ReMINDS team. A review of the literature has allowed us to suggest a novel ReMINDS ecosystem as a solution for reusing returned prescribed medicines [24]. This system relies on active sensing technologies integrated with the Internet of Things platform to validate the quality and safety of medicines while interconnecting the relevant stakeholders. Additionally, we have developed the prototype for a novel digital time, temperature and humidity indicator using smart sensors with cloud connectivity as the key technology for verifying and enabling the reuse of returned medicines [25]. The past year has also seen a global pandemic impacting on the supply of medicines which in the UK has resulted in the temporary approval of medicines reuse within the hospice and care home sectors [26]. Our challenge now is to learn from the reuse of medicines within these settings and continue to explore the technological ways in which medicines reuse can be further progressed.

Author Contributions: P.D. prepared, reviewed and revised the manuscript. R.M., T.K.L.H. and R.S.S. critically reviewed and revised the manuscript. All authors have read and agreed to the published version of the manuscript.

Funding: This research was funded through the University of Reading Research Endowment Trust Fund (RETF), and the Building Outstanding Impact Support Programme (BOISP).

Acknowledgments: We would like to thank our stakeholders who have engaged with us on the topic of medicines reuse over the past 24 months. We specifically thank Tracey Duncombe for facilitating one of the stakeholder meetings we held in 2019.

Conflicts of Interest: The authors declare no conflict of interest.

References

1. Bekker, C.; van den Bemt, B.; Egberts, T.C.G.; Bouvy, M.; Gardarsdottir, H. Willingness of patients to use unused medication returned to the pharmacy by another patient: A cross-sectional survey. *BMJ Open* **2019**, *9*, e024767. [CrossRef] [PubMed]
2. Bekker, C.L.; Gardarsdottir, H.; Egberts, T.C.G.; Bouvy, M.L.; van den Bemt, B.J.F. Redispensing of medicines unused by patients: A qualitative study among stakeholders. *Int. J. Clin. Pharm.* **2017**, *39*, 196–204. [CrossRef] [PubMed]
3. Alhamad, H.; Patel, N.; Donyai, P. How do people conceptualise the reuse of medicines? An interview study. *Int. J. Pharm. Pract.* **2018**, *26*, 232–241. [CrossRef] [PubMed]
4. Alhamad, H.; Donyai, P. Intentions to "Reuse" Medication in the Future Modelled and Measured Using the Theory of Planned Behavior. *Pharmacy* **2020**, *8*, 213. [CrossRef] [PubMed]
5. Dean, B. Guide to POD Schemes and One-Stop Dispensing. Available online: https://hospitalpharmacyeurope.com/news/editors-pick/guide-to-pod-schemes-and-one-stop-dispensing/ (accessed on 27 February 2021).
6. TerraCycle. The Medicine Packet Recycling Programme. Available online: https://www.terracycle.com/en-GB/brigades/medicine-packet-uk (accessed on 27 February 2021).
7. The UK Government. Novel Coronavirus (COVID-19) Standard Operating Procedure: Running a Medicines Reuse Scheme in a Care Home or Hospice Setting. Available online: https://www.gov.uk/government/publications/coronavirus-covid-19-reuse-of-medicines-in-a-care-home-or-hospice/novel-coronavirus-covid-19-standard-operating-procedure-running-a-medicines-re-use-scheme-in-a-care-home-or-hospice-setting (accessed on 25 February 2021).
8. Dicomidis, J.; Kirby, A. Reuse of medicines: Looking beyond the waste blame game. *Prescriber* **2012**, *23*, 13–17. [CrossRef]
9. Royal Pharmaceutical Society. *Medicines, Ethics and Practice*; Royal Pharmaceutical Society: London, UK, 2019.
10. Department of Health [ARCHIVED CONTENT] Repeat Prescribing Systems: Department of Health—Publications. Available online: https://webarchive.nationalarchives.gov.uk/+/http://www.dh.gov.uk/en/Publicationsandstatistics/Publications/PublicationsPolicyAndGuidance/Browsable/DH_4892136 (accessed on 26 February 2021).
11. House of Commons—Public Accounts—Minutes of Evidence Supplementary memorandum from the Department of Health 2009. Available online: http://webarchive.parliament.uk/20160609130754/http://www.publications.parliament.uk/pa/cm200809/cmselect/cmpubacc/99/8121708.htm (accessed on 15 April 2021).
12. Berterö, C. Guidelines for writing a commentary. *Int. J. Qual. Stud. Health Well-Being* **2016**, *11*. [CrossRef] [PubMed]
13. GIVMED. Available online: https://givmed.org/en/ (accessed on 9 January 2020).
14. Cauchi, R.; Berg, K. State Prescription Drug Return, Reuse and Recycling Laws. Available online: https://www.ncsl.org/research/health/state-prescription-drug-return-reuse-and-recycling.aspx (accessed on 9 January 2020).
15. Trueman, P.; Lowson, K.; Blighe, A.; Meszaros, A. *Evaluation of the Scale, Causes and Costs of Waste Medicines*; York Health Economics Consortium: York, UK, 2011; Volume 17.
16. Layton, J.L.; Lewis, B.; Ryan, C.; Beer, T.M.; Sartor, O. Recycling Discarded Drugs: Improving Access to Oral Antineoplastic Drugs. *Oncologist* **2019**, *24*, 291–292. [CrossRef] [PubMed]
17. Neelam, S.; Vipula; Monica, K.; Mohini, K. Reusing Medicines-An Unexplored Concept in India. *Indian J. Pharm. Pract.* **2014**, *7*, 1–6.
18. Toh, M.R.; Chew, L. Turning waste medicines to cost savings: A pilot study on the feasibility of medication recycling as a solution to drug wastage. *Palliat. Med.* **2017**, *31*, 35–41. [CrossRef] [PubMed]

19. Nicoli, F.; Paudel, D.; Bresciani, G.; Rodi, D.; Siniscalchi, A. Donation programme of returned medicines: Role of donors and point of view of beneficiaries. *Int. Health* **2018**, *10*, 133–136. [CrossRef] [PubMed]
20. Donyai, P. Prescription Charging Must Balance Health and Budget Benefits. Available online: https://theconversation.com/prescription-charging-must-balance-health-and-budget-benefits-27080 (accessed on 9 April 2021).
21. Liou, J.; Clyne, K.; Knapp, D.; Snyder, J. Establishing a quality control program: Ensuring safety from contamination for recycled metered-dose inhalers. *Hosp. Pharm.* **2014**, *49*, 437–443. [CrossRef] [PubMed]
22. McRae, D.; Allman, M.; James, D. The redistribution of medicines: Could it become a reality? *Int. J. Pharm. Pract.* **2016**, *24*, 411–418. [CrossRef] [PubMed]
23. Mackridge, A.J.; Marriott, J.F. Returned medicines: Waste or a wasted opportunity? *J. Public Health* **2007**, *29*, 258–262. [CrossRef] [PubMed]
24. Hui, T.K.L.; Mohammed, B.; Donyai, P.; McCrindle, R.; Sherratt, R.S. Enhancing Pharmaceutical Packaging through a Technology Ecosystem to Facilitate the Reuse of Medicines and Reduce Medicinal Waste. *Pharmacy* **2020**, *8*, 58. [CrossRef] [PubMed]
25. Hui, T.K.L.; Donyai, P.; McCrindle, R.; Sherratt, R.S. Enabling Medicine Reuse Using a Digital Time Temperature Humidity Sensor in an Internet of Pharmaceutical Things Concept. *Sensors* **2020**, *20*, 3080. [CrossRef] [PubMed]
26. Donyai, P.; McCrindle, R.; Sherratt, R.S.; Hui, T.K.L. COVID-19 Pandemic is Our Chance to Learn How to Reuse Old Medicines. Available online: https://theconversation.com/covid-19-pandemic-is-our-chance-to-learn-how-to-reuse-old-medicines-137671 (accessed on 22 February 2020).

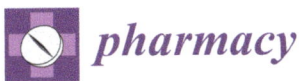

Article

Public Attitudes towards Medicinal Waste and Medicines Reuse in a 'Free Prescription' Healthcare System

David McRae [1,*], Abigail Gould [2], Rebecca Price-Davies [3], Jonathan Tagoe [3], Andrew Evans [4] and Delyth H. James [2]

1. Pharmacy Department, Prince Charles Hospital, Medicines Management Directorate, Cwm Taf Morgannwg University Health Board, Merthyr Tydfil CF47 9DT, UK
2. Cardiff School of Sport and Health Sciences, Cardiff Metropolitan University, Cardiff CF5 2YB, UK; A.Gould4@cardiffmet.ac.uk (A.G.); dhjames@cardiffmet.ac.uk (D.H.J.)
3. School of Pharmacy and Pharmaceutical Sciences, Cardiff University, Cardiff CF10 3NB, UK; PriceR@cardiff.ac.uk (R.P.-D.); TagoeJA@Cardiff.ac.uk (J.T.)
4. Health and Social Services Group, Welsh Government, Cardiff CF10 3NQ, UK; Andrew.Evans@gov.wales
* Correspondence: David.McRae@wales.nhs.uk

Abstract: This study investigates public attitudes towards medicinal waste and medicines reuse within a 'free prescription' healthcare system. A quantitative online survey was employed in a sample drawn from the population of Wales, where prescription medicines have been 'free' since 2007. Qualitative interviews informed the content of the attitude statements with categorical or ordinal response options assigned. The questionnaire was hosted on the HealthWise Wales platform for 1 year from October 2017. Of the 5584 respondents, 67.2% had at least one medicine on repeat prescription. Overall, 89.1% held strong concerns about medicinal waste. High acceptance for the reuse of prescription medicines which have been returned unused by patients to pharmacies was reported for tablets (78.7%) and capsules (75.1%) if the medicine is checked by a pharmacist first (92.4% rated essential). Concerns identified related to tampering of packs (69.2%) and the need for hygienic storage (65.4%). However, those working in healthcare had less concern about the safety of reusing medicines. The level of public acceptance for the reuse of medication was higher than previously reported. This is the largest survey to capture these views to date, which has implications for the future design of medicines reuse schemes.

Keywords: medicines reuse; medicinal waste; re-dispensing; re-issuing; redistribution; recycling; public views; public attitudes; medicines storage

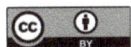

1. Introduction

Medicinal waste can be produced at all points in the pharmaceutical supply chain. However, it is the waste generated when prescription medicines are returned to healthcare providers by patients, many of which remain unopened with packaging intact, which has, over the last decade, received increased interest from both researchers [1,2] and mainstream British news outlets [3–6]. These returned medicines are currently prohibited from re-entering the pharmaceutical supply chain in most healthcare systems and are, consequently, destroyed. This is considered by many stakeholders to represent an unacceptable and costly waste of limited healthcare resources [7,8].

One potential solution to reduce the amount of waste is for returned medicines to be re-dispensed to other patients. This practice, which has been referred to previously as medicines reuse [9], re-dispensing [7], re-issuing [10], redistribution [8], and recycling [2] (reuse and re-dispensing are used interchangeably in this paper), is prohibited due to concerns that returned medicines may have been stored inappropriately in patients' homes (i.e., stored at temperatures which would cause the active pharmaceutical ingredient to degrade) or that they may have been tampered with [11].

In 2015, however, our research group identified that some pharmacists—the healthcare professionals charged with ensuring the quality of medication supplied to the public—would consider re-dispensing returned medicines if certain criteria were met [8]. These criteria included incorporating newer packaging technologies (which could alert pharmacists if medicines have been stored incorrectly or tampered with) and the need for public engagement prior to any such scheme commencing, due to concerns about how the public would accept medicines reuse [8].

At the time this study was conceptualised, little research had been conducted into how the public perceive the issue of medicines reuse. In 2011, the National Health Service (NHS) Sustainability Development Unit in the United Kingdom (UK) found that 52% of a sample of 1101 people living in England would accept medicines returned by other patients if they have been checked for safety [10]. Unfortunately, no further questions were asked to elicit the details of what would be expected to be included in a safety check or whether there were any other criteria participants would require before they would accept returned medicines. Following this, Hendrick and colleagues conducted a small survey of hospital in-patients and out-patients, which found that 66% (of the 59 respondents) would accept reused medicines, but that few (specific figures not provided) would do so unconditionally [9].

Medicines reuse schemes exist in some private healthcare systems, such as Greece and the United States of America (USA), where reuse allows members of the public to access medicines which they would not otherwise be able to afford [12,13]. To date, no research had been conducted with the aim of sampling public attitudes towards medicines reuse and medicinal waste drawn solely from a healthcare system where prescription medicines are 'free'. Some policy makers may share the belief expressed by primary care professionals, in interviews conducted by Truman and colleagues, that people receiving free medicines do not value them [14]. Anchored by that belief, policy makers may also take the view that there would be little incentive for the public to accept medicines reuse (in a free medicines healthcare system) and that concerns about medicinal waste would be low.

The aim of this study was, therefore, to determine public attitudes towards medicinal waste and medicines reuse in a large sample of the general population, within a 'free prescription medicine' healthcare system, through the use of a web-based platform where members of the public register to receive health related questionnaires. This study sought to identify whether the public has concerns about the reuse of medicines and what criteria, if any, would need to be met for medicines reuse to be accepted. In addition, the suitability of returned medicines for reuse may depend on how they have been stored and, therefore, this study also aimed to capture information on domiciliary medicines storage practices. Furthermore, it has been suggested that to sustain a reuse scheme the public would need to be encouraged to return their medicines to healthcare facilities [15,16]. Previous research, conducted in 2006, found that only one in three respondents disposed of their medicines appropriately (by returning to healthcare facilities) [17] and as such, this study also seeks to establish current medicines disposal practices of the public and whether the public would be more likely (or not) to return medicines to pharmacies if medicines started to be reused. This study was predominantly exploratory in nature. However, one hypothesis was tested, which arose from previous research relating to pharmacists' positive views about a re-dispensing scheme [8]. Our hypothesis was:

Healthcare professionals hold stronger concerns about medicinal waste and less perceived concerns about the safety of medicines reuse than non-healthcare workers.

2. Materials and Methods

2.1. Overview of Study

A predominantly quantitative approach was adopted to meet the aims of this study. A questionnaire was developed and hosted on a web-based platform (HealthWise Wales, Cardiff, UK). The questionnaire was designed to capture participants' attitudes towards medicinal waste, medicines reuse and to identify contemporary domiciliary medicines storage and disposal practices.

2.2. Study Setting

Wales is a country in the UK with a population of 3.1 million people [18]. Prescription charges were abolished by the Welsh Assembly Government in April 2007 [19]. Prior to this, prescriptions were only free for people under 25 and over 60 years of age or for those who had certain medical conditions [19].

The questionnaire was hosted on the HealthWise Wales' platform which is the survey's virtual online interface comprising the HealthWise Wales Website and Web Application (data collection tool) [20]. People over the age of sixteen years of age living in Wales or using health services in Wales have been eligible to register with the HealthWise Wales platform since it was launched in 2016. Registered platform users are contacted every six months and asked to complete a suite of questions of which the present questionnaire was one.

2.3. Data Collection

HealthWise Wales participants provide demographic data (see Table 1) as part of a core module when registering with the platform. Educational attainment is not collected. Employment status is measured using a 4-category classification of employment (higher occupations; intermediate occupations; lower occupations; students or long-term unemployment).

Table 1. Characteristics of the population of Wales and HealthWise Wales participants.

Demographic Variable	Population of Wales	HealthWise Wales Participants [1]
Gender [2]	Female = 51% Male = 49%	Female = 75% Male = 25%
Age (in years) [3]		
16–24	11%	12%
25–44	24%	30%
45–64	26%	41%
>65	21%	16%
Occupational Class [4]		
Professional	27%	50%
Intermediate	21%	18%
Routine and Manual	37%	11%
Other	15%	21%

[1] Information taken from: HealthWise Wales: Resource Access Guidance for Researchers [21]. The characteristics of HealthWise Wales participants presented in Table 1 are those of the first 10,000 participants recruited to the platform. [2] Gender categories for other/prefer not to say were also available, but responses for these were too small to report. The gender breakdown presented is for persons aged 16 years and older to aid comparison with HealthWise Wales participants [22]. [3] Mid-year estimates for 2019 used for breakdown of population by age for Wales [22]. [4] Occupational Class breakdowns for Wales and HealthWise Wales participants taken from HealthWise Wales: Resource Access Guidance for Researchers [21]. Occupational classes come from the National Statistics Socio-economic Classification (NS-SEC) [23]. Professional occupations include higher managerial, higher administrative and traditional professional occupations. Intermediate occupations include secretary, personal assistant, clerical worker, office clerk. Routine and manual occupations include HGV driver, van driver, cleaner, porter, packer, sewing machinist, messenger, labourer and waiter/waitress.

The Welsh Index of Multiple Deprivation (WIMD), the Welsh Government's official measure of relative deprivation, is determined for each HealthWise Wales participant from the address entered when registering. Deprivation, within the WIMD, refers to the degree to which the needs associated with each indicator (income, employment, health, education, access to services, housing, community safety and physical environment) are met [24]. All areas in Wales (n = 1909, average population of 1600) are ranked from 1 (most deprived) to 1909 (least deprived) [20]. Areas are then divided into five relative deprivation categories (or quintiles): 10% most deprived (areas 1–191); 10–20% most deprived (area

192–382); 20–30% (areas 383–573); 30–50% (areas 574–955) and 50% least deprived (areas 956–1909) [24].

2.4. Questionnaire Design

Qualitative interview data from an MPharm undergraduate student project [JT] conducted in 2014 informed the content of the questionnaire. The questionnaire items were developed following analysis of the transcripts of eleven interviews conducted to gather views on medicinal waste and medicines reuse with members of the public between 30 and 70 years of age recruited via GP practices in one healthcare authority in Wales. All interview participants were in receipt of repeat medications from the GP surgery. Content analysis of 32 comments made by the general public under a web article about the potential for reuse of medicines [25] was also utilised. The questionnaire was subsequently piloted on a convenience sample of ten members of the public from South East Wales and community pharmacy users from South West Wales. Following feedback, several questions were removed in an attempt to improve face and content validity (these questions focused on the role of medicines cost to the NHS) and a definition of regular medicines use added (those medicines which are on 'repeat prescription'). The resultant questionnaire (Supplementary Materials Data S1) comprised twelve questions (question 11 having two parts).

Question 1 asked participants whether they considered themselves to work in healthcare, with question 2 providing a list of healthcare roles to choose from for those answering in the affirmative to question 1.

Question 3 sought to determine whether participants were prescribed medication regularly (on repeat prescription).

Question 4 aimed to determine whether respondents were concerned about 'the amount of prescription medicines' wasted in the healthcare system. Respondents were asked to rate their agreement on a 5-point Likert scale (Strongly Agree, Agree, Neither Agree or Disagree, Disagree, Strongly Disagree) plus a response option for Don't Know.

Question 5 asked respondents where they stored medicines within their home. Respondents were able to select one or more location from a pre-generated list (Living room, Kitchen, Bathroom, Entrance hall, Other, I don't have medicines). If 'Other' was selected, participants were provided with space to enter the location.

Question 6 asked participants what they did with medicines they no longer needed. Participants were provided with a list of possible ways of dealing with medicines which they no longer needed (throw out with household waste, keep just in case I need in future, return to pharmacy, return to GP, I don't use medicines or other) from which they were able to select more than one option. If 'Other' was selected, participants were provided with space to enter how they dealt with these medicines.

Question 7 asked participants what they believed currently happened with medicines that were returned to pharmacies. Participants were provided with a list of options from which they could choose one (re-dispensed to other people, sent to developing countries (or 'third world'), destroyed, not sure, other). If 'Other' was selected, participants were provided with space to enter what they believed happened to these medicines.

Question 8 was presented as a table that included a list of pharmaceutical forms. Participants were asked which of the types of medicine they would accept if they were re-dispensed. Participants were able to select "yes", "no" or "unsure" for each form.

Question 9 was presented as a table that included statements that sought to determine factors (or conditions) that participants would need to be in place for them to accept a medicine that had been returned to a pharmacy by someone else. Participants were able to select a response of: 'Essential', 'Desirable', 'Unsure' or 'Not Needed', for each statement.

Question 10 was presented as a table that included statements which sought to determine participant's beliefs about the safety of reused medicines and concerns about reuse schemes. Participants were asked to indicate their agreement (or disagreement) with each statement on a 5-point Likert scale (Strongly Agree, Agree, Neither Agree or Disagree, Disagree, Strongly Disagree). Participants were also provided with a 'Don't Know' option.

Question 11 had two parts. Part A asked participants whether they would be more or less likely to return medicines that they no longer needed to a pharmacy if medicines started to be reused. Participants could choose one of the following statements "More likely to return to a pharmacy", "Less likely to return to a pharmacy" or "Would not change how I get rid of medicines". Part B asked how participants return their unused medicines to a pharmacy. Participants were provided with the following options to select from: 'Always', 'Often', 'Sometimes', 'Rarely' or 'Never'.

Question 12 asked participants whether they thought all medicines should be considered for re-dispensing or only those which were expensive. Participants were able to select from one of the following options: 'Only expensive medicines (perhaps costing the NHS greater than £20) should be considered for re-dispensing', 'all medicines should be considered for re-dispensing', or 'not sure'.

2.5. Sampling and Recruitment

The questionnaire was made available on the HealthWise Wales platform between October 2017 and October 2018. The number of registered users in October 2017 was 12,818, and 26,198 in October 2018. Due to the dynamic nature of the number of platform users, it was not possible to calculate a response rate for this study.

2.6. Analysis

The data were accessed and analysed via the HealthWise Wales Information Repository (SAPPHIRe), which is implemented on the UK Secure eResearch Platform (UKSeRP) [26] using IBM Statistical Package for Social Sciences (SPSS) version 26 ©.

Basic descriptive statistical analyses were undertaken for the demographic characteristics, i.e., gender, age, ethnicity, health board, level of employment, level of deprivation, and whether they worked in healthcare. Categorical data such as participant storage practices, disposal of medicines, current fate of medicines returned to the pharmacy and level of acceptance for twelve formulations of medicines considered for re-dispensing were summed and percentages calculated. Frequency distributions were calculated for Likert scale responses for the 'concerns about medicinal waste' item, nine 'factors affecting acceptance for reuse' items (Question 9) and nine items to measure 'concerns about the safety of re-dispensing prescribed medicines' (Question 10).

2.6.1. Factor Analysis, Cronbach's Alpha and Scale Score Analysis

All items relating to 'beliefs about the safety of medicines reuse' were negatively worded apart from one—'It is safe for other people to use medicines that I have returned' (Q10b). This item was reverse scored prior to analysis to ensure that 5-point Likert scale response were in the same direction as all other items. 'Don't know' responses were treated as missing data and removed from the analysis. Principal Component Factor Analysis was conducted for all nine items using Varimax Rotation with Kaiser Normalisation and the Eigen value was set to 1 [27]. This yielded a two-component matrix where 59.8% of the variance was explained by two factors (see Supplementary Materials Data S2). For the purpose of this analysis one 5-item scale (Q10a, b, d, e, f) was used to represent concerns about the safety of medicines reuse and this was labelled 'perceived safety of medicines reuse'. Cronbach's alpha analysis was undertaken to check for the internal consistency of the scale. A Cronbach's alpha value above 0.70 is acceptable [28] and in this case was calculated as 0.817 indicating excellent internal reliability. Individual item scores were therefore summed to produce a total scale score for 'perceived safety of medicines reuse' with a minimum possible score of 5 and maximum possible score of 25 and mid-point of the scale of 15. Higher scores indicate stronger beliefs that the concept of medicines reuse is unsafe.

2.6.2. Relationships with Beliefs about Safety of Medicines Reuse Scale Scores

Parametric tests such as independent sample *t*-tests and one-way Analysis of Variance (ANOVA) were used to test for statistically significant differences between scale scores which were normally distributed (e.g., perceived safety of medicines reuse scale) and dichotomous variables (e.g., healthcare vs. non-healthcare worker). Non-parametric tests (i.e., Mann–Whitney) were used to test for statistically significant differences in scores where data were not normally distributed (e.g., concerns for medicinal waste) and dichotomous variables (i.e., healthcare vs. non-healthcare workers). A probability level of $p < 0.05$ was set as a benchmark for reaching statistical significance.

3. Results

3.1. Participants

Table 2 summarises the participant demographic characteristics. Of the 5584 Health-Wise Wales members who completed the questionnaire, over two-thirds were female. Participants' age ranged from 16 to 96 years (mean age = 53.1 years; SD = 16.059).

One-fifth of participants (19.9%, $n = 1109/5584$) indicated that they worked in a healthcare setting, with nearly half (47.9%) working in non-clinical roles and 52.1% in patient-facing roles.

Table 2. Participant demographic characteristics ($n = 5584$ unless otherwise stated [1]).

Demographic Variable	n (%)
Gender	Female = 3877 (69.5)
	Male = 1703 (30.5)
	Other/Prefer not to say = 4 (<0.001)
Age (in years)	
16–24	288 (5.2)
25–44	1411 (25.3)
45–64	2273 (40.7)
>65	1610 (28.8)
Ethnicity	$n = 5107$; *missing data* = 477
Welsh	2921 (57.2)
Other British	1979 (38.8)
Irish	43 (0.8)
Other White background	89 (1.7)
Mixed/Multiple ethnic background	39 (0.7)
Asian background	<27 (0.7)
Black/African/Caribbean ethnic background	<15 (0.1)
Arab and other ethnic group	<16 (0.2)
University Health Board (UHB)	$n = 5458$; *missing data* = 126
Cardiff and Vale	1053 (18.9)
Aneurin Bevan	816 (14.6)
Abertawe Bro Morgannwg [2]	780 (14.0)
Cwm Taf [2]	750 (13.4)
Betsi Cadwaladr	738 (13.2)
Powys [3]	705 (12.6)
Hywel Dda	616 (11.0)
Level of Employment	$n = 5180$; *missing data* = 404
Higher occupations	2659 (51.2)
Intermediate occupations	974 (18.8)
Lower occupations	489 (9.4)
Students or long-term unemployment	1058 (20.6)

Table 2. Cont.

Demographic Variable	n (%)
Level of deprivation	n = 5458; missing data = 126
1—Most deprived	617 (11.3)
2	883 (16.2)
3	1107 (20.3)
4	1423 (26.1)
5—Least deprived	1428 (26.2)
Urban and rural classification	n = 5458; missing data = 126
Urban > 10 k	3290 (60.3)
Town and fringe	1018 (18.7)
Village, hamlet and isolated dwellings	1150 (21.1)
Currently prescribed one or more medicines regularly (repeat prescription) by your doctor (Question 3)	n = 5555; missing data = 29 3733 (67.2)

[1] Missing data are quantified in individual sections as the HealthWise Wales platform permits participants to submit incomplete questionnaires, both in core modules and researcher-led modules (such as this). [2] These two UHBs have been restructured since this study was undertaken. [3] Powys is a Teaching Health Board, not a University Health Board.

3.2. Concerns about Medicinal Waste (Question 4)

Responders reported strong concerns about medicinal waste (mean score = 4.46; SD = 0.719), where 89.1% strongly agreed or agreed with the statement shown in Table 3 and therefore these scores were not normally distributed.

Table 3. Concerns about medicinal waste (n = 5573).

	Strongly Agree n (%)	Agree n (%)	Neither Agree nor Disagree n (%)	Disagree n (%)	Strongly Disagree n (%)	Don't Know n (%)
Q4. I am concerned by the amount of prescription medicines which are wasted in the NHS	3143 (56.3)	1826 (32.8)	428 (7.7)	67 (1.2)	18 (0.3)	91 (1.6)

3.3. Medicines Storage and Disposal (Questions 5–7)

Table 4 details participants' storage and disposal practices. The majority of participants reported keeping their prescribed medicines in either the kitchen, bedroom or bathroom. Over half said they returned unwanted medicines to the pharmacy and over one-quarter reported keeping unused medicines for the future. Over three-quarters of participants were aware that returned, unused medicines are currently destroyed.

3.4. Views about Medicines Reuse (Question 8)

Table 5 reports the formulation of medicines which the participants would be prepared to accept if they were re-dispensed, indicating that tablets and capsules have the highest acceptance for reuse.

Table 4. Storage, disposal and return of medicines (n = 5584).

Question	Response Option	n = (%)
Q5. In your home, where do you store medicines that have been prescribed for you? (Can select more than one option)	Kitchen	2775 (49.7)
	Bedroom	1601 (28.7)
	Bathroom	1094 (19.6)
	Living room	244 (4.4)
	Entrance hall	25 (0.4)
	Other specific cupboard/cabinet/box or drawer	39 (0.7)
	utility/laundry room	24 (0.4)
	handbag, gym or work bag	12 (0.2)
	upstairs landing	10 (0.2)
	under the stairs	8 (0.1)
	dining room	7 (0.1)
	fridge	7 (0.1)
	hallway	6 (0.1)
	study or home office	6 (0.1)
	store room	5 (0.1)
	larder/pantry	5 (0.1)
Q6. What do you do with prescription medicines that you no longer need? (Can select more than one option)	Return to a pharmacy	3032 (54.3)
	Keep just in case I need in future	1492 (26.7)
	Throw out with household waste	759 (13.6)
	Return to GP	134 (2.4)
	Other	365 (6.5)
Q7. What do you think currently happens to prescription medicines that are returned unused to the community pharmacy?	Destroyed	4330 (77.7)
	Not sure	979 (17.6)
	Re-dispensed to other people	129 (2.3)
	Sent to developing countries or third world	125 (2.2)
	Other	7 (0.1)

Table 5. Formulation of prescription medicine preparation accepted for re-dispensing.

Which of the Following Types of Prescription Medicines Would You Accept If They Were Re-Dispensed? (Question 8)	No n = (%)	Yes n = (%)	Unsure n = (%)
Tablet	647 (11.7)	**4371 (78.7) ***	533 (9.6)
Capsule	792 (14.3)	**4147 (75.1) ***	583 (10.6)
Skin patch	1852 (33.9)	2710 (49.6)	904 (16.5)
Liquid	**2731 (50.0) ***	1568 (28.7)	1164 (21.3)
Cream/ointment	2387 (43.6)	2113 (38.6)	971 (17.7)
Ear drop	2469 (45.2)	2033 (37.2)	956 (17.5)
Injection	2558 (46.8)	1848 (33.8)	1065 (19.5)
Eye drop	2723 (49.7)	1801 (32.8)	960 (17.5)
Nasal spray	2704 (49.4)	1763 (32.2)	1002 (18.3)
Suppository **	**2743 (50.1) ***	1754 (32.1)	974 (17.8)
Pessary **	**2776 (51.8) ***	1517 (28.3)	1069 (19.9)
Inhaler	**2791 (51.3) ***	1533 (28.2)	1121 (20.6)

* >50% acceptance or otherwise in bold. ** These questions contained an explanation of these forms of medicine.

3.5. Attitudes towards the Possible Reuse of Medicines (Questions 9)

Table 6 summarises factors affecting the acceptance of a medicines reuse scheme. The most important factor was the checking of the medicine by a pharmacist, with this being reported as the most important criterion. The next most essential factors were that the medicine is still in date, that the medicine has been returned unopened and with an intact tamper proof seal to confirm that they were unopened.

Table 6. Factors affecting acceptance for reuse.

If You Were Given a Prescription Medicine Which Had Been Returned to the Pharmacy by Someone Else (Question 9)	Essential	Desirable	Unsure	Not Needed
The medicine has been checked by a pharmacist ($n = 5522$)	**5103 (92.4)** *	281 (5.1)	89 (1.6)	49 (0.9)
The medicine is still 'in date' ($n = 5534$)	**4914 (88.8)** *	470 (8.5)	99 (1.8)	49 (0.9)
The medicine has been returned unopened ($n = 5536$)	**4750 (85.8)** *	610 (11)	104 (1.9)	72 (1.3)
The medicine has been returned with an intact tamper proof seal ($n = 5514$)	**3923 (71.1)** *	1179 (21.4)	220 (4.0)	192 (3.5)
I am informed that I am receiving a re-dispensed medicine ($n = 5522$)	3393 (61.4)	1154 (20.9)	333 (6.0)	642 (11.6)
I have the opportunity to give my consent to receive a re-dispensed medicine ($n = 5517$)	3343 (60.6)	1249 (22.6)	315 (5.7)	610 (11.1)
None of the tablets or capsules in the blisters have been used ($n = 5521$)	3028 (54.9)	1527 (27.7)	374 (6.8)	584 (10.6)
The medicine has been returned in packaging that has not been damaged ($n = 5532$)	2861 (51.8)	1999 (36.2)	225 (4.1)	436 (7.9)
The packaging of the medicine has been cleaned ($n = 5490$)	2842 (51.8)	1709 (31.1)	545 (9.9)	394 (7.2)

* >70% essential or otherwise in bold.

With regards to whether the cost of the medicine should dictate which medicines are considered for re-dispensing, the majority said that all medicines should be considered (79.5% agreement), not only the expensive ones (7.6% disagreement, 12.8% not sure). Respondents indicated that they would be more likely to return unused medicines to the pharmacy if a re-dispensing scheme were initiated (Table 7).

Table 7. Intentions to change medicines disposal practices if prescription medicines start to be reused and current disposal practices.

	More Likely to Return to a Pharmacy	Less Likely to Return to a Pharmacy	Would Not Change How I Get Rid of Medicines
Q11a. If prescription medicines did start to be re-dispensed, would you be more or less likely to return your unused prescription medicines to a pharmacy?	3143 (56.3)	1826 (32.8)	428 (7.7)

A total of 2531 respondents reported that they do not return their unused prescriptions medicines to the pharmacy. Of these, 84.5% ($n = 2128/2519$ who answered the question) indicated that they were more likely to return their medicines to a pharmacy in the future if a medicine reuse scheme was in place. Only 1.9% said they would be less likely to return medicines to the pharmacy and 13.6% would not change their current practice of disposing medicines.

Table 8 presents participants' concerns about the safety of introducing a re-dispensing scheme. The strongest concern related to the possibility that returned medicine packs could have been tampered with or that they may not have been stored hygienically. In contrast, most agreed that medicines they had returned themselves would be safe for others to use.

Table 8. Concerns about the safety of re-dispensed medicines.

Statement	Agree or Strongly Agree n = (%)	Neither Agree or Disagree n = (%)	Disagree or Strongly Disagree n = (%)	Don't Know n = (%)
Q10c—Returned medicines could have been tampered with ($n = 5514$)	3817 (69.2)	1110 (20.1)	402 (7.3)	246 (4.5)
Q10b—It is safe for other people to use medicines that I have returned ($n = 5522$) [1]	3814 (69.1)	957 (17.3)	457 (8.3)	294 (5.3)
Q10f—Returned medicines may have not been stored hygienically ($n = 5513$)	3604 (65.4)	1212 (22.0)	424 (7.7)	273 (5.0)
Q10a—Medicine packs that have been returned partly used should be destroyed ($n = 5513$)	2633 (47.9)	1118 (20.2)	1545 (28.0)	217 (3.9)
Q10h—Pharmacists may use re-dispensed medicines as an opportunity to commit fraud by charging the NHS for 'new' medicines when a re-dispensed medicine has been used ($n = 5525$)	1434 (26.0)	1700 (30.8)	1671 (30.2)	720 (13.0)
Q10i—Re-dispensing medicines could spread disease ($n = 5499$)	1119 (20.4)	1558 (28.3)	2203 (41.1)	619 (11.3)
Q10e—Returned medicines may be ineffective ($n = 5507$)	909 (16.5)	1207 (21.9)	3033 (55.1)	358 (6.5)
Q10g—It is not safe for medicines that have been returned by other people to be re-dispensed ($n = 5503$)	827 (16.0)	1359 (24.7)	2916 (52.9)	401 (7.3)
Q10d—Returned medicines are not safe to be re-dispensed ($n = 5513$)	744 (13.3)	1430 (25.9)	2999 (55.7)	340 (6.2)

[1] Item reverse scored for scaling.

Scale scores for the 5-item scale 'perceived concerns about the safety of medicines reuse' ranged from 5 to 25, utilising the full range of possible scale scores and were normally distributed (median = 17.0; mean = 16.2, SD = 4.359, $n = 5383$) with 36.7 scoring up to and including the mid-point of the scale (MP = 15). A higher scale score indicated less concern about the safety of medicine reuse suggesting that the majority of respondents considered the reuse of medicines to be safe.

Differences in Healthcare Professionals' Concerns about Medicinal Waste and Perceived Safety of Reuse.

Hypothesis: Healthcare professionals hold stronger concerns about medicinal waste and less perceived concerns about the safety of medicines reuse than non-healthcare workers.

Healthcare workers reported a significantly more concern for medicinal waste than non-healthcare participants (U = -6.937, $n = 5455$, $p < 0.001$). There was a significant difference in 'perceived safety concerns for reusing medicines' scale scores for those who worked in healthcare (mean = 16.57, SD = 4.315, n = 1085) and those who did not (mean = 16.11, SD = 4.365, n = 4257) (mean difference = -0.462, df = 5340, $p < 0.01$), with those working in healthcare being less concerned about the safety of a medicines reuse scheme.

4. Discussion

This study has found a large proportion of respondents (78.7% for tablets and 75.1% for capsules), in a sample drawn entirely from a 'free prescription' medicines healthcare system, indicating that they would accept the reuse of oral solid pharmaceutical dosage forms. However, this acceptance is caveated by strong concerns, held by the same respondents, about the quality and safety of these medicines. The results of this study also provide support for our hypotheses that healthcare workers would have stronger concerns about medicinal waste and less concern about the safety of a medicines reuse scheme compared to individuals not working in healthcare.

This questionnaire was designed and piloted in 2016. At that point in time, little research had been undertaken into how the public viewed medicines reuse, and, of the research which had been conducted, none had sought the views of individuals residing in a 'free prescription' medicines healthcare system. Since 2016, the number of researchers working in the area of medicines reuse has increased and significant gains have been made in understanding the public perspective of this issue [7,29–32]. The results of this study support the findings of other researchers [7,29–32]. Additionally, when considering public attitudes towards medicines reuse in the UK, this study has provided insight into the views of the Welsh public and provides an indication of how medicines reuse may be perceived within the other 'free prescription' medicines healthcare systems of the Union, namely Scotland and Northern Ireland. The recruitment strategy employed in the present study was effective in that it was able to harness the views of the general public, rather than more conventional approaches to recruitment in pharmacy settings using customer surveys [33].

The hypothesis that healthcare professionals would have stronger concerns about medicinal waste and fewer concerns about medicines reuse was derived from our previous study with healthcare professionals [8]. In the qualitative interviews which informed our Delphi study, we noted strong concerns at the amount of medicinal waste amongst the healthcare professionals (doctors, nurses and pharmacists) interviewed. We also identified, through the Delphi study, that pharmacists could support re-dispensing returned medicines if certain criteria in place, which led us to believe that healthcare professionals may have fewer concerns than the general public. We speculate that the support for medicines reuse amongst healthcare professionals may be influenced, at least in part, by a desire to ease the tight budgetary conditions in which they operate (in the UK)—through saving money which they see as currently being wasted—to allow for increased spending on direct patient care. Additionally, while the proportion of respondents identifying as working in healthcare in the present study should be viewed as a limitation to our findings (discussed below), we also believe that capturing the views of so many healthcare professionals is an important finding in the field of medicines reuse research. Alhamad and colleagues, who have evaluated a Theory of Planned Behaviour-based questionnaire (their Medicines Reuse Questionnaire (MRQ)), found that the views of doctors and pharmacists would play an important role in norm-based intentions to accept reused medicines [32]. A conclusion from Alhamad's study based on this finding being that interventions which encourage doctors and pharmacists to endorse medicines reuse being needed to help the public embrace reuse schemes. Our findings suggest such interventions would be welcomed by these professional groups.

It is of interest that the present study has found higher levels of acceptance towards medicines reuse than two other large quantitative surveys undertaken with a similar aim [29,30,32]. Alhamad and colleagues developed and validated the MRQ which was distributed to a representative sample of the UK public, drawn from its different regions [29,32]. Participants were presented with a precise definition of reuse behaviour:

"...would [you] personally consider reusing medication in the future. We define reusing medication as the idea that you would accept for your own personal use a prescription medication that has been previously given out to another patient but then returned to a pharmacy, where the pharmacist has verified that the medication: has been kept by the other patient for less than three months, has more than six months of shelf-life remaining, has not been tampered with, has been kept under normal storage conditions, and has been kept in an original sealed blister pack (i.e., medication strip). When we refer to reusing medication, we are interested in prescribed medication that an individual/patient may use for a long-term illness. The individual/patient would be well enough to make their own healthcare decisions." Of the 1003 valid responses received, 54.5% 'intended to', 56.5% 'wanted to' and 56.5% 'expected to' reuse medicines in the future [32]. Bekker and colleagues administered a medicines reuse questionnaire to community pharmacy users in a region of the Netherlands [30]. Of the 2215 participants, 61.2% indicated that they would personally be willing to "reuse medication returned unused to the pharmacy by another patient if the quality was guaranteed" [30]. There are a number of possible reasons for the difference in the rates of willingness, acceptance or intention to reuse observed in this study. One reason for the difference may be the relatively high proportion of healthcare workers participating in our survey, who, we have identified, have less concern about medicines reuse than non-healthcare workers. Another potential reason could be due to Bekker and colleagues asking participants about reusing medication in general as opposed to specific pharmaceutical dosage forms [30]. As our current study and a qualitative interview study by Alhamad previously identified, the public exhibit different levels of acceptance towards medicines reuse dependent on pharmaceutical forms [31]. In their study, Alhamad and colleagues found that this preference was influenced by beliefs about the protection against tampering afforded by the more traditional packaging associated with dosage forms ('creams come in a tube') and beliefs about the ease with which such tampering could be to detected.

Respondents in the present study reported concerns about the quality and safety of reused medicines which have been found by other researchers working in the area [7,30–32]. While respondents were concerned about how hygienically medicines had been stored by others, few respondents were concerned that the reuse of medicines could spread disease or believed that medicines returned by others would be ineffective. It is of note that Alhamad and colleagues found, in their qualitative interview study, that participants had concerns about the logistics of a potential medicines reuse scheme [31]. Our focus, when designing the questionnaire for the present study, was on the quality and safety of reused medicines, but, it appears that, based on Alhamad and colleagues' findings, that the public have concerns which extend beyond what is dispensed to them [31]. Indeed, we were surprised that over three-quarters of respondents' number of respondents in the present study who knew that medicines returned to pharmacies were destroyed. Taken together, concerns about the logistics of a potential reuse system and awareness of the current fate of medicines returned to pharmacies, it is apparent that a proportion of the public are well informed about the issues which surround medicinal waste and medicines reuse and this should be considered when medicines reuse schemes are designed.

We have also found similar requirements of medicines reuse to other questionnaires that have been conducted in this area [30–32]. One exception to this was the finding that over 90% of respondents in the current study considered that a pharmacist check of the returned medicine was essential. This finding may indicate high levels of public trust in pharmacists in the healthcare system sampled.

Most respondents reported storing medicines in kitchens and bathrooms, which is contrary to guidance on the correct storage of medicines in the home [34]. It is believed that storage in kitchens and bathrooms may expose medicines to temperatures above those which manufacturers recommend and that this could lead to the medicine having reduced efficacy and an increased potential to cause side effects [35]. Providing support for this concern, Hewson found maximum temperatures in bathrooms and kitchens of 31.5 and 32.8 °C, respectively [36]. However, mean temperatures for the areas were much lower (18.4–23.6 °C) [36] and the potential for isolated or regular but transient high temperatures to negatively affect medicines, particularly when considering storage periods of 3–6 months, is disputed [15]. Indeed, when researchers have assessed all temperatures that medicines have been exposed to over a pre-determined period in the home environment, they have found that the majority of patients store their medicines in acceptable temperature conditions (both studies looking at medicines which needed to be stored either below 25 or 30 °C) [37,38]. As medicines which are sensitive to humidity are stored in protective packaging, it is temperature that remains the primary storage concern when considering medicines reuse. Researchers (including ourselves) interested in medicines reuse have proposed digital solutions [39], pointed to the existence of smart temperature labels [15] and envisaged the use of temperature monitors as part of reuse schemes [8,40] as a solution to identifying medicines which have been stored at inappropriate temperatures within homes. However, we find ourselves persuaded, in agreement with the conclusions of Mackridge and Marriot and Donyai and colleagues [41], that future work aiming to overcome the barrier which storage temperature in the home has posed towards medicines reuse should focus on improving the packaging in which medicines are supplied (by the manufacturer). It is essential, not just for medicines reuse, but for the primary recipient (from the first dispensing) that medicines are supplied in packaging that are able to tolerate reasonable domiciliary temperature conditions (including those encountered in bathrooms and kitchens) in the home.

Over half of respondents in the current study reported returning medicines to pharmacies for disposal. This contrasts with other studies which have found that only small proportions of respondents disposed of medicines in this way, with the majority disposing of medicines in household waste or via wastewater systems [17,42]. This finding may be due to greater public awareness of the harm that inappropriate medicines disposal can have on the environment or because of campaigns to increase awareness of the risk that unused medicines in the home create for accidental ingestion by children or deliberate ingestion as part of suicide attempts in the sample population.

The present study has several limitations which must be considered when interpreting the results. Only one question about concerns about medicinal waste concern was included in the questionnaire. As with any single item measure, this approach is not robust in terms of psychometric properties and we advise caution in the interpretation of this finding.

While this study captures a large sample from the population of Wales, the sample is self-selecting in nature which has introduced sampling bias into this study. We are unable to provide assurance that non-responders (or non-registrants with the platform) would share the views of those we have captured. Females, aged between 45 and 64 years old and professional occupational class are over-represented in the Healthwise Wales population compared to the population of Wales and this was also the case in our study sample. Similarly, those over 65 years of age and in routine and manual occupational classes are under-represented in both the HealthWise Wale population and our study sample. Nevertheless, a wide range of demographic characteristics and geographical locations of Wales are represented in the findings, but the findings should not be taken as being generalisable to the population of Wales as a whole.

Proportionally, ethnic minorities are poorly represented in the sample and further work must attempt to increase participation of these groups in further research on the subject so that views form these groups can be captured. While the HealthWise Wales platform has provided us with access to a large, geographically dispersed sample with a mix of demographics (apart from minority groups) it is also important to acknowledge that a proportion of the public, 13% in Wales at the time this study was conducted, did not have home internet access and that the views of this group have also not have been captured [43].

We have also noted that the proportion of respondents identifying as working in healthcare (approximately one-fifth) is greater than the proportion of the population that work in healthcare (approximately 2%) and, as such, that the views of healthcare workers are over-represented in the findings [44]. Moreover, over two-thirds of respondents had at least one medicine on repeat prescription and therefore had some level of familiarity with the healthcare system in Wales. Proportionally, it is likely that this constitutes an over representation of repeat medicines users when compared to the population of Wales (previous estimates of the proportion of population in receipt of at least one repeat item from the UK being 43–48% [45,46]). These limitations should be considered when interpreting these findings and when applying the results to other settings.

Further research is needed to establish whether medicines that are returned to pharmacies are suitable for reuse. We see this as a sequential piece of research which would commence with a multidisciplinary panel (including pharmaceutical scientists) identifying commonly dispensed medicines which are likely to remain stable in the presence of temperature fluctuations likely to be experienced in the home. The next stage would seek to identify whether a questionnaire, designed to establish the storage conditions a returned medicine has been exposed to, administered at the point of a medicine being returned to pharmacy, could be validated to identify medicines which are suitable for reuse (through the pharmaceutical analysis of returned medicines).

5. Conclusions

A growing body of research is highlighting that the majority of the general public would favourably receive reused medicines for their personal use. This study contributes to how medicines reuse is viewed amongst a large sample of the public from a 'free prescription' healthcare system. Importantly, it also contributes that medicines reuse appears to be supported by healthcare professionals, whose views on the matter would play a significant role in influencing the general public's attitudes towards reuse when it becomes a reality.

Supplementary Materials: The following are available online at https://www.mdpi.com/article/10.3390/pharmacy9020077/s1, Supplementary Materials Data S1: Participant Medicines Reuse Questionnaire. Supplementary Materials Data S2: Factor analysis of 9 items measuring views about the safety of medicines reuse.

Author Contributions: Conceptualisation, D.M. and D.H.J.; methodology, D.M., D.H.J. and R.P.-D.; software, D.H.J., A.G. and D.M.; formal analysis, A.G. and D.H.J.; investigation, J.T. and A.G.; writing—original draft preparation, D.M. and D.H.J.; writing—review and editing, D.M., D.H.J., R.P.-D., A.E., J.T. and A.G.; supervision, D.H.J. and R.P.-D.; project administration, D.M. All authors have read and agreed to the published version of the manuscript.

Funding: This research received no external funding.

Institutional Review Board Statement: Ethical approval for this study was obtained from this NHS Wales Research Ethics Committee-REC 3 on 28 July 2017 (REC reference: 15/WA/0076).

Informed Consent Statement: Informed consent is obtained from all subjects who register with the HealthWise Wales Platform.

Data Availability Statement: Restrictions apply to the availability of these data. Application for access to the data can be made to HealthWise Wales.

Acknowledgments: This study was facilitated by HealthWise Wales, the Health and Care Research Wales initiative, which is led by Cardiff University in collaboration with SAIL, Swansea University and the Medicines Management Directorate of Cwm Taf Morgannwg University Health Board.

Conflicts of Interest: The authors declare no conflict of interest.

References

1. Dicomidis, J.; Kirby, A. Reuse of Medicines: Looking Beyond the Waste Blame Game. *Prescriber* **2012**, *23*, 13–17. Available online: http://onlinelibrary.wiley.com/doi/10.1002/psb.962/pdf (accessed on 28 August 2020). [CrossRef]
2. Pomerantz, J.M. Recycling expensive medication: Why not? *MedGenMed* **2004**, *6*, 4.
3. James, D. Pharmacists May Accept Re-Dispensing Medication, But Will Patients? The Conversation. 2016. Available online: https://theconversation.com/pharmacists-may-accept-re-dispensing-medication-but-will-patients-63897 (accessed on 28 August 2020).

4. British Broadcasting Corporation. Drug Wastage Costing NHS Millions. 2011. Available online: http://www.bbc.co.uk/news/health-13042794 (accessed on 1 August 2020).
5. British Broadcasting Corporation. Are You Willing to Swallow a Recycled Pill? 2012. Available online: http://www.bbc.co.uk/news/health-17219584 (accessed on 1 August 2020).
6. British Broadcasting Corporation. World Hacks: Putting Your Leftover Pills Back to Work. 2018. Available online: https://www.bbc.com/news/av/stories-43155451 (accessed on 1 August 2020).
7. Bekker, C.L.; Gardarsdottir, H.; Egberts, T.C.G.; Bouvy, M.L.; van den Bemt, B.J. Redispensing of medicines unused by patients: A qualitative study among stakeholders. *Int. J. Clin. Pharm.* **2017**, *39*, 196–204. [CrossRef]
8. McRae, D.; Allman, M.; James, D. The redistribution of medicines: Could it become a reality? *Int. J. Pharm. Pract.* **2016**, *24*, 411–418. [CrossRef]
9. Hendrick, A.; Baqir, W.; Barrett, S.; Campbell, D. Prescribing Mrs Smith's Medication To Mr Jones: The Views Of Patients And Professionals On The Reuse Of Returned Medicines. *Pharm. Manag.* **2013**, *29*, 25–26.
10. NHS Sustainable Development Unit (SDU) Survey. Topline Results and Summary Report December 2011. Available online: https://www.sduhealth.org.uk/documents/resources/Ipsos_MORI_Survey.pdf (accessed on 1 August 2020).
11. Sejpal, P.R. Reasons for Society's no-returns policy. *Pharm. J.* **2007**, *278*, 249.
12. Cauchi, R.; Berg, K. State Prescription Drug Return, Reuse and Recycling Laws. National Conference of State Legislatures. Available online: https://www.ncsl.org/research/health/state-prescription-drug-return-reuse-and-recycling.aspx (accessed on 8 March 2021).
13. GIVMED. Available online: https://givmed.org/en/ (accessed on 8 March 2021).
14. Trueman, P.; Taylor, D.; Lowson, K.; Newbould, J.; Blighe, A.; Bury, M.; Maszeros, A.; Barber, N.; Wright, D.; Jani, Y.; et al. Evaluation of the Scale, Causes and Costs of Waste Medicines, Technical Report. 2010. Available online: https://discovery.ucl.ac.uk/id/eprint/1350234/1/Evaluation_of_NHS_Medicines_Waste__web_publication_version.pdf (accessed on 28 August 2020).
15. Mackridge, A.J.; Marriott, J.F. Returned medicines: Waste or a wasted opportunity? *J. Public Health* **2007**, *29*, 258–262. [CrossRef]
16. Annear, B.; Sinclair, K.; Robbé, I.J. Response to returned medicines: Waste or a wasted opportunity? *J. Public Health* **2008**, *30*, 209. [CrossRef] [PubMed]
17. Mackridge, A.; Marriott, J. Unused medicines in primary care: A postal questionnaire. *Int. J. Pharm. Pract.* **2006**, *14*, A23–A24.
18. Office of National Statistics. Wales Population Mid-Year Estimate. Available online: https://www.ons.gov.uk/peoplepopulationandcommunity/populationandmigration/populationestimates/timeseries/wapop/pop (accessed on 6 September 2020).
19. Welsh Assembly Government. Helping to Improve Wales' Health: Free Prescriptions Three Years on 2010. Available online: http://www.wales.nhs.uk/documents/prescriptions-report-three-years.pdf (accessed on 6 September 2020).
20. Hurt, L.; Ashfield-Watt, P.; Townson, J.; Heslop, L.; Copeland, L.; Atkinson, M.D.; Horton, J.; Paranjothy, S. Cohort profile: HealthWise Wales. A research register and population health data platform with linkage to National Health Service data sets in Wales. *BMJ Open* **2019**, *9*, e031705. [CrossRef] [PubMed]
21. HealthWise Wales. Resource Access Guidance for Researchers. 2020. Available online: https://www.healthwisewales.gov.wales/files/Reseacher_Access_Guide_January_2020.pdf (accessed on 6 September 2020).
22. Welsh Government. StatsWales. Available online: https://statswales.gov.wales/Catalogue (accessed on 22 November 2020).
23. Office of National Statistics. Standard Occupational Classification 2010: Volume 3, The National Statistics Socio-economic Classification: (Rebased on the SOC2010) User Manual. Available online: https://www.ons.gov.uk/file?uri=/methodology/classificationsandstandards/standardoccupationalclassificationsoc/soc2010/soc2010volume3thenationalstatisticssocioeconomicclassificationnssecrebasedonsoc2010/soc2010vol31amendedjanuary2013tcm77179133.pdf (accessed on 10 March 2021).
24. Welsh Government. Welsh Index of Multiple Deprivation (WIMD) 2019: Guidance. 2019. Available online: https://gov.wales/sites/default/files/statistics-and-research/2020-06/welsh-index-multiple-deprivation-2019-guidance.pdf (accessed on 6 September 2020).
25. Which? Conversation. Would You Re-Use Medicines Returned to the NHS? 2012. Available online: https://conversation.which.co.uk/health/reuse-reissue-medicines-prescription-nhs-medication-wastage/ (accessed on 6 September 2020).
26. Jones, K.H.; Ford, D.V.; Jones, C.; Dsilva, R.; Thompson, S.; Brooks, C.J. A case study of the Secure Anonymous Information Linkage (SAIL) Gateway: A privacy-protecting remote access system for health-related research and evaluation. *J. Biomed. Inform.* **2014**, *50*, 196–204. [CrossRef]
27. Field, A. *Discovering Statistics Using IBM SPSS Statistics*, 4th ed.; SAGE Publications Ltd.: London, UK, 2013.
28. Tavakol, M.; Dennick, R. Making sense of Cronbach's alpha. *Int. J. Med. Educ.* **2011**, *2*, 53–55. [CrossRef] [PubMed]
29. Alhamad, H.; Patel, N.; Donyai, P. Beliefs and intentions towards reusing medicines in the future: A large-scale, cross-sectional study of patients in the UK. *Int. J. Pharm. Pract.* **2018**, *26*, 4–36.
30. Bekker, C.; Bemt, B.V.D.; Egberts, T.C.; Bouvy, M.; Gardarsdottir, H. Willingness of patients to use unused medication returned to the pharmacy by another patient: A cross-sectional survey. *BMJ Open* **2019**, *9*, e024767. [CrossRef]
31. Alhamad, H.; Patel, N.; Donyai, P. How do people conceptualise the reuse of medicines? An interview study. *Int. J. Pharm. Pract.* **2018**, *26*, 232–241. [CrossRef]
32. Alhamad, H.; Donyai, P. Intentions to "Reuse" Medication in the Future Modelled and Measured Using the Theory of Planned Behaviour. *Pharmacy* **2018**, *8*, 213. [CrossRef] [PubMed]

33. Eades, C.; Ferguson, J.S.; O'Carroll, R. Public health in community pharmacy: A systematic review of pharmacist and consumer views. *BMC Public Heal.* **2011**, *11*, 582. [CrossRef] [PubMed]
34. Royal Pharmaceutical Society of Great Britain. 2007. Available online: https://www.rpharms.com/Portals/0/RPS%20document%20library/Open%20access/Support/toolkit/handling-medicines-socialcare-guidance.pdf (accessed on 28 August 2020).
35. Wieczorkiewicz, S.M.; Kassamali, Z.; Danziger, L.H. Behind Closed Doors: Medication Storage and Disposal in the Home. *Ann. Pharmacother.* **2013**, *47*, 482–489. [CrossRef]
36. Hewson, C.; Shen, C.C.; Strachan, C.; Norris, P. Personal medicines storage in New Zealand. *J. Prim. Health Care* **2013**, *5*, 146–150. [CrossRef]
37. Vlieland, N.D.; Bemt, B.V.D.; Van Riet-Nales, D.; Bouvy, M.L.; Egberts, A.; Gardarsdottir, H. Actual versus recommended storage temperatures of oral anticancer medicines at patients' homes. *J. Oncol. Pharm. Pract.* **2019**, *25*, 382–389. [CrossRef]
38. Vlieland, N.D.; van den Bemt, B.J.F.; Bekker, C.L.; Bouvy, M.L.; Egberts, T.C.; Gardarsdottir, H. Older Patients' Compliance with Drug Storage Recommendations. *Drugs Aging* **2018**, *35*, 233–241. [CrossRef] [PubMed]
39. Hui, T.K.L.; Donyai, P.; McCrindle, R.; Sherratt, R.S. Enabling Medicine Reuse Using a Digital Time Temperature Humidity Sensor in an Internet of Pharmaceutical Things Concept. *Sensors* **2020**, *20*, 3080. [CrossRef] [PubMed]
40. Bekker, C.L.; Gardarsdottir, H.; Egberts, A.C.; Molenaar, H.A.; Bouvy, M.L.; van den Bemt, B.J.; Hövels, A.M. What does it cost to redispense unused medications in the pharmacy? A micro-costing study. *BMC Health Serv. Res.* **2019**, *19*, 243. [CrossRef]
41. The Pharmaceutical Journal. The COVID-19 Pandemic Has Forced the Government to Allow Medicines Reuse: We Must Not Waste This Opportunity to Counter Our Throwaway Culture. Available online: https://pharmaceutical-journal.com/article/opinion/the-covid-19-pandemic-has-forced-the-government-to-allow-medicines-reuse-we-must-not-waste-this-opportunity-to-counter-our-throwaway-culture (accessed on 12 March 2021).
42. Makki, M.; Hassali, M.A.; Awaisu, A.; Hashmi, F. The Prevalence of Unused Medications in Homes. *Pharmacy* **2019**, *7*, 61. [CrossRef] [PubMed]
43. Welsh Government. Statistical Bulletin: National Survey for Wales, 2018–19 Internet Use and Digital Skills. Available online: https://gov.wales/sites/default/files/statistics-and-research/2019-09/internet-use-and-digital-skills-national-survey-wales-april-2018-march-2019-207.pdf (accessed on 6 September 2020).
44. Welsh Government. StatsWales. NHS Staff by Staff Group and Year. Available online: https://statswales.gov.wales/Catalogue/Health-and-Social-Care/NHS-Staff/NHS-Staff-Summary/nhsstaff-by-staffgroup-year (accessed on 22 November 2020).
45. Petty, D.R.; Zermansky, A.G.; Alldred, D.P. The scale of repeat prescribing—Time for an update. *BMC Health Serv. Res.* **2014**, *14*, 76. [CrossRef]
46. Harris, C.M.; Dajda, R. The scale of repeat prescribing. *Br. J. Gen. Pract.* **1996**, *46*, 649–653. [PubMed]

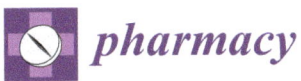

Review

The Validity of the Theory of Planned Behaviour for Understanding People's Beliefs and Intentions toward Reusing Medicines

Hamza Alhamad [1,2,*] and Parastou Donyai [1,*]

1 Department of Pharmacy, University of Reading, Reading RG6 6DZ, UK
2 Department of Pharmacy, Zarqa University, P.O. Box 132222, Zarqa 13132, Jordan
* Correspondence: halhamad@zu.edu.jo (H.A.); p.donyai@reading.ac.uk (P.D.)

Abstract: Background: many factors can impact a person's behaviour. When the behaviour is subject to prediction, these factors can include, for example, the perceived advantages and disadvantages of performing the behaviour, normative beliefs, and whether the behaviour is thought to be achievable. This paper examines intentions to engage in medicines reuse, i.e., to accept medicines that are returned unused to a pharmacy to be reused. The paper aims to outline the validity of the Theory of Planned Behaviour (TPB) for understanding people's intentions to engage in medicines reuse by examining this against other long-standing health-related psychological theories of behavioural change. Thus, the Health Belief Model (HBM), Protection Motivation Theory (PMT), Trans-Theoretical Model of Health Behaviour Change (TTM/SoC), Theory of Reasoned Action (TRA), and TPB are examined for their application in the study of medicines reuse. Discussion: the HBM, PMT, TTM/SoC, TRA, and TPB were assessed for their relevance to examining medicines reuse as a behaviour. The validity of the TPB was justified for the development of a Medication Reuse Questionnaire (MRQ) to explore people's beliefs and intention toward reusing medicines. Conclusion: TPB has been widely used inside and outside of health-related research and it was found to have more accurately defined constructs, making it helpful in studying medicines reuse behaviour.

Keywords: medicines reuse; medication waste; psychological theories; theory of planned behaviour; people's belief; people's intentions

Citation: Alhamad, H.; Donyai, P. The Validity of the Theory of Planned Behaviour for Understanding People's Beliefs and Intentions toward Reusing Medicines. *Pharmacy* 2021, 9, 58. https://doi.org/10.3390/pharmacy9010058

Received: 11 September 2020
Accepted: 3 March 2021
Published: 9 March 2021

Publisher's Note: MDPI stays neutral with regard to jurisdictional claims in published maps and institutional affiliations.

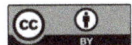

Copyright: © 2021 by the authors. Licensee MDPI, Basel, Switzerland. This article is an open access article distributed under the terms and conditions of the Creative Commons Attribution (CC BY) license (https://creativecommons.org/licenses/by/4.0/).

1. Introduction

A multitude of factors can influence people's behaviour. The behaviour of interest here is whether people will accept medicines that are returned unused to a pharmacy for their own use (i.e., take part in medicines reuse). The influencing factors for medicines reuse could include, for example, the perceived advantages and disadvantages of performing the behaviour, views about the therapeutic classes and safety [1,2], and storage conditions [3] of returned unused medicines, and social pressure or normative belief regarding reusing medicines. Understanding the precise nature and significance of these factors is not straightforward, but could be explored using psychological theory. Additionally, as well as providing a generalisable organising framework for studying and predicting potentially foreseeable behaviour [4], psychological theory can also provide a mechanism for changing people's behaviour, which is of added interest to health practitioners and policy-makers.

Arguably, then, the application of a framework to study people's thoughts and behavioural responses to medicines reuse could not only help to explain, but also enable relevant stakeholders to predict and influence medicines reuse behaviour [5]. However, while there are many different and overlapping health-related psychological theories and models available in the literature [6–8], none have been examined for applicability in relation to medicines reuse until our own research. The lack of guidance regarding how to select a suitable theory for a particular research interest [4,9] meant this was not a straightforward task. One suggestion to improve the selection of theory across relevant disciplines is to consider all of those psychological theories that could be of potential use in informing public health questions, and then narrow down according to the particular behaviour, population, and context of the research [10]. This review aims to do that by providing an overview of common health-related behavioural change theories, justifying the selection of a particular theory and then briefly describing steps that were required to manage the development of a Medication Reuse Questionnaire (MRQ) to explore people's beliefs and intention toward reusing medicines based on the selected theory. An argument is made for the validity of the Theory of Planned Behaviour (TPB) to predict *medicines reuse* behaviour. Subsequent to the work described in this paper, the TPB was successfully applied to understand people's conceptualization of this behaviour [11] and model and measure their intention to reuse medicines in the future [12].

2. Overview of the Common Health-Related Behavioural Change Theories

Many psychological theories and models attempt to explain the relationship between people's thoughts, beliefs, decisions, and behaviours; however, not all are unconditionally helpful, health-related, or, in fact, evidenced-based [13]. Additionally, numerous theories have been criticised based on their (in)effectiveness and lack of predictive power, unclear construct development, and lack of guidelines on how exactly they could be used to measure behaviour or intention toward a behaviour [13]. The more common and frequently-used health-related behavioural change theories that are potentially relevant to medicines reuse as a behaviour are reviewed [7,8,14]; these include, the Health Belief Model (HBM), Protection Motivation Theory (PMT), Trans-Theoretical Model of Health Behaviour Change (TTM/SoC), Theory of Reasoned Action (TRA), and the Theory of Planned Behaviour (TPB). The majority of these theories focus on behaviours that relate directly to health, e.g., smoking cessation, but there is also a precedence for applying these theories to other behaviours, such as those that are linked to the environment and waste reduction, meaning that these theories could potentially be relevant to studying medicines reuse as a behaviour.

2.1. Health Belief Model (HBM)

The Health Belief Model (HBM) is one of the earliest psychological health models, developed in the 1950s to predict preventive health behaviours and the behavioural reaction to treatment in acutely and chronically ill patients [15]. Over recent years, the HBM has been used to try and improve many health-related interventions by predicting a wide variety of health-related behaviours [8,16]. The HBM constructs consist of; *perceived susceptibility*, including a person's perception regarding the risk of the (maladaptive) health behaviour (e.g., susceptibility to lung cancer because of a behaviour such as smoking); *perceived severity* of the threat to health via the behaviour (e.g., severity of lung cancer as an illness); *perceived benefits* from taking action to change the behaviour (e.g., stopping smoking will save money and reduce my illness); *perceived barriers* towards the behaviour or the costs that are involved in performing the behaviour (e.g., stopping smoking will make me irritable); *cues to actions*, which might be internal (e.g., family member illness due to smoking) or external (e.g., television news and reports about the ill effects of smoking); and, *demographics and socio-economic values* (e.g., age, ethnicity, education, and income) [7,8]. Each of the individual constructs or in combination can theoretically be used to predict the likelihood that the behaviour change will occur (Figure 1). Yet, the HBM has received many criticisms, including that it has weak predictive power in most areas of health-related behaviour [7,14], poor construct definition, and that other core psychological factors are missing from the model, including environmental or economic issues that might also impact behaviours [7,14]. Variables, such as intentions to carry out a specific behaviour and the influence of social pressure, which can be highly predictive of behaviour, are also absent from the HBM [17]. Importantly, the HBM does not include clear guidelines on how its variables might be combined and operationalised, especially the constructs of benefits and barriers [14]. The literature on the usefulness of the HBM is contradictory, but studies utilising this model or different aspects of the model's constructs report it to predict some health-related behaviours, such as taking part in screening for hypertension, screening for cervical cancer, genetic screening, exercise behaviour, decreased alcohol use, changes in diet, and smoking cessation [7,8]. The HBM was considered here, because of its prevalence in health psychology research and because medicines reuse could arguably be perceived as a preventive behaviour (e.g., helping to prevent environmental waste through reuse could improve health indirectly). Indeed, some of the constructs of the HBM could be seen as relatable to medicines reuse behaviour (e.g., perceived benefits, perceived barriers, and cues to action). However, because medicines reuse is not a health condition or behaviour that can directly impact on a person's health, some of the other constructs of the HBM cannot be judged as applicable at all (e.g., perceived susceptibility and perceived severity), which renders this theory ineffective for our purposes. To explain, in the HBM the construct, perceived susceptibility relates to a person's perception regarding the risk of the maladaptive behaviour and perceived severity relates to how bad this health threat would be. However, for our purposes, medicines reuse would be defined as the 'favoured' behaviour, which would make these constructs redundant as the act of reusing medicines is not directly *preventing* a condition.

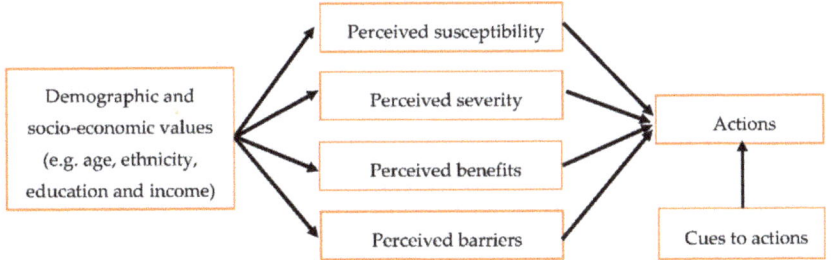

Figure 1. A graphical representations of the Health Belief Model (HBM) [8].

2.2. Protection Motivation Theory (PMT)

The Protection Motivation Theory (PMT) is considered to be a revised version and expansion to HBM to include additional constructs. According to PMT, the primary determinant to carry out a health-related behaviour is protection motivation or intention to carry out the behaviour, and the behaviour change may be achieved by engaging with an individual's fears [18]. Protection motivation is determined by *threat appraisal* and the *coping appraisal process*. *Threat appraisal* is referred to as a cognitive process that the individual uses to assess the level of threat (including severity, susceptibility, and fear), while the *coping appraisal process* refers to the individual's assessment of their ability to carry out risk preventive behaviour which influences the protection motivation (including response effectiveness and self-efficacy) (Figure 2) [19]. Together, the outcome of the appraisal processes is classified into either adaptive (adopting health behaviour) or maladaptive responses (avoidance or denial of health threat) [8,17]. The PMT has been successfully applied to predict several health behaviours and it is less widely criticised when compared to HBM [20]. Nonetheless, PMT does not account for habitual behaviours (e.g., brushing teeth), nor does it include social (e.g., what others think/do) and environmental factors (e.g., opportunities to exercise or eat appropriately at work) [8]. However, the main reason it lacks utility for studying medicines reuse behaviour, similar to the HBM, is because medicines reuse does not pose a direct health threat to individuals, which means that the main constructs (e.g., threat appraisal) are not valid for application to medicines reuse.

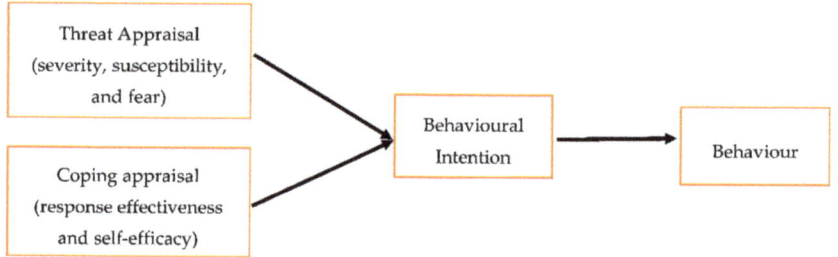

Figure 2. A graphical representation of the Protection Motivation Theory (PMT) [8].

2.3. Trans-Theoretical Model of Behaviour Change or Stages of Change (TTM/SoC)

The TTM/SoC was specifically designed to facilitate behavioural change [7]. TTM/SoC provides information regarding different target groups and how they should be approached. It has received empirical support with regard to different health-related behaviours and is a widely used cognitive model [7]. TTM/SoC divides individuals into five stages that represent different levels of motivational willingness to change their behaviour. These stages were first developed about smoking and include; *pre-contemplation* (e.g., the person might think "I am happy being a smoker and intend to continue"), *contemplation* (e.g., "recently, I have been coughing a lot, maybe I should think about stopping smoking"), *preparation* (e.g., "I will buy fewer cigarettes"), *action* (e.g., "I have stopped smoking"), and maintenance (e.g., "I have stopped smoking for five months now") [8,21]. The model allows for people to exit and re-enter, including cases of relapse. In some versions of the TTM/SoC, the final stage, *termination,* is added. In this stage, the new behaviour is seen as being entirely determined after a period of five or more years (see Figure 3) [7].

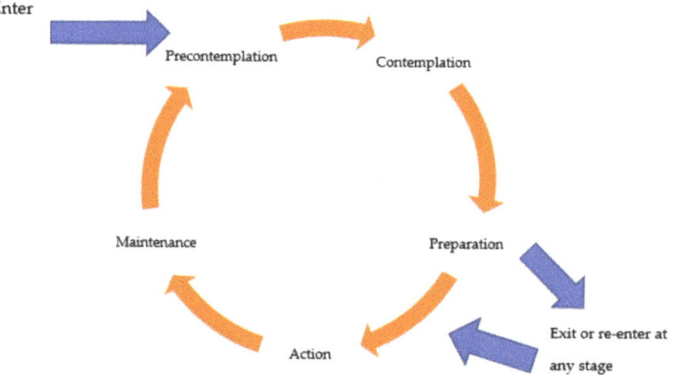

Figure 3. A graphical representation of the Trans-Theoretical Model of Behaviour Change or Stages of Change (TTM/SoC).

The transition between stages is thought of as being controlled by self-efficacy and decisional balance constructs. Self-efficacy (which is also included in the HBM and TPB) is expected to increase as individuals move toward action and maintenance stages. Decisional balance measures the individual's relative balancing of the advantages and disadvantages of changes that combine to form a decision. This balance between advantages and disadvantages mainly depends on which stage of change the individual is in [22]. There are many criticisms regarding the complexity of the TTM/SoC model, how distinct the stages really are, and whether an individual would actually move through each stage. Moreover, movement between the stages can occur so quickly as to make the distinction between stages less valuable [8]. Consequently, the TTM/SoC model is less clear on how individuals change or the reasons some change more efficiently than others [21]. Another criticism of the TTM/SoC model is that the effectiveness of a stage-based intervention differs based on the behaviour [23]. Some have called for a more coherent definition of the stages in the TTM/SoC model, as well as some level of standardisation [24].

Having considered the TTM/SoC model and its potential advantages and disadvantages, its use for studying medicines reuse was discounted, as explained here. Because the practice of medicines reuse does not currently take place in the UK, there was no experience of this behaviour to draw on in order to delineate the difference between the distinct stages unique to the TTM/SoC. Thus, neither an interview study nor an observational study could have possibly elicited relevant information against these very specific constructs that rely on actual experience.

2.4. The Theory of Reasoned Action (TRA) and the Theory of Planned Behaviour (TPB)

Fishbein and Ajzen developed the TRA in 1967 to examine the relationship between beliefs, attitudes, intentions, and behaviour [25]. The TRA assumes that an individual's intention to perform a behaviour is the most proximal antecedent of that behaviour. Individuals' intentions are, in turn, influenced by their attitudes toward performing the behaviour and the subjective/social norms relating to behavioural performance (Figure 4). Therefore, the TRA is a model in which the individual is positioned within the social context [8]. Ajzen later expanded the TRA to develop the TPB by taking account of what people believe stops or facilitates their behaviour.

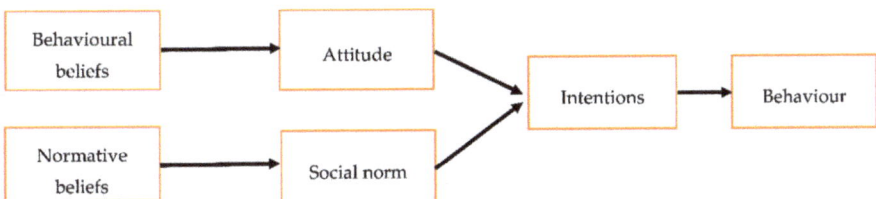

Figure 4. A graphical representation of the Theory of Reasoned Action (TRA) model [26].

In the TPB, Ajzen attempted to evolve and extend the TRA by adding the perceived behavioural control (PBC) construct. PBC is a construct describing the factors that control the individual's decision to carry out the behaviour. PBC is considered to be representative for actual control, as it is expected to moderate the effect of intention on behaviour [26]. The intention to perform the behaviour is considered the key determinant of behaviour in the TPB [6]. Here, the stronger the intentions to engage in behaviour, the more likely behaviour will be performed [27]. The TPB proposes a framework in which cognitions (i.e., behavioural, normative, and control beliefs) and broader constructs (i.e., attitude toward the behaviour, subjective norm, and perceived behavioural control) influence behaviour [28] via intentions [8,29]. Moreover, in this model, the PBC construct itself could predict behaviour without the effect of intention [8]. The TPB could make the following predictions if TPB is applied to medication reuse: if a person believes that reusing their medicines would benefit the economy and environment, and would be useful to their own health (i.e., attitude toward the behaviour), that essential people in their life would like them to reuse medicine (i.e., subjective norm), and that they have the ability to reuse medicines in the future after evaluating the internal and external factors that allow or preclude medicine reuse (i.e., PBC), then this could predict a high intention to reuse medicines in the future. On the face of it, then, the constructs of the TPB could all be relevant in determining medicines reuse behaviour, albeit via the intention construct. Additionally, Ajzen recognised the importance of demographics variables and later added the background factors to the TPB [30,31]. The background factors impact intentions and behaviour indirectly by affecting behavioural, normative, and/or control beliefs [30,31].

That is, background factors can supply useful information regarding possible precursors of behavioural, normative, and control beliefs (Figure 5).

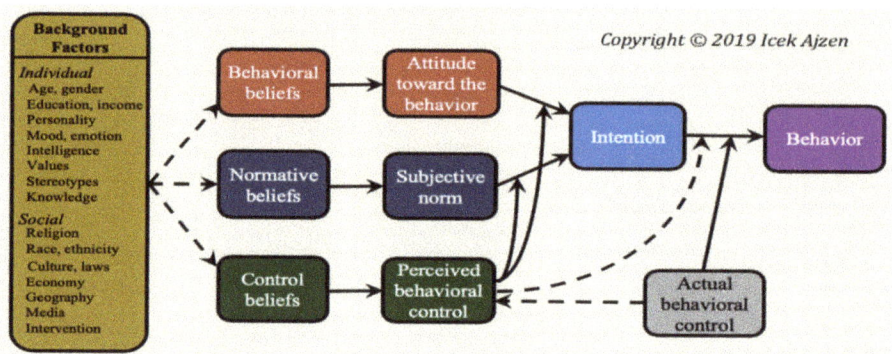

Figure 5. A graphical presentation of the Theory of Planned Behaviour Model (TPB) with background factors [30].

3. Discussion

The main focus of this discussion is to assess, support, and argue for the validity of the TPB to predict people's behavioural beliefs and their intentions to reuse medicines in the future. The steps that are used to develop a TPB Medication Reuse Questionnaire (MRQ) to explore people's beliefs and intention toward reusing medicines are also described.

3.1. The TPB Compared to the TRA, HBM, PMT, and TTM/SoC

The TPB, TRA, HBM, PMT, and TTM/SoC are particular models that have a number of constructs relating to behaviour in common [14,15,21]. The construct commonalities involve components relating to how individuals balance the perceived costs and benefits of alternative behaviours; beliefs about others' expectations and values relating to health behaviours; the formation of intentions to act (except for the HBM); and, individuals' self-efficacy perceptions regarding taking behavioural action (except for the TRA) [7,32,33]. For example, self-efficacy, perceived barriers and benefits described within the HBM, could be seen as being very similar to control beliefs and behavioural beliefs described in the TPB [34]. However, some of these constructs are only unique to a particular theory [13,32,33]. For example, the perceived threat construct of HBM described as perceived seriousness and perceived susceptibility to the illness does not appear in the TRA, TPB, and TTM/SoC models. This can be seen as an advantage in which the perceived threat construct can describe the consequences of reusing medicines that have been tampered with or contaminated. Moreover, the HBM includes objective demographics and cue to action constructs that are not included in the TRA, TPB, and TTM/SoC models, which can be seen as a another potential advantage [7]. However, the evidence indicates that the HBM's objective demographics and cue to action constructs, although perceived as potential strengths, have not been effectively used in practice [7]. In any case, the HBM is more health-behaviour focused as compared to the TRA and TPB, which are designed to be applicable to more general behaviours; thus, the TRA and the TPB can be applied outside as well as inside the health discipline [5–7,10,16,26,32,34–48]. The combination of TPB and the TTM/SoC has been tested with good results. For instance, TPB adds to our understanding of what motivates the behaviour, whereas TTM/SoC provides information regarding different target groups and how they should be approached. TTM/SoC has also received empirical support with regard to different health-related behaviours and it is a widely used cognitive mode. The TRA and the TPB have identical attitudinal and social norm constructs in common; however, the TPB, contains a PBC construct relating to control related beliefs and self-efficacy [26,27,31]. With the help of the revised TPB, it becomes possible to examine why a given background factor influences, or fails to influence, behaviour by following its effects through the more proximal antecedents of the behaviour [30,31]. The TRA and the TPB have fewer, but more accurately defined, constructs and they are mathematically better specified than the HBM and the TTM/SoC models. This promotes the adequacy and consistency of the use of TRA and TPB [7]. The TPB is more successful in predicting behaviour and it has been widely used inside and outside health-related research [6,7,21,26,32,35–48]. There is meta-analytic and systematic review evidence that the predictive performance of both the TRA and the TPB is superior to the HBM [7]. Moreover, the additional constructs that are contained in the TPB allow it to have a more significant predictive percentage of the overall behavioural variance than the TRA [7]. The available evidence suggests that the application of the TPB in countries, such as USA and UK, can predict around 20–30% of the observed variance of health behaviours [7]. Additionally, there is a strong correlation between behaviour and both attitudes towards the behaviour and PBC constructs of TPB [7]. However, the correlation between behaviour and subjective norms is less and is sometimes referred to as a weak correlation [21]. The issue of the weak correlation was argued to be probably methodological, as a small number of studies that measured subjective norms fairly reported strong relationships with behaviour [6,21].

3.2. Support for the Application of TPB to Predicts People's Behaviour and Intention towards Reusing Medicines

The TPB is a framework that has been widely applied in a variety of domains for predicting and explaining behaviour and increasingly for conducting behaviour change interventions [27,28,49]. There have been several reviews and meta-analyses describing the generalisability of the TPB in different behavioural domains and its effectiveness to predict a range of health behaviours [6–8]. The generalisability of TPB-based interventions is illustrated in a recent meta-analysis [28]. The studies reviewed were concerned with reducing alcohol consumption [50,51], smoking cessation [36,47], predicting adherence to medicines [48,52], promoting hand hygiene [53], nutrition-related intervention, such as promoting whole-grain foods by dieticians [37], and food safety [38], physical activity [39], and weight control [40,54], sexual behaviour related interventions, such as promoting safer sex practices [41,55,56], traffic-related interventions, such as promoting school-age cyclists to wear safety helmets [42], and promoting drivers' compliance with speed limits [43], and work-related interventions, such as promoting work health and safety [57]. In addition to the above, TPB-based interventions have been applied in other domains, such as environment and sustainability [44,58,59], reuse [60], recycling [35,45], and intention to donate to charity [61]. The effectiveness of TPB-based interventions in predicting behavioural changes is illustrated in the quantitative meta-analysis review of 185 independent studies published up to the end of 1997, where it was found that across all behaviours, the average multiple correlations of intention and PBC with behaviour was 0.52, accounting for 27% of the variance, and the average multiple correlations of attitude, subjective norm, and PBC with intention was 0.63, accounting for 39% of the variance [6]. Finally, the correlation between subjective norms and the behavioural intention was found to be weaker than those between attitudes and the behavioural intention and between PBC and behavioural intention [6]. In 1991, Ajzen conducted a review of 16 studies involving the TPB to examine the effectiveness of TPB-based interventions in predicting the behavioural changes and found that attitude, subjective norm, and PBC accounted for a significant amount (20% to 78%) of variance in behavioural intention [27]. The multiple correlations between behavioural intention and its three predictors (i.e., attitude, subjective norm, and PBC) ranged from (0.43 to 0.94), with an average correlation of 0.71. Moreover, Ajzen added that PBC, together with intention, were significant predictors of behaviour, with the average multiple correlations being 0.51 [27]. Finally, in a review of 56 studies, the variance in behavioural intention that was explained by TPB constructs was 40.9%, and PBC was a significant predictor of behavioural intention in 85.5% of health-related studies, followed by attitude (81.5%) and subjective norm (74.4%) [46]. PBC contributed a mean additional 13% of variance to the prediction of behavioural intentions, over and above the attitude and subjective norm constructs, and 12% to the prediction of behaviour [46]. The PBC figures that were reported in this review [46] were higher than those reported by the study of Armitage and Conner [6]. Subjective norm was a strong predictor of the behaviour in the study by Godin and Kok [46] as compared to the Armitage and Conner study [6], which was reported to be a weak predictor of the behaviour. Ajzen stated that intentions are heavily influenced by personal factors, such as attitudes and perceived behavioural control [27]; however, Ajzen recommends the inclusion of injunctive (i.e., expectation or subjective probability that a referent individual or group, such as friends, family, spouse, coworkers, one's physician, or supervisor approves or disapproves of performing the behaviour under consideration) and descriptive (i.e., beliefs as to whether important others themselves perform the behaviour) norms as a solution to improve the correlation between subjective norm and intention [31,62]. These reviews and meta-analyses support the empirical applicability and popularity of TPB, and demonstrate that TPB, overall, is quite a successful model in explaining and predicting behavioural intentions and actual behaviours. Despite the addition of PBC to the TPB, other variables that may control the actual behaviour, such as desire, need, and emotion, are still lacking [31,63]. These factors may affect the actual behaviour, regardless of the expressed attitude [31,63]. For example, a person may have a positive attitude towards reusing medicine, but do not need, or do not have, a desire to reuse medicine. Based on the above strength and limitation, TPB was chosen to be applied to understand people's beliefs and intentions to reuse medicines in the future.

3.3. Steps to Manage the Development of a TPB Medication Reuse Questionnaire (MRQ) to Explore People's Beliefs and Intention toward Reusing Medicines

When the TPB as a psychological framework is applied, specific steps are followed to enhance the validity of the research. These steps are according to the recommendations made by Francis and Ajzen [29,64]. The first step would then be to define medicines reuse as behaviour an select the population of interest. The TACT principle is used, by which the behaviour is defined according to target, action, context, and time. For example, for the behaviour "capturing people's beliefs and intention to reuse medication that is returned to pharmacies by another patient", the target is people in general, the action is their beliefs and intentions to reuse medication, the context is reusing medication that is returned to pharmacies by another patient, and the time is in the future. Medicine reuse as behaviour was primarily defined as "accepting prescribed medication with more than six months of shelf-life remaining that, as verified by a pharmacist, had been kept untampered for less than three months, under normal storage conditions and in an original sealed blister pack, by another patient before being returned to a community pharmacy" [11]. A sample of the population of interest for an elicitation (i.e., qualitative) study then needs to be determined. The sample size for an elicitation study is aimed to be between 15–20 participants. The second step is to complete the elicitation study to develop the indirect measures (behavioural beliefs, normative beliefs, and control beliefs) for all of the predictor constructs of the TPB (attitude, subjective norms, and PBC). An elicitation study was indeed completed with a sample of 19 participants that were interviewed face to face. Themes obtained from the elicitation study were classified according to the TPB constructs and they were used to develop the questions related to the indirect measures of the TPB [11]. The third step was to develop the MRQ. The MRQ questions are of three types; first, the questions developed from the elicitation study that are related to the indirect measures of TPB, second, the question related to the direct measures of TPB, and third, the questions related to the background factors that are important and related to medicines reuse. All of the MRQ questions were indeed developed according to Francis and Ajzen recommendations [29,64]. The fourth step was to pilot and validate the MRQ. Validity and reliability testing were also applied. Content validity is applied by asking cognitive questions, and questions at the end of the interview, such as: are any items difficult to answer or ambiguous; does the questionnaire feel too repetitive; does it feel too long; does it feel superficial; and, are there any annoying features of the wording or formatting? Reliability testing was applied, including internal consistency for the direct measures of TPB and test-retest reliability for the indirect measures of the TPB [12]. Fifth, Confirmatory Factory Analysis (CFA) was applied to the MRQ in order to confirm that the questions measuring each construct are considered indicators of the same latent variable; and, the TPB model in which the attitude, subjective norm, PBC, and intention items are treated, as assessing separate constructs is superior to a model in which all questions are considered to measure the same underlying construct [12]. The sixth step was to use the MRQ to capture the representative views regarding people's beliefs and willingness to reuse medicines in the future [12]. The data about the development, validation, and evaluation of a TPB model used to predict medicines reuse behavioural intentions were successfully used to understand people's intention to reuse medicines in the future [12].

4. Conclusions

This review summarised the common and frequent health-related behavioural change theories that might be potentially relevant to medicines reuse behaviour. The need for the psychological framework was described and the rationale presented for selecting TPB as an appropriate theory to develop the MRQ to explore people's beliefs and intention toward reusing medicines in the future. The TPB has been widely used inside and outside health-related research, and it has been found to have more accurately defined constructs and be better mathematically specified than the HBM and the TTM/SoC. The TPB was found to be more useful in studying medicines reuse behaviour because of its wider use outside of health behaviours and the apparent relevance of its constructs. The theory has since been applied in both an elicitation study as well as a large-scale questionnaire study measuring people's attitudes to medication reuse.

Author Contributions: P.D.: Conceptualization, Supervision, Project administration, Validation Visualisation, Writing—Reviewing and Editing Resources; H.A.: Conceptualization, Methodology, Investigation, Data Curation, Formal analysis, Validation, Visualisation, Writing—Original draft preparation All authors have read and agreed to the published version of the manuscript.

Funding: This research was part of a PhD project sponsored and funded by Al-Zarqa University (under the regulation of the Jordanian Ministry of Higher Education).

Acknowledgments: We thank Zarqa University for the funding of the PhD project.

Conflicts of Interest: The Authors declare that they have no conflicts of interest to disclose.

References

1. Alhamad, H.; Patel, N.; Donyai, P. Towards Medicines Reuse: A Narrative Review of the Different Therapeutic Classes and Dosage Forms of Medication Waste in Different Countries. *Pharmacy* **2020**, *8*, 230. [CrossRef]
2. Hui, T.K.L.; Mohammed, B.; Donyai, P.; McCrindle, R.; Sherratt, R.S. Enhancing pharmaceutical packaging through a technology ecosystem to facilitate the reuse of medicines and reduce medicinal waste. *Pharmacy* **2020**, *8*, 58. [CrossRef]
3. Hui, T.K.L.; Donyai, P.; McCrindle, R.; Sherratt, R.S. Enabling Medicine Reuse Using a Digital Time Temperature Humidity Sensor in an Internet of Pharmaceutical Things Concept. *Sensors* **2020**, *20*, 3080. [CrossRef]
4. Michie, S.; Johnston, M.; Abraham, C.; Lawton, R.; Parker, D.; Walker, A. Making psychological theory useful for implementing evidence based practice: A consensus approach. *BMJ Qual. Saf.* **2005**, *14*, 26–33. [CrossRef]
5. Godin, G.; Bélanger-Gravel, A.; Eccles, M.; Grimshaw, J. Healthcare professionals' intentions and behaviours: A systematic review of studies based on social cognitive theories. *Implement. Sci.* **2008**, *3*, 36. [CrossRef] [PubMed]
6. Armitage, C.J.; Conner, M. Efficacy of the theory of planned behaviour: A meta-analytic review. *Br. J. Soc. Psychol.* **2001**, *40*, 471–499. [CrossRef] [PubMed]
7. Taylor, D.; Bury, M.; Campling, N.; Carter, S.; Garfied, S.; Newbould, J.; Rennie, T. *A Review of the Use of the Health Belief Model (HBM), the Theory of Reasoned Action (TRA), the Theory of Planned Behaviour (TPB) and the Trans-Theoretical Model (TTM) to Study and Predict Health Related Behaviour Change*; The National Institute for Health and Clinical Excellence: London, UK, 2006; pp. 1–215.
8. Ogden, J. *Health Psychology: A Textbook: A textbook*; McGraw-Hill Education: London, UK, 2012.
9. Michie, S. Designing and implementing behaviour change interventions to improve population health. *J. Health Serv. Res. Policy* **2008**, *13* (Suppl. S3), 64–69. [CrossRef] [PubMed]
10. Davis, R.; Campbell, R.; Hildon, Z.; Hobbs, L.; Michie, S. Theories of behaviour and behaviour change across the social and behavioural sciences: A scoping review. *Health Psychol. Rev.* **2015**, *9*, 323–344. [CrossRef]

11. Alhamad, H.; Patel, N.; Donyai, P. How do people conceptualise the reuse of medicines? An interview study. *Int. J. Pharm. Pract.* **2018**, *26*, 232–241. [CrossRef]
12. Alhamad, H.; Donyai, P. Intentions to "Reuse" Medication in the Future Modelled and Measured Using the Theory of Planned Behavior. *Pharmacy* **2020**, *8*, 213. [CrossRef] [PubMed]
13. Donyai, P. *Social and Cognitive Pharmacy: Theory and Case Studies*; Pharmaceutical Press: London, UK, 2012.
14. Armitage, C.J.; Conner, M. Social cognition models and health behaviour: A structured review. *Psychol. Health* **2000**, *15*, 173–189. [CrossRef]
15. Rosenstock, I.M. Historical origins of the health belief model. *Health Educ. Monogr.* **1974**, *2*, 328–335. [CrossRef]
16. Carpenter, C.J. A meta-analysis of the effectiveness of health belief model variables in predicting behavior. *Health Commun.* **2010**, *25*, 661–669. [CrossRef] [PubMed]
17. Conner, M. Cognitive determinants of health behavior. In *Handbook of Behavioral Medicine*; Springer: Berlin/Heidelberg, Germany, 2010; pp. 19–30.
18. Munro, S.; Lewin, S.; Swart, T.; Volmink, J. A review of health behaviour theories: How useful are these for developing interventions to promote long-term medication adherence for TB and HIV/AIDS? *BMC Public Health* **2007**, *7*, 104. [CrossRef]
19. Janmaimool, P. Application of protection motivation theory to investigate sustainable waste management behaviors. *Sustainability* **2017**, *9*, 1079. [CrossRef]
20. Norman, P.; Boer, H.; Seydel, E.R. Protection motivation theory. *Predict. Health Behav.* **2005**, *81*, 126.
21. Morris, J.; Marzano, M.; Dandy, N.; O'Brien, L. *Theories and Models of Behaviour and Behaviour Change*; Forest Research: Surrey, UK, 2012; pp. 1–27.
22. Prochaska, J.O.; Velicer, W.F. The transtheoretical model of health behavior change. *Am. J. Health Promot.* **1997**, *12*, 38–48. [CrossRef]
23. West, R. Time for a change: Putting the Transtheoretical (Stages of Change) Model to rest. *Addiction* **2005**, *100*, 1036–1039.
24. Friman, M.; Huck, J.; Olsson, L.E. Transtheoretical model of change during travel behavior interventions: An integrative review. *Int. J. Environ. Res. Public Health* **2017**, *14*, 581. [CrossRef]
25. Fishbein, M. *Leek Ajzen (1975), Belief, Attitude, Intention, and Behavior: An Introduction to Theory and Research. Reading*; Addison-Wesley: Boston, MA, USA, 1981.
26. Ajzen, I. Perceived behavioral control, self-efficacy, locus of control, and the theory of planned behavior 1. *J. Appl. Soc. Psychol.* **2002**, *32*, 665–683. [CrossRef]
27. Ajzen, I. The theory of planned behavior. *Organ. Behav. Hum. Decis. Process.* **1991**, *50*, 179–211. [CrossRef]
28. Steinmetz, H.; Knappstein, M.; Ajzen, I.; Schmidt, P.; Kabst, R. How effective are behavior change interventions based on the theory of planned behavior? *Zeitschrift für Psychol.* **2016**, *224*, 216–233. [CrossRef]
29. Francis, J.; Eccles, M.P.; Johnston, M.; Walker, A.E.; Grimshaw, J.M.; Foy, R.; Kaner, E.F.S.; Smith, L.; Bonetti, D. *Constructing Questionnaires Based on the Theory of Planned Behaviour: A Manual for Health Services Researchers*; Centre for Health Services Research, University of Newcastle upon Tyne: Newcastle upon Tyne, UK, 2004.
30. TPB with Background Factors. Available online: https://people.umass.edu/aizen/tpb.background.html (accessed on 4 December 2020).
31. Ajzen, I. The theory of planned behavior: Frequently asked questions. *Hum. Behav. Emerg. Technol.* **2020**, *2*, 314–324. [CrossRef]
32. Armitage, C.J.; Christian, J. From attitudes to behaviour: Basic and applied research on the theory of planned behaviour. *Curr. Psychol.* **2003**, *22*, 187–195. [CrossRef]
33. Noar, S.M.; Zimmerman, R.S. Health behavior theory and cumulative knowledge regarding health behaviors: Are we moving in the right direction? *Health Educ. Res.* **2005**, *20*, 275–290. [CrossRef]
34. Orji, R.; Vassileva, J.; Mandryk, R. Towards an effective health interventions design: An extension of the health belief model. *Online J. Public Health Inf.* **2012**, *4*. [CrossRef] [PubMed]
35. Davis, G.; Morgan, A. Using the Theory of Planned Behaviour to Determine Recycling and Waste Minimisation Behaviours: A Case Study of Bristol City, UK. *Aust. Community Psychol.* **2008**, *20*, 105–117.
36. Topa, G.; Moriano, J.A. Theory of planned behavior and smoking: Meta-analysis and SEM model. *Subst. Abus. Rehabil.* **2010**, *1*, 23. [CrossRef] [PubMed]
37. Chase, K.; Reicks, M.; Jones, J.M. Applying the theory of planned behavior to promotion of whole-grain foods by dietitians. *J. Am. Diet. Assoc.* **2003**, *103*, 1639–1642. Available online: https://pubmed.ncbi.nlm.nih.gov/14647092/ (accessed on 5 December 2020). [CrossRef]
38. Milton, A.C.; Mullan, B.A. An application of the theory of planned behavior—A randomized controlled food safety pilot intervention for young adults. *Health Psychol. Off. J. Div. Health Psychol. Am. Psychol. Assoc.* **2012**, *31*, 250–259. [CrossRef]
39. Hagger, M.S.; Chatzisarantis, N.L.D.; Biddle, S.J.H. A meta-analytic review of the theories of reasoned action and planned behavior in physical activity: Predictive validity and the contribution of additional variables. *J. Sport Exerc. Psychol.* **2002**, *24*, 3–32. [CrossRef]
40. McConnon, Á.; Raats, M.; Astrup, A.; Bajzova, M.; Handjieva-Darlenska, T.; Lindroos, A.K.; Martínez, J.A.; Larson, T.M.; Papadaki, A.; Pfeiffer, A.F.H.; et al. Application of the Theory of Planned Behaviour to weight control in an overweight cohort. Results from a pan-European dietary intervention trial (DiOGenes). *Appetite* **2012**, *58*, 313–318. [CrossRef]

41. Armitage, C.J.; Talibudeen, L. Test of a brief theory of planned behaviour-based intervention to promote adolescent safe sex intentions. *Br. J. Psychol.* **2010**, *101*, 155–172. [CrossRef]
42. Quine, L.; Rutter, D.R.; Arnold, L. Persuading school-age cyclists to use safety helmets: Effectiveness of an intervention based on the Theory of Planned Behaviour. *Br. J. Health Psychol.* **2001**, *6*, 327–345. [CrossRef] [PubMed]
43. Elliott, M.A.; Armitage, C.J. Promoting drivers' compliance with speed limits: Testing an intervention based on the theory of planned behaviour. *Br. J. Psychol.* **2009**, *100*, 111–132. [CrossRef]
44. de Leeuw, A.; Valois, P.; Schmidt, P.; Ajzen, I. Using the theory of planned behavior to identify key beliefs underlying pro-environmental behavior in high-school students: Implications for educational interventions. *Artic. J. Environ. Psychol.* **2015**, *42*, 128–138. [CrossRef]
45. Pakpour, A.H.; Zeidi, I.M.; Emamjomeh, M.M.; Asefzadeh, S.; Pearson, H. Household waste behaviours among a community sample in Iran: An application of the theory of planned behaviour. *Waste Manag.* **2014**, *34*, 980–986. [CrossRef] [PubMed]
46. Godin, G.; Kok, G. The theory of planned behavior: A review of its applications to health-related behaviors. *Am. J. Health Promot.* **1996**, *11*, 87–98. [CrossRef]
47. Bledsoe, L.K. Smoking cessation: An application of theory of planned behavior to understanding progress through stages of change. *Addict. Behav.* **2006**, *31*, 1271–1276. [CrossRef] [PubMed]
48. Chisholm, M.A.; Williamson, G.M.; Lance, C.E.; Mulloy, L.L. Predicting adherence to immunosuppressant therapy: A prospective analysis of the theory of planned behaviour. *Nephrol. Dial. Transplant.* **2007**, *22*, 2339–2348. [CrossRef] [PubMed]
49. Perkins, M.B.; Jensen, P.S.; Jaccard, J.; Gollwitzer, P.; Oettingen, G.; Pappadopulos, E.; Hoagwood, K.E. Applying theory-driven approaches to understanding and modifying clinicians' behavior: What do we know? *Psychiatr. Serv.* **2007**, *58*, 342–348. [CrossRef] [PubMed]
50. Hagger, M.S.; Lonsdale, A.; Chatzisarantis, N.L.D. A theory-based intervention to reduce alcohol drinking in excess of guideline limits among undergraduate students. *Br. J. Health Psychol.* **2012**, *17*, 18–43. [CrossRef]
51. Armitage, C.J.; Rowe, R.; Arden, M.A.; Harris, P.R. A brief psychological intervention that reduces adolescent alcohol consumption. *J. Consult. Clin. Psychol.* **2014**, *82*, 546. [CrossRef] [PubMed]
52. Abraham, C.; Clift, S.; Grabowski, P. Cognitive predictors of adherence to malaria prophylaxis regimens on return from a malarious region: A prospective study. *Soc. Sci. Med.* **1999**, *48*, 1641–1654. [CrossRef]
53. Yardley, L.; Miller, S.; Schlotz, W.; Little, P. Evaluation of a Web-based intervention to promote hand hygiene: Exploratory randomized controlled trial. *J. Med. Internet Res.* **2011**, *13*, e107. [CrossRef]
54. Schifter, D.E.; Ajzen, I. Intention, perceived control, and weight loss: An application of the theory of planned behavior. *J. Pers. Soc. Psychol.* **1985**, *49*, 843–851. [CrossRef] [PubMed]
55. Booth, A.R.; Norman, P.; Goyder, E.; Harris, P.R.; Campbell, M.J. Pilot study of a brief intervention based on the theory of planned behaviour and self-identity to increase chlamydia testing among young people living in deprived areas. *Br. J. Health Psychol.* **2014**, *19*, 636–651. [CrossRef]
56. Asare, M. Using The Theory of Planned Behavior to Determine the Condom Use Behavior Among College Students. *Am. J. Health Stud.* **2015**, *30*, 43–50.
57. Sheeran, P.; Silverman, M. Evaluation of three interventions to promote workplace health and safety: Evidence for the utility of implementation intentions. *Soc. Sci. Med.* **2003**, *56*, 2153–2163. [CrossRef]
58. Understanding Individuals' Environmentally Significant Behavior | Environmental Law Reporter. Available online: https://elr.info/news-analysis/35/10785/understanding-individuals-environmentally-significant-behavior (accessed on 5 December 2020).
59. Koger, S.M. *The Psychology of Environmental Problems*; Psychology Press: East Sussex, UK, 2011; Available online: http://www.copyright.com/ (accessed on 5 December 2020).
60. Sumaedi, S.; Yarmen, M.; Bakti, I.G.M.Y.; Rakhmawati, T.; Astrini, N.J.; Widianti, T. The integrated model of theory planned behavior, value, and image for explaining public transport passengers' intention to reuse. *Manag. Environ. Qual.* **2016**, *27*, 124–135. [CrossRef]
61. van der Linden, S. Charitable Intent: A Moral or Social Construct? A Revised Theory of Planned Behavior Model. *Curr. Psychol.* **2011**, *30*, 355–374. Available online: https://link.springer.com/article/10.1007/s12144-011-9122-1 (accessed on 5 December 2020). [CrossRef]
62. Ham, M.; Jeger, M.; Frajman Ivković, A. The role of subjective norms in forming the intention to purchase green food. *Econ. Res. Istraživanja* **2015**, *28*, 738–748. [CrossRef]
63. Heuckmann, B.; Hammann, M.; Asshoff, R. Advantages and disadvantages of modeling beliefs by single item and scale models in the context of the theory of planned behavior. *Educ. Sci.* **2019**, *9*, 268. [CrossRef]
64. Ajzen, I. TPB Questionnaire Construction 1. Constructing a Theory of Planned Behavior Questionnaire. Available online: https://people.umass.edu/aizen/pdf/tpb.measurement.pdf (accessed on 19 February 2021).

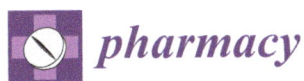

Article

Intentions to "Reuse" Medication in the Future Modelled and Measured Using the Theory of Planned Behavior

Hamza Alhamad [1,2,*] **and Parastou Donyai** [2,*]

1. Department of Pharmacy, University of Reading, Reading RG6 6AP, UK
2. Department of Pharmacy, Zarqa University, Zarqa 132222, Jordan
* Correspondence: halhamad@zu.edu.jo (H.A.); p.donyai@reading.ac.uk (P.D.)

Received: 16 September 2020; Accepted: 16 October 2020; Published: 12 November 2020

Abstract: Background: A range of pro-environmental behaviors are recognized, promoted, and investigated, but urgent action is also needed to tackle the direct and indirect environmental impact of medication waste. One solution is to reissue medicines, returned unused to pharmacies (i.e., reuse medicines). Yet, if medicines reuse is to be formally introduced in the UK, it is imperative also to understand people's willingness to take part in such a scheme and importantly, the underpinning drivers. This study aimed to develop, validate, and evaluate a Theory of Planned Behavior model aimed at predicting medicines reuse behavioral intentions. Methods: The behavior of interest, medicines reuse, was defined according to its Target, Action, Context, and Time. Then themes from an existing qualitative study were used in order to draft, validate and pilot a Theory of Planned Behavior-based questionnaire before its completion by a representative sample (n = 1003) of participants from across the UK. Results: The majority expressed pro-medicines reuse intentions. The three direct measures accounted for 73.4% of the variance in relation to people's intention to reuse medicines in the future, which was statistically significant at $p < 0.001$. People's specific beliefs about medicines reuse and how they evaluate other people's expectations of them had a substantial impact on their intentions to reuse medication in the future, mediated in an intricate way via attitudes, subjective norms and perceived behavioral control (PBC). Conclusions: This study shows how people could embrace medicines reuse via practical measures that illustrate the safety and quality assurance of reissued medicines, educational interventions that bolster beliefs about the pro-environmental benefits, and norm-based interventions encouraging doctors and pharmacists to endorse the practice. The findings add to the emerging work on medicines reuse and, significantly, provide a theoretical framework to guide policymakers and other organizations looking to decrease the impact of medication waste through medicines reuse schemes.

Keywords: medicine reuse; theory of planned behavior; questionnaire; recycle; medicine waste; unused medicines; attitudes; intentions

1. Introduction

Waste associated with prescribed medicines cost NHS England an estimated £300 million a year in 2009, £110 million of which related to medicines returned to community pharmacies for disposal [1]. A decade on, all medicines returned to community pharmacies in the UK continue to be branded as waste and earmarked for disposal [2]. Even if unused, unopened, and still in date, medicines thus returned are not allowed to re-enter the pharmaceutical supply chain, an often-cited reason being the possible loss of potency from unknown storage conditions outside a pharmacy [3] or the threat of tampering and falsification. However, some countries including the United States (US) [4] and

Greece (GIVMED) [5] do operate "medication reuse" schemes, mainly for benevolent reasons—the idea being, briefly, that suitable medicines can re-enter the supply chain and be reissued to others in need. Furthermore, researchers have found that around 20–25% of medicines returned for disposal to community pharmacies in the UK and the Netherlands are potentially eligible for reuse [6,7], 90% of donations to a pilot recycling scheme in Singapore were reusable [8] and 10 million unused prescription medication discarded by long-term care facilities such as nursing homes in the US could be reused [9]. These studies form part of a global drive, including in the UK [10], to examine the evidence for medicines reuse as a plausible arrangement for tackling medication waste. Although an internationally agreed definition of medicines reuse remains to be developed, further description is outlined in a previous study [11].

Medicines reuse concurs with ideas on sustainable pharmacy [12] because, in addition to the economic impact of medication waste, accruing unused medicines can also produce deleterious environmental effects. For example, according to a systematic review [13], globally people are more likely to dispose of their unwanted residential medication in the household bin than use any other method, with disposal down the drain also taking place especially with liquid formulations and, in the US, with dangerous substances. These practices can contribute to water and ground contamination [14]. In fact, disposal via the drain is considered to be the most harmful route as it leads to direct input into the aquatic system via effluent released from wastewater treatment works [15] where pharmaceutical traces have been shown to withstand standard treatment methods [16]. The environmental impact of disposing of medicines into garbage also poses a risk especially where landfilling (versus, say, incineration) is a key waste management route (e.g., 42% of waste ends up in landfill in Ireland, and 35% in the UK) or where landfills act as dumping areas rather than being engineered sites (e.g., in Malaysia, Thailand, India, Bangladesh) [13]. Prescribed medication waste can also impact negatively on the environment through the "carbon footprint" [17]. Thus, logically reusing prescribed medicines could reduce the economic and environmental cost of medication waste provided a workable scheme exists, and people can be motivated to use it.

In the UK the logistics of a credible scheme for reusing medication have been largely academic [18]. For patients, most NHS medicines are supplied free of charge or at a fixed cost (£9 per product in 2020) [19], weakening the humanitarian impetus. Regardless, the professional and regulatory bodies express no appetite to explore opportunities or a change in the law to enable medicines reuse, citing concerns over medicinal quality as the main rationale [10]. Yet, the UK government has relaxed its position on medicines reuse sporadically in the past, meaning the concept is not altogether implausible. In 2008 the Department of Health proposed the reuse of patient-returned and date-expired medicines when it anticipated supply-chain problems amid a flu pandemic [20]. More recently, in 2018, a drug company was allowed to extend the expiry date of adrenaline auto-injectors by four months, including for products already in circulation, when the supply chain was disrupted [21]. With medication shortages now a recognized problem in the UK [22], alongside the general urgency to halt the further environmental decline, a formal scheme for reusing medication becomes increasingly plausible. Yet, if medicines reuse is to be formally introduced, it is imperative to understand both pharmacist and people's views and willingness about the medicine reuse idea. A UK study reported that pharmacists of one Health Board in South-East Wales are willing to redistribute returned unused medicines if certain criteria were met such as medicines being solid dosage forms only, with tamper evident seals in place [23]. This study focused on understanding people's willingness to take part in such a scheme by accepting reissued medicines, and importantly, the underpinning drivers. There is evidence to suggest that environmental knowledge is positively linked with pro-environmental behavior regarding medicines disposal practices [24,25]. In addition, although a qualitative study in the UK suggests people could accept medicines in their original packaging if these are considered to be safe for reuse by the pharmacist [11], large-scale beliefs and intentions to personally take part in a medication reuse scheme in the future remain unexplored.

This study aimed to address this gap by measuring people's views on personally taking part in medicines reuse (by accepting reissued medicines) with the Theory of Planned Behavior (TPB) [26] as the underpinning framework. The TPB has been shown to be relevant to studying environmental problems and pro-environmental behaviors [27,28], including managing household waste and recycling [29,30]. According to the TPB, people's intentions to personally take part in any particular behavior (e.g., smoking, eating healthy food, or, in this paper, taking part in medicines reuse) is the most proximal determinant of that behavior. In this model, behavioral intention is predicted by the psychological constructs "attitude" toward the behavior (which is a person's overall evaluation of the behavior), "subjective norm" (which is a person's own estimate of social pressure to perform the behavior or not), and "perceived behavioral control" (PBC) (the extent to which a person feels able to enact the behavior). Although each predictor of intention could be measured directly (by asking respondents, for example, about their overall attitude toward the behavior in question), the TPB approach to measurement also encompasses indirect questions. The indirect questions relating to *attitude*, measure specific beliefs about the likely consequences of the behavior (behavioral beliefs) and corresponding outcome evaluation for each behavioral belief. The indirect questions relating to the *subjective norm*, measure beliefs about how other important people would like them to behave (normative beliefs/social pressure) and their motivation to comply with each of these reference groups or individuals. The indirect questions relating to *PBC*, measure beliefs about how much a person has control over the behavior (control beliefs) and the power of the factors that facilitate or inhibit the behavior. The model has been shown to be robust and effective [31].

Taking account of these constructs, a Medicines Reuse Questionnaire (MRQ) was developed, validated and then used to survey a representative sample of just over 1000 people in the UK. We theorized:

Hypothesis 1 (H1). *There will be a positive relationship between medicines reuse attitudes and intention to reuse medication in the future.*

Hypothesis 2 (H2). *There will be a positive relationship between medicines reuse subjective norms and intention to reuse medication in the future.*

Hypothesis 3 (H3). *There will be a positive relationship between medicines reuse PBC and intention to reuse medication in the future.*

Hypothesis 4 (H4). *There will be a positive relationship between medicines reuse behavioral beliefs and medicines reuse attitudes.*

Hypothesis 5 (H5). *There will be a positive relationship between medicines reuse normative beliefs, and medicines reuse subjective norms.*

Hypothesis 6 (H6). *There will be a positive relationship between medicines reuse control beliefs and medicines reuse PBC.*

The rest of this paper is organized as follows. The methods for the development and validation of the MRQ are discussed as well as for the conduct of the survey. Then the descriptive and statistical analyses of the data are discussed followed by a wider discussion which includes the limitation of this work. The article concludes with a summary of the findings and final statements.

2. Materials and Methods

2.1. Compliance with Ethical Standards

This study was approved by the University of Reading's Research Ethics Committee through the School Exemptions process (reference number 30/15) with an amendment approved 2/2017.

2.2. Questionnaire Development

The development of a TPB questionnaire requires a methodical approach that unearths both the direct and indirect measures of intention. Accordingly, the MRQ was developed in eight stages consistent with the procedure set out by Francis et al. (2004), as briefly described below and shown in (Figure S1).

First, the behavior of interest, taking part in medicines reuse, was defined in terms of its Target, Action, Context, and Time (TACT) [32]. Here the target was prescription medication previously given out to another individual but then returned to a pharmacy. The action was accepting medication for one's own personal use. The context was a situation where the pharmacist has verified that the medication has been kept by the other individual for less than three months, has more than six months of shelf-life remaining, has not been tampered with, has been kept under normal storage conditions, and has been kept in an original sealed blister pack (i.e., medication strip). In addition, the time was in the future when collecting own medication from a pharmacy for the management of a long-term illness. See (Box S2) for the presentation of this information to the participants at the start of the MRQ.

Second, to construct the indirect questions, the themes obtained from an elicitation study [11] were mapped against the constructs in the TPB model [32] in order to identify the behavioral beliefs, normative beliefs, and control beliefs. As medicines reuse does not currently take place in the UK, the normative beliefs encompassed injunctive norms only. Third, a draft questionnaire was produced to include items covering at all these constructs (see Figure S3). Likert scales for the indirect measures were unipolar and graded from 1 to 7 for the behavioral belief items, motivation to comply items and control belief items. The Likert scales were recoded into bipolar scales from -3 to +3 for the outcome evaluation items, normative belief items, and power of control factors, as per published recommendations [32]. The recoding allowed a composite score to be obtained for each of the indirect measures by multiplying scores on the relevant unipolar scale by those on the respective bipolar scale so that positive scores reflect favorable attitudes, more social pressure to perform the behavior (i.e., reuse medication), and control factors that make medicines reuse more likely, and vice versa with negative scores (see Tables S4–S6).

In addition, 12 items in total were initially developed for the "direct" measures of attitude, subjective norm, and perceived behavioral control. Where appropriate, a mix of positive and negative endpoints was used to intermittently prompt respondents to further contemplate their answers. The endpoints of the direct measures of attitude were constructed using bipolar adjectives on a 7-point Likert scale with both instrumental (whether reusing medication achieves something, e.g., worthless-worthwhile) and experiential items (how it would feel to reuse medication, e.g., satisfying-dissatisfying, good-bad). The endpoints of the direct measures of subjective norms prompted respondents either to complete an otherwise incomplete sentence or to agree or disagree with a complete sentence. The endpoints of the direct measures of PBC were developed to assess the person's "self-efficacy", using both an incomplete sentence and a complete sentence prompting respondents to either agree or disagree, and to assess beliefs about the "controllability" of the behavior using complete sentences prompting respondents to either agree or disagree. The composite scores for each of the direct measures were obtained by calculating the mean of the item scores (see Tables S7–S9). Three items related directly to the intention construct were developed using a generalized intention method with positive (strongly disagree/strongly agree) endpoints. The composite score for the three intention items was obtained by calculating the mean score (see Table S10). Finally, seven items were developed to measure respondents' demographic/background characteristics (i.e., age, gender, religion, ethnicity, the level of education, whether currently using medication and having any long-term conditions) using a multiple-choice response format. This generated 50 items initially.

Fourth, the content validity (CV) (i.e., how well the items cover and assess the constructs of interest) of the first set of 50 questions was determined by interviewing a panel of 11 service users who had taken part in a previous elicitation study. This was carried out using the process of cognitive interviewing, which involved asking each participant four questions about each item on the questionnaire [33]. As a result, three of the items on the questionnaire (Q11, Q12, Q37) were reworded (see Table S11). This produced the first version (V1) of the MRQ (see Table S12). Fifth, MRQ (V1) was transferred to the Bristol Online Survey (as then known) platform and pilot tested with 46 participants recruited by emailing staff and students within the School of Pharmacy. Responses were subjected to construct validity analysis using confirmatory factor analysis (CFA) and the Statistical Package for Social Sciences (SPSS) software version 23. Data screening for multicollinearity and singularity was performed. To explain, first, principal component analysis (PCA) with orthogonal rotation (varimax), Bartlett's test, and the Kaiser–Meyer–Olkin (KMO) measure were completed. The R matrix (the correlation matrix), an SPSS output produced using the coefficient and significant levels options, showed that multicollinearity was not a problem. Sampling adequacy was verified by an overall KMO of 0.735 (with all KMO values for the individual items being >0.59). Finally, the value of Bartlett's test of sphericity χ^2 (253) was = 1287.947, $p < 0.001$, indicating that correlations between the items were sufficiently large for completion of the analysis. As a result, CFA was performed with a sample of 46 responses using Analysis of a Moment Structures (Amos) SPSS software (v. 23). For the factor loadings for each item of the indirect and direct measures, see Table S12. Items with low factor loading were later deleted (Q38 and Q43 in MRQ V1) (a question pair relating to PBC) or rephrased (Q5, Q14, Q15, Q26, Q27, Q30, and Q31), as described below.

In addition, two methods were used to measure the reliability of the MRQ items. Cronbach's alpha (α) coefficient was used as a measure of internal consistency of the "direct" measures of TPB using the responses obtained from the 46 participants. The Cronbach's α coefficient of the different constructs (relating to the direct measures) of the TPB are shown in Table S13. These were found to be excellent apart from the Cronbach's α coefficient value of the PBC construct, which was below 0.5, but improved first by deleting Q15 (the Cronbach's α value increased from 0.303 into 0.562), then further improved by also deleting Q14 (the Cronbach's α value further increased from 0.562 into 0.830). These two questions related to PBC ("controllability") and as noted above, were already flagged for rewording due to low factor loadings as part of CFA. Pearson correlation was used as a measure of the test-retest reliability of the "indirect" measures of TPB. Therefore, as a sixth step, 24 of the participants recompleted the same survey after two weeks, and this allowed the test-retest reliability of the indirect measures of MRQ (V1) to be determined (using Pearson's coefficient) (see Table S12). Of the 28 items that were the indirect measures, 22 had correlations that met the threshold for reliability (>0.5). The Pearson correlation of 6 items (Q26, Q30, Q27, Q31, Q38, Q43) was <0.5. This provided further the rationale for removing two items (Q38, Q43) (a question pair relating to PBC) and rephrasing four items (Q26, Q27, Q30, Q31) as described below.

Seventh, MRQ (V1) was reworded by working with ten service users, recruited through the original elicitation study to produce the second version of the MRQ (V2). Two items (Q38, Q43) which related to the idea that a reward system may encourage people to reuse medicines in the future, had low factor loading (0.026) for the composite behavioral belief, and low Pearson's correlation coefficients (<0.5). The service users expressed that a reward system would not affect their decision to reuse medicines. These two items were therefore removed. Four items for the composite normative beliefs (Q26, Q30 and Q27, Q31) with low factor loadings (0.358 and 0.356, respectively) and low Pearson's correlation coefficients (<0.5) were reworded. These items related to normative beliefs (injunctive norms) and motivation to comply with the expectations of environmentalists and the pharmaceutical industry, respectively. On speaking with the service users about this, they expressed that their own decisions about medicines reuse would be affected by social pressure from pharmacists and doctors and not the groups listed above—Q26, Q30 and Q27, Q31 were modified accordingly. Finally, one item relating to the direct measures of subjective norms (Q5) and two items relating to the direct measures of PBC (Q14 and Q15) which all had low factor loadings (0.262, 0.258 and 0.019, respectively) were reworded with the help of the ten service users (see Table S12).

Eight, MRQ (V2) was administered to a further set of 46 participants recruited by emailing staff and students from the wider university community. Responses for this second pilot were subjected again to validity (CFA) and reliability (internal consistency of the direct measures using Cronbach's α) tests. The result of the second pilot showed good factor loading for all the items except for two items from the PBC construct (Q14, Q15) which measured the controllability of medicines reuse behavior (factor loading −0.068 and −0.052, respectively) (see Table S12). Also, the Cronbach's α coefficient values of the direct measures of the TPB constructs were consistent and better compared to the previous pilot testing (see Table S14), again except for the PBC construct which had a Cronbach's α coefficient value of only 0.425. As Q14 and Q15 had been reworded previously, they were deleted at this stage, meaning that the PBC items that remained measured only self-efficacy in relation to medicines reuse behavior.

The above steps resulted in the refinement of MRQ (V3) with 46 items as a stable and accurate questionnaire ready for dissemination to a larger sample of the population.

2.3. Questionnaire Distribution

The final version of the questionnaire, MRQ (V3), was transferred to the Qualtrics online platform and disseminated to a panel of participants via a market research company (Research Now®, Plano, TX, USA). The aim was to recruit a sample of over 1000 participants with a long-term health condition, from different regions in the UK, and across all age groups and genders. Thus, as well as using a sampling technique that targeted those with a long-term condition, three additional questions were added to MRQ (V3), namely: "We are interested in the views of people with a long-term health condition only, do you currently have a long-term health condition?", "Which of the following (or another) long-term health condition(s) do you have?", and "In which region of the UK do you currently live?". The question about participants' religion was removed as it was considered a sensitive question in hindsight and its inclusion could not be justified.

The intended sample size was divided into participants with long-term conditions who were using medicines ($n = 800$), or not currently using medicines but had used medication for their condition in the past ($n = 100$) or had never taken any medicines for their long-term condition ($n = 100$). The recruitment was, therefore mainly targeting people with a long-term condition who were using medicines, as they might reasonably be expected to consider reusing medication in the future if the practice became a reality. However, it was important not to miss the viewpoints of those not presently using medicines (10% of the sample size), or those who have never taken any medicines for their long-term condition (10% of the sample size), as they too might require medicines in the future and thus have a view on medicines reuse.

A soft launch (10% of the total sample, $n = 100$) of MRQ (V3) was undertaken to review and quality-check the data before the full launch. Data obtained during the soft launch were included in the main study analysis. During the two-week data collection period, the representativeness of the sample was monitored for geographical spread, age groups, and gender balance, but no adjustment to the recruitment strategy was found to be necessary. Descriptive analysis was completed with the anonymized dataset using SPSS (V23).

2.4. Questionnaire Sample

A total of 1,181 people was invited to complete the MRQ (V3), with 178 potential respondents excluded because they reported not to have a long-term condition, resulting in 1003 useable responses. A summary of the background factors including gender, age, ethnicity, educational level, participants' geographical areas in the UK, and if participants were taking medicines for their long-term conditions is all shown in Table S15, Supplementary material. There was an almost equal number of female ($n = 509$) to male ($n = 494$) participants. Figure 1 shows the age distribution of the participants.

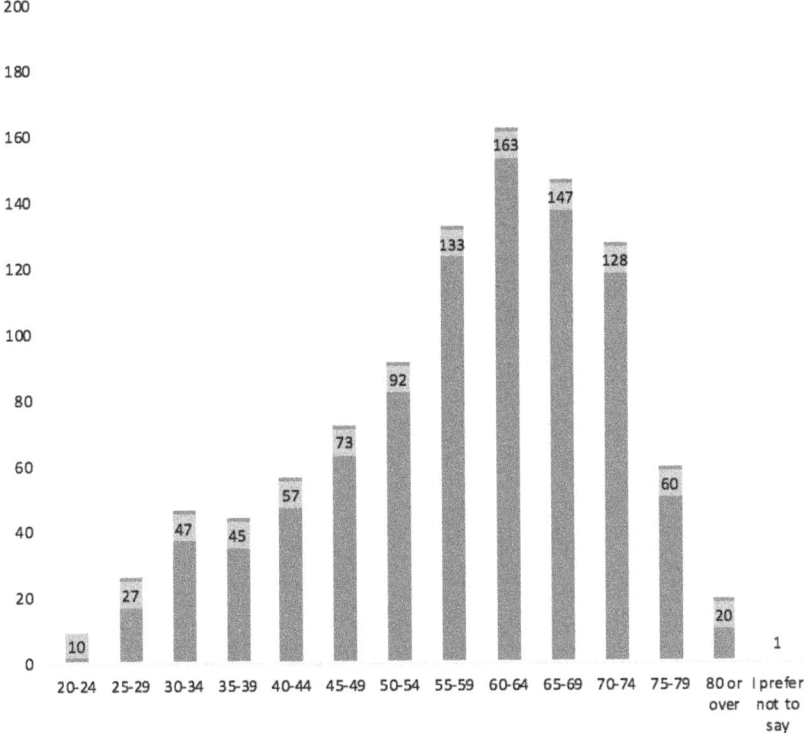

Figure 1. The number of participants in each age group.

In addition, there was an excellent spread of responses from across the UK (see Table S15). The majority of the participants were taking medicines for their long-term condition (86.4%) ($n = 867$), 10% ($n = 100$) were not taking medicines but did take medicines in the past, and 3.6% ($n = 36$) were not taking medicines and had never taken any medicines for their long-term condition(s).

2.5. Analysis of Survey Results

Several assumptions were checked before performing multiple regression analysis, namely to ensure that there was no violation of the assumptions on normality, linearity, and multicollinearity. Accordingly, it was found that the relationship between the independent variables and dependent variables was linear; there was no multicollinearity in the data; the values of residuals were independent and uncorrelated; the values of the residuals were normally distributed; there were no influential cases biasing the model.

Multiple regression was used to analyze the relationships between the main constructs of MRQ (V3). First, the intention to reuse medicines in the future construct was treated as the dependent (outcome) variable, and the three direct measures of attitude, subjective norm, and PBC constructs were each treated as the independent (predictor) variables. We also examined the relationship between the indirect and the direct measures using bivariate correlation, where each directly measured score was treated as the dependent variable, and the sum of the corresponding weighted indirect measure was treated as the independent variable.

To avoid interpretation problems encountered in or associated with multiple regression procedures, Structural Equation Modelling (SEM) with the standardized path coefficient was then applied using analysis of a moment structures (AMOS) SPSS to test six main hypotheses about the relationships between the main constructs of the TPB-based model. SEM allows for variables to correlate and accounts for measurement error, while multiple regression adjusts for variables in the model and assumes perfect measurement.

SEM was also used to assess the TPB-based model's overall goodness-of-fit. This was completed to check whether the standard relationship between the different constructs of the TPB proposed by the original model applies in relation to the data obtained in this study. These tests included chi-square, Root Mean Square Error of Approximation (RMSEA), Normalized Fit Index (NFI), Tucker Lewis Index (TLI) and the Comparative Fit Index (CFI), which are standard modification indices offered by AMOS SPSS. A new model with additional relationships between the constructs was created accordingly by calculating the modification indices (MI) using AMOS SPSS. The modification indices were checked to be at least five before the model was considered to be modified as recommended by Jöreskog and Sörbom [34]. The suggested relationships were checked carefully, and the logical relationships between constructs (i.e., only where the new relationships between the constructs made sense in relation to reusing medication as the behavior) were used to improve the model fit.

Finally, an independent t-test (for gender) or a one-way analysis of variance (ANOVA) (for age, ethnicity, level of education, and geography) was performed to test any relationship between participant characteristics and their intention (using mean intention scores) to reuse medicines in the future, to test a further 5 hypotheses:

Hypothesis 7 (H7). *There will be a difference in the intention to reuse medicines in the future according to the participants' gender.*

Hypothesis 8 (H8). *There will be a difference in intention to reuse medicines in the future according to the participants' age.*

Hypothesis 9 (H9). *There will be a difference in intention to reuse medicines in the future according to the participants' ethnicity.*

Hypothesis 10 (H10). *There will be a difference in intention to reuse medicines in the future according to the participants' level of education.*

Hypothesis 11 (H11). *There will be a difference in intention to reuse medicines in the future according to the participants' geographical location.*

3. Results

3.1. Description of Findings

The majority of respondents intended to (i.e., scored 5 or more on the Likert scale, with 7 being strongly agree) ($n = 547$; 54.5%; Mean 4.67, SD 1.90), wanted to ($n = 567$; 56.5%; Mean 4.69, SD 1.98) or expected to ($n = 570$; 56.5%; Mean 4.67, SD 1.90) reuse medication in the future, while 19.7%, 19.8% and 22.9%, respectively, were unsure (scored 4 on the Likert scale) and 23.4%, 23.6% and 22.5%, respectively, disagreed (3 or less on the Likert scale, with 1 being strongly disagree) (see Figure 2).

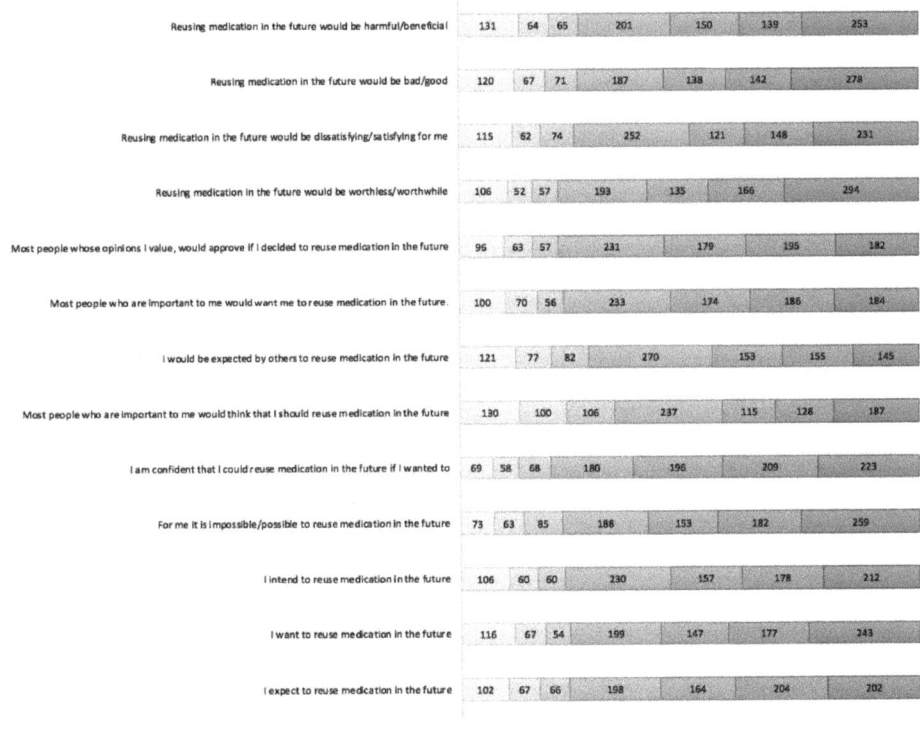

Figure 2. The distribution of responses to the direct questions and intention questions on the Likert scales. Key: Responses on each Likert scale, with seven indicating strongest agreement/pro-medicines-reuse sentiment and 1 indicating strongest disagreement/anti-medicines-reuse sentiment.

In terms of the direct measures of attitude, the majority of respondents (i.e., scored 5 or more on the Likert scale, with 7 being strongly agree) thought reusing medication in the future would be beneficial (n = 542; 54%; Mean 4.60, SD 2.03), good (n = 558; 55.6%; Mean 4.69, SD 2.03), satisfying for them (n = 500; 49.9%; Mean 4.56, SD 1.95), or worthwhile (n = 595; 59.3%; Mean 4.87, SD 1.97), while 20%, 18.6%, 25.1% and 19.2%, respectively, were unsure (scored 4 on the Likert scale), and 25.9%, 25.7%, 25% and 21.4%, respectively, disagreed (scored 3 or less on the Likert scale, with 1 being strongly disagree) (see Figure 2).

In terms of the direct measures of subjective norm, the majority of respondents thought most people whose opinion they value would approve if they decided to (n = 542; 54%; Mean 4.64, SD 1.83), most people important to them would want them to (n = 553; 54.1%; Mean 4.60, SD 1.85), they would be expected by others to (n = 453; 45.2%; Mean 4.30, SD 1.85), or that most people important to them would think that they should (n = 430; 42.9%; Mean 4.23, SD 1.98) reuse medication in the future, while 23%, 23.2%, 26.9% and 23.6%, respectively, were unsure, and 21.5%, 22.5%, 27.9% and 33.5%, respectively, disagreed (see Figure 2).

In terms of the direct measures of PBC (measuring self-efficacy), the majority of respondents felt confident they could reuse medication in the future if they wanted to, (n = 628; 62.6%; Mean 4.89, SD 1.78), or thought it would be possible for them to reuse medication in the future (n = 594; 59.2%;

Mean 4.86, SD 1.86), while 17.9%, and 18.7%, respectively, were unsure, and 19.4%, and 22%, respectively, disagreed (see Figure 2).

In terms of the indirect measures of attitude, the majority of respondents thought reusing medication will help them contribute toward reducing the harmful effects of medication on the environment (*n* = 732; 73%; Mean 5.57, SD 1.48) [with 73.9% agreeing this was good] or toward reducing the amount of money spent by the NHS on medication (n = 784; 78.2%; Mean 5.84, SD 1.43) [with 79.2% agreeing this was good], but the majority also thought that reusing medication is likely to result in them receiving low-quality medication (*n* = 579; 57.7%; Mean 5.84, SD 1.63) [with 79.3% agreeing this was bad], unsafe medication (*n* = 575; 57.3%; Mean 6.40, SD 1.36) [with 88.3% agreeing this was bad], or incorrect medication (*n* = 603; 60%; Mean 6.40, SD 1.46) [with 88% agreeing this was bad], while 16.2%, 13.4%, 21.8%, 20.7% and 18.3%, respectively, were unsure, and 10.8%, 8.5%, 20.4%, 21.9%, and 21.4%, respectively, disagreed (see Figure 3).

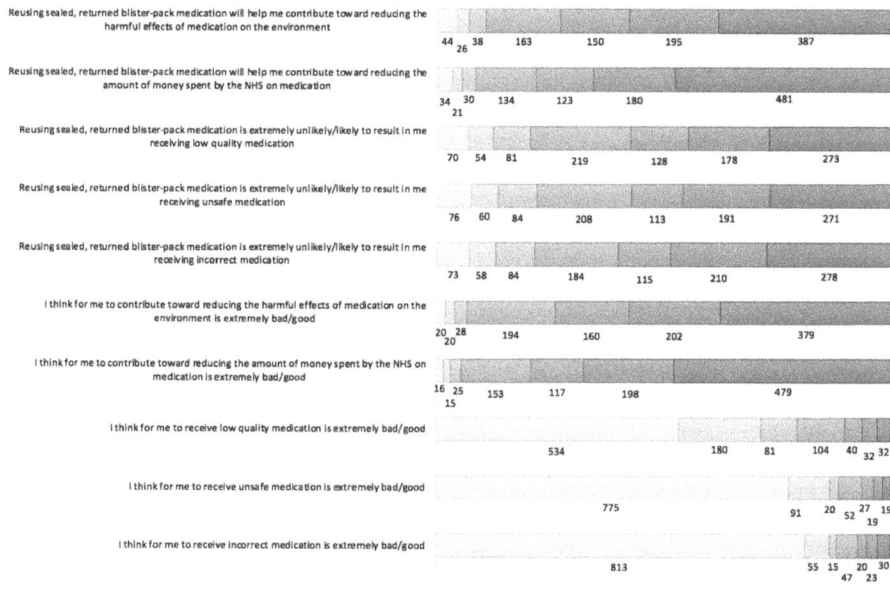

Figure 3. The distribution of responses to the indirect questions about behavioral beliefs and outcome evaluation, on the Likert scales. Key: Responses on each Likert scale, with 7 indicating strongest agreement/best outcome evaluation and 1 indicating strongest disagreement/worst outcome evaluation.

In terms of the indirect measures of subjective norm, the majority of respondents thought that their doctor (*n* = 455; 45.4%; Mean 4.58, SD 1.67), pharmacist (*n* = 501; 50%; Mean 4.58, SD 1.77), close friends (*n* = 457; 45.6%; Mean 4.45, SD 1.79), or family (*n* = 497; 49.6%; Mean 4.48, SD 1.90) would believe they should reuse medication in the future, while 36.7%, 29.2%, 31.6% and 23.7%, respectively, were unsure, and 17.9%, 20.7%, 22.8%, and 26.8%, respectively, disagreed (see Figure 4). Overall, 77.6% agreed they would generally want to do what their doctor says, 68.5% what their pharmacist says, 44.3% what their close friends say, and 61.1% what their family says.

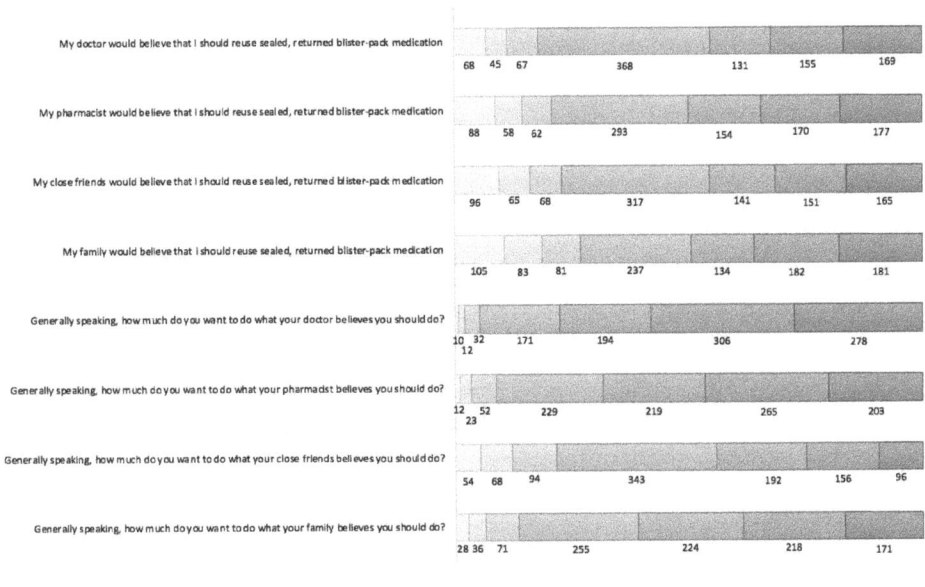

Figure 4. The distribution of responses to the indirect questions about normative beliefs and motivation to comply on 7-point Likert scales. Key: Responses on each Likert scale, with 7 indicating strongest agreement/motivation to comply and 1 indicating strongest disagreement/least motivation to comply.

In terms of the indirect measures of PBC, the majority of respondents expected any medication offered to them for reuse will be in the original, sealed, blister packaging ($n = 872$; 86.9%; Mean 6.19, SD 1.29), would have been quality-checked ($n = 920$; 91.7%; Mean 6.48, SD 1.03), or safety-checked ($n = 928$; 92.5%; Mean 6.55, SD 0.97), will have more than six months of shelf-life remaining ($n = 854$; 85.1%; Mean 6.10, SD 1.29), while 9.6%, 6.5%, 6.1% and 11.5%, respectively, were unsure, and 3.5%, 1.8%, 1.4%, and 3.4%, respectively, disagreed (see Figure 5). On the whole, 84.4% agreed it would make it easier for them to reuse medication if they could see that it was in the original, sealed, blister packaging, 90.6% if it had been quality-checked, 91.2% if safety-checked, and 83.6% if it had more than six months of shelf-life remaining (see Figure 5).

3.2. Regression Analysis

As shown in Table 1, intentions to reuse medicines in the future based on attitudes, subjective, norm, and PBC, returned a statistically significant regression equation: $F(3, 999) = 920.645$, $p < 0.001$, with an R square of 0.734 (i.e., the three independent variables accounted for 73.4% of the variance in intention to reuse medicines in the future). In addition, each of the direct measures of attitude, subjective norm, and PBC about the behavior was a positive and (statistically) significant predictor of intentions to reuse medicines in the future ($B = 0.212$, $p < 0.001$), ($B = 0.497$, $p < 0.001$), and ($B = 0.326$, $p < 0.001$), respectively (see Table 1).

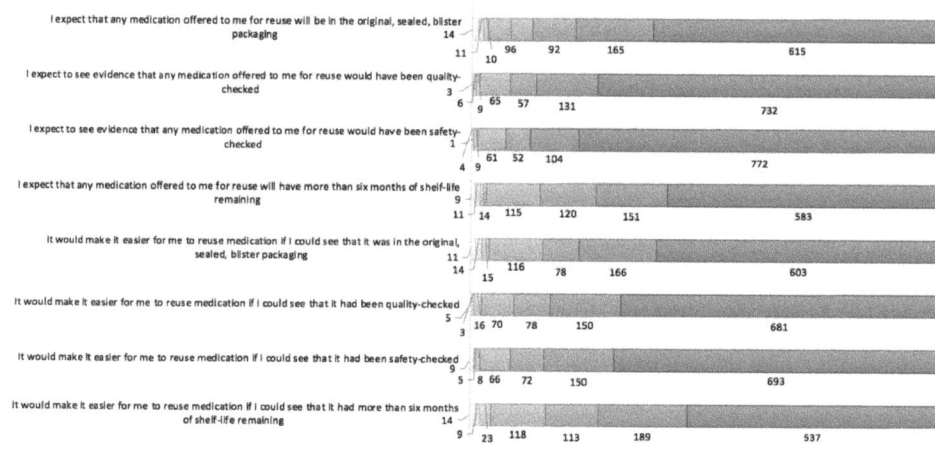

Figure 5. The distribution of responses to the indirect questions about control beliefs and power of control factors on 7-point Likert scales. Key: Responses on each Likert scale, with 7 indicating strongest agreement and 1 indicating strongest disagreement with the statement.

Table 1. Results of multiple regression analysis of TPB constructs using both direct and indirect measures.

Predictor Variable	B	SE	Beta (β)	t	p
Direct Measures					
Attitude	0.212	0.025	0.217	8.545	<0.001
Subjective norm	0.497	0.029	0.445	16.900	<0.001
PBC	0.326	0.025	0.296	12.941	<0.001
N = 1003 participants, F = 920.645, df = 3, p < 0.001, R = 0.857, R2 = 0.734, Adjusted R2 = 0.734					
Indirect Measures					
Behavioral belief .... Attitudes F = 512.301, df = 1, p < 0.001, R = 0.582, R2 = 0.339, Adjusted R2 = 0.339	0.024	0.001	0.591	2.18	<0.001
Normative beliefs .... Subjective norms F = 512.301, df = 1, p < 0.001, R = 0.591, R2 = 0.349, Adjusted R2 = 0.349	0.027	0.001	0.582	22.634	<0.001
Control beliefs .... PBC F = 50.507, df = 1, p < 0.001, R = 0.219, R2 = 0.048, Adjusted R2 = 0.047	0.013	0.002	0.219	7.107	<0.001

The correlation between the indirect and the direct measures were all statistically significant ($p < 0.001$) with a correlation between behavioral beliefs and attitude (β 0.591), and normative beliefs and subjective norm (β 0.582) being good, and the correlation between control beliefs and PBC being poor (β 0.219).

3.3. Construction of a TPB-based Model and Hypothesis Testing

As shown in Table 2, SEM with the standardized path coefficient returned a positive and statistically significant relationship between each of the direct measures of attitude, subjective norm, and PBC, and intention to reuse medicines in the future, upholding the first three hypotheses. Also, there were positive and statistically significant relationships between behavioral beliefs and attitude toward reusing medicines in the future, between normative beliefs and subjective norms about reusing medicines in the future, and between control beliefs and PBC about reusing medicines in the future, upholding hypotheses four to six. Figure 6 shows the complete TPB-based model using SEM with standardized path analysis.

Table 2. The testing of study hypotheses relating to the TBP-based model using SEM.

Hypotheses	Standardized Path Coefficient
H1	0.27 ($p < 0.001$, $n = 1003$)
H2	0.55 ($p < 0.001$, $n = 1003$)
H3	0.37 ($p < 0.001$, $n = 1003$)
H4	0.59 ($p < 0.001$, $n = 1003$).
H5	0.58 ($p < 0.001$, $n = 1003$)
H6	0.22 ($p < 0.001$, $n = 1003$)

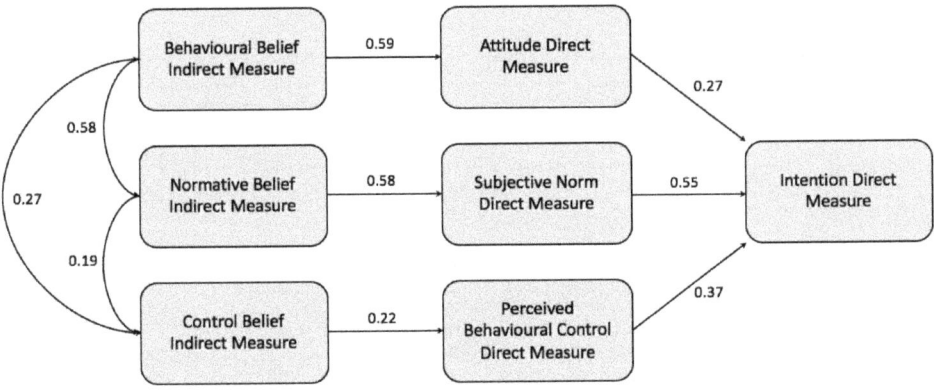

Figure 6. The TPB model created using SEM with standardized path analysis results.

3.4. Model Modification

An additional set of tests on the model (Table 3), however, showed the assumed relationships to be a poor fit in terms of their predictive power (i.e., to predict intention to reuse medicines), necessitating the exploration of other, potentially stronger relationships between the constructs.

Table 3. Measures of model fit value which indicate poor model fit.

TEST	RECOMMENDED VALUE	MODEL VALUE	DEGREE OF MODEL FIT
Chi-square	$p \geq 0.05$	1298.857 *	Poor fit
Chi-square/df	≤ 5	108.238	
RMSEA	≤ 0.08	0.327	Poor fit
NFI	≥ 0.9	0.676	Poor fit
TLI	≥ 0.9	0.435	Poor fit
CFI	≥ 0.9	0.677	Poor fit

df = degree of freedom; * $p \leq 0.001$.

The use of MI suggested 11 new relationships between the construct of the TPB model as presented in Table 4. Five of these relationships, emboldened in Table 4, were judged by the authors to be logical in relation to medicines reuse and therefore added sequentially to the model to improve the fit (Table 5).

Table 4. All the new relationships between the model constructs suggested by MI.

The New Relationships between the Constructs		MI
Normative belief →	PBC	191.137
Behavioral belief →	PBC	241.787
Subjective norm →	PBC	430.755
Attitude →	PBC	372.591
Behavioral belief →	Subjective norm	53.964
PBC →	Subjective norm	238.809
Attitude →	Subjective norm	312.129
Normative belief →	Attitude	37.007
PBC →	Attitude	156.050
Subjective norm →	Attitude	288.170
Normative belief →	Intention	7.701

Table 5. Measures of model fit achieved after MIs were applied to make improvements.

TEST	RECOMMENDED VALUE	MODEL VALUE	DEGREE OF MODEL FIT
Chi-square	$p \geq 0.05$	* 16.755	Good fit (considering a large sample)
Chi-square/df	≤5	108.238	
RMSEA	≤0.08	0.037	Good fit
NFI	≥0.9	0.996	Good fit
TLI	≥0.9	0.993	Good fit
CFI	≥0.9	0.998	Good fit

df = degree of freedom; * $p \leq 0.001$.

Briefly, the AMOS model analysis indicated that the chi-square would drop dramatically and other model values would also improve if a path was drawn from subjective norms to attitude, which seemed reasonable: people's own attitudes could be affected by their perception of the opinion of key people in their lives, as reported in other studies using TPB [35,36]. Second, the AMOS model indicated a further improvement if a path was drawn from subjective norms to PBC; the idea that people's confidence to reuse medication in the future could reasonably be influenced by the opinion of key people. Third, the AMOS model indicated model values would again improve if a path was drawn from behavioral beliefs to PBC; the idea that people's self-confidence to reuse medication in the future could also be influenced by their individual beliefs about the behavior (e.g., how they might save the environment). Fourthly, the AMOS model indicated another improvement if a path is drawn from PBC to attitude; the idea that a person's confidence to reuse medicines would influence their attitude to reuse medicines. Finally, the AMOS model indicated the model values would also improve if a path is drawn from behavioral beliefs to the subjective norm; the idea that someone's own specific beliefs about the value of reusing medicines would influence what they considered people important to them would also believe.

The modified model is shown in Figure 7. Although the value of the standardized path coefficient for subjective norms reduced from 0.55 to 0.45 ($p < 0.001$, $n = 1003$) as a result of the new relationships between the construct, it remained the strongest predictor of intention to reuse medicines compared to the attitude and PBC constructs.

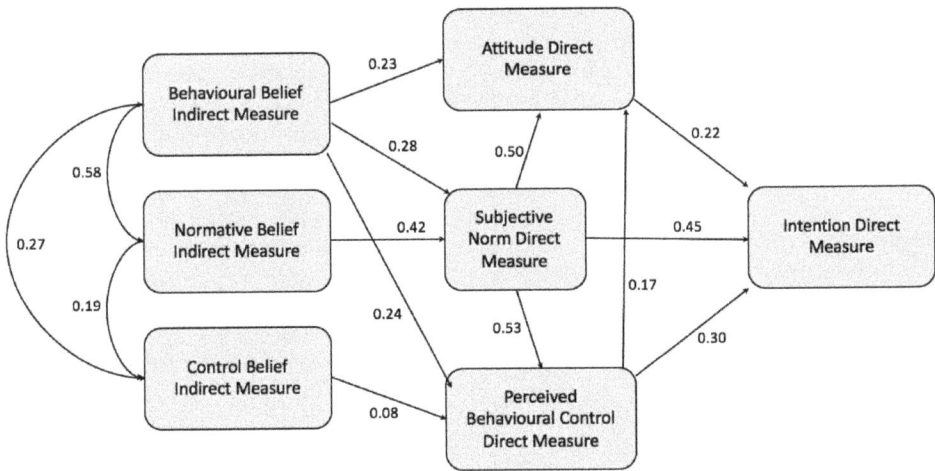

Figure 7. TPB model after modification showing the new relationships between the constructs.

3.5. Participant Characteristics

There was no statistically significant difference between any of the participant characteristics and the mean intention score, leading to the rejection of hypotheses 7–11 (see Table 6).

Table 6. Participant characteristics and intention to reuse medicines in the future.

HYPOTHESES	STATISTIC
H7	$t = -1.506$, df = 1001, $p = 0.132$
H8	$F = 0.971$, df = 13, 1002, $p = 0.478$
H9	$F = 0.954$, df = 17, 1002, $p = 0.509$
H10	$F = 1.665$, df = 16, 1002, $p = 0.480$
H11	$F = 0.989$, df = 12, 1002, $p = 0.457$

4. Discussion

The data support our premise that the direct measures of attitude toward medicines reuse, subjective norms, and PBC would positively and significantly predict intentions to reuse medication in the future and that these, in turn, would be predicted by specific behavioral, normative, and control beliefs, respectively (the latter with a proviso, explained below). The three direct measures accounted for 73.4% of the variance in relation to people's intention to reuse medicines in the future, which was statistically significant at $p < 0.001$. The construct of subjective norms was the strongest predictor of intentions to reuse medication, with PBC also predicting intentions but attitude being a less powerful predictor. The specific indirect measures showed statistically significant correlation with the respective direct measures, but the relationship between control beliefs and PBC, although statistically significant, was poor. A modified model also provided a significant path from behavioral beliefs to subjective norms and PBC, and from the subjective norm to attitudes and PBC (but further minimized the path from control beliefs to PBC). Thus, we have shown how specific beliefs about reusing medication and what people think others would expect of them, mediated in an intricate way via attitudes, subjective, norms, and PBC, work to influence intentions to reuse medication in the future.

The convincing effect of behavioral and normative beliefs, mainly via subjective norms and PBC, on intention is worth considering. In terms of behavioral beliefs, the findings highlight the importance of creating conditions that will first, bolster people's beliefs about the environmental and economic benefits of medicines reuse, and second, illustrate to them that medicines reuse would not expose them to additional medication-related risks. The first point could be addressed through an educational intervention while the second could reasonably be tackled through the creative use of existing systems, and the advent of new technologies, to demonstrate safety. For example, to tackle the unwanted entry of counterfeit medicines into the supply chain, the European Union has already introduced the falsified medicines directive which specifies that manufacturers should embed specific safety features on the packaging of prescription medicines [37]. This includes a physical anti-tampering device that confirms the product had remained sealed as well as a two-dimensional barcode which when scanned authenticates the product via the unique identifier. For our purposes, this technology could be repurposed to prevent the inadvertent reissuing of low quality or unsafe medicines by eliminating counterfeit/tampered with packs. There would, however, still be a gap in the market for other technologies, for example, sensors to measure and track the interaction of the storage conditions (e.g., temperature, light, humidity) with the medicinal pack when kept outside of the formal pharmacy supply chain. Sensors that work in this way could reassure people, and reasonably regulators, about the continued quality of reused medicines, with such technology likely having the most influence on experts and health professionals who might better understand them. In terms of normative beliefs, the included injunctive norms had a significant effect on intentions to engage in medicines reuse in the future, meaning that what others would say about medicines reuse is important to people. This appears to be particularly so in terms of what doctors and pharmacists would say, and therefore a norm-based intervention could focus on encouraging doctors and pharmacists to endorse medicines reuse, which again could be achieved via sensor-based technology.

This study did not include any items relating to descriptive social norms, simply because medicines reuse is not currently a reality—accordingly, it is suggested that any future study incorporates descriptive norms if at the time medicines reuse is in place. In addition, during the validation stage, we deleted PBC items relating to controllability (i.e., situational/external factors), which is also explained by the fact that medicines reuse is not currently in place (i.e., not externally controlled), so again we would recommend that this element is revisited in any future study. Finally, we found the relationship between control beliefs and PBC to be poor, especially in the modified model. Control beliefs ask specific questions on what facilitates or impedes the uptake of a given behavior. This finding is puzzling, especially since PBC itself was found to predict intention to reuse medication in the future, albeit by mediating the effects of behavioral beliefs and subjective norms. It is possible that the predefined context (see Section 2.2) for offering medicines for reuse (encompassing the physical characteristics and quality assurance of medicines offered for reuse) was too closely aligned to the control belief questions, creating complexity by first defining the physical characteristics and quality checks as pre-requisites to medicines reuse and then asking if they are important to control issues. Nonetheless, it is also possible that the specific control factors in MRQ (V3), although valid and reliable, did not capture the entirety of relevant ideas.

Referring back to the original elicitation study [11], as well as physical characteristics and quality assurance of medicines offered for reuse, expectations about returned medicines encompassed ideas about the logistics of medicines reuse; collecting and redistributing medicines either "on-site" within a pharmacy or "off-site", as well as incentives for taking part in medicines reuse. The logistics of collecting and redistributing medicines for reuse logically fall outside of the control of individual patients, and while we did include a control belief question about incentives, this was deleted during the validation stage. A potential limitation of this study therefore is our inability to shed light on specific control beliefs that could be addressed through future interventions. However, read alongside our discussion about behavioral beliefs, it is reasonable to suggest that demonstrating the continued quality and safety of reissued medicines should be a pre-requisite to any future medicines reuse scheme introduced in the UK.

Despite the poor relationship between the included control beliefs and PBC, the latter was nonetheless an important mediator of intentions to reuse medicines in the future. However, since our questions focus on people's perceived confidence in their ability (self-efficacy), it is possible that what people stated on the questionnaires might not translate into reality in the future. This is a recognized problem with using hypothetical questions [38] and further highlights the importance of recognizing the interrelationship between all of the constructs in our TPB-based model so that pro-medicines reuse behaviors could be encouraged effectively in the future through a multipronged approach.

Most of our respondents expressed pro-medicines-reuse intentions. This concurs with the recent findings of researchers in the Netherlands, who reported that 61.2% of their respondents "were willing to use medication returned unused to the pharmacy by another patient" [39]. Based on their further analyses, those authors also conclude that guaranteeing the quality of returned medicines should facilitate people's willingness to reuse medicines. However, by their own admission, Bekker et al. [39] did not identify in-depth information on patient barriers and facilitators to medicines reuse. In contrast, our paper provides a theoretical framework with detailed insights to guide future work.

The online MRQ distribution to a panel of participants via a market research company (Research Now®) allowed us to have a representative, large and national UK sample, with ease of data gathering afforded at lower costs. Although it is possible that a face-to-face survey might have allowed further explanation of relevant points to participants, the online nature of this survey allowed a large and national sample to be reached without the risk of bias that a face-to-face survey might have inadvertently have introduced. This (not being face-to-face) could be a possible limitation to this study.

A systematic review that quality appraised TPB-based questionnaire studies highlighted the main problems with these to relate to sample size estimation, omitting some of the direct and indirect measures or questions on demographics, as well as lack of detail on the questionnaire development processes [40]. The current paper illustrates in detail the process of questionnaire development, including the entirety of the validity and reliability testing following the step-by-step guidelines recommended by Ajzen [26] and Francis [32]. Thus, as a strength, our paper is the first to employ the TPB and its entire framework to measure intentions to reuse medication in the future. Another strength is that our paper is the first to systematically measure people's views on medicines reuse via a representative sample in the UK. Our work adds to the emerging global research on medicines reuse. Finally, the discussions above show the practical implications of our findings which can be taken forward by other researchers, pharmacy regulators, government policymakers, and all others looking to decrease the impact of medication waste through medicines reuse schemes.

This study is the first to highlight public perception and willingness to take part in medicines reuse using a validated questionnaire and a large representative sample in the UK setting. In this study, most people surveyed reported positive sentiments toward medicines reuse if the safety and quality assurance of reissued medicines can be shown. By using the TPB as an underpinning theoretical framework, our paper provides detailed insights that will allow others to design specific interventions for helping the public engage with medicines reuse in the future.

5. Conclusions

The problem of medication waste has been recognized for decades, and there is now an emerging field of study looking at medicines reuse as a plausible solution to the ensuing economic and environmental impact of this waste. As the new decade sees the rise of a global pro-environmental movement inspired by a 16-year old, it would be a mistake to dismiss the importance of ordinary people's opinion on the topic of medicines reuse. Although we are not suggesting that people's views alone should be the driver for change, it is nonetheless important to understand the beliefs and willingness of people in the UK to take part in medicines reuse, especially as this is a practice that already takes place in other countries including in Greece and the US.

To understand the factors leading to medicines reuse intent, we developed, validated, and used the TPB-based MRQ. Our results show most people expressing pro-medicines-reuse intentions. Our paper shows how people could be encouraged embrace medicines reuse via practical measures that illustrate the safety and quality assurance of reissued medicines, educational interventions that bolster beliefs about the pro-environmental benefits, and norm-based interventions encouraging doctors and pharmacists to endorse the practice.

Supplementary Materials: The following are available online at http://www.mdpi.com/2226-4787/8/4/213/s1, Figure S1: A schematic illustrating the eight steps taken in the development of the MRQ, Figure S3: The number of the items developed for each construct of the TPB, Table S4: Calculating the composite score of attitude (via the indirect measures) by multiplying scores on a unipolar scale of behavioural beliefs items by scores on a bipolar scale of outcomes evaluation (MRQ V1), Table S5: Calculating the composite score of subjective norm (via the indirect measures) by multiplying scores on a bipolar scale of normative beliefs items by scores on a unipolar scale of motivation to comply items (MRQ V1), Table S6: Calculating the composite score of PBC (via the indirect measures) by multiplying scores on a unipolar scale of control beliefs items by scores on a bipolar scale of power of control factors items (MRQ V1), Table S7: Calculating the mean of the item scores to give an overall attitude score (MRQ V1), Table S8: Calculating the mean of the item scores to give an overall subjective norm score (MRQ V1), Table S9: Calculating the mean of the item scores to give an overall PBC score (MRQ V1), Table S10: Calculating the mean of the item scores to give an overall intention score (MRQ V1), Table S11: Panel responses obtained for the content validity exercise completing before finalising MRQ V1, Table S12: The testing and modification of the MRQ (V1-3), showing the factor loadings using confirmatory factor analysis (CFA) and the test re-test reliability of the indirect measures of the MRQ items using Pearson's correlation (r), Table S13: The internal consistency (Cronbach's alpha) of the direct measures in MRQ V1, Table S14: The internal consistency (Cronbach's alpha) of the direct measures in MRQ V2, Table S15: The summary of the background factors.

Author Contributions: P.D.: Conceptualization, Supervision, Project administration, Validation Visualization, Writing—Reviewing and Editing, Resources; H.A.: Conceptualization, Methodology, Investigation, Data Curation, Formal analysis, Validation, Visualization, Writing—Original draft preparation. All authors have read and agreed to the published version of the manuscript.

Funding: This research was part of a PhD project sponsored and funded by Zarqa University.

Acknowledgments: The authors acknowledge Zarqa University, Jordan for funding the PhD of the first author, the participants who contributed to the study, and Nilesh Patel for pastoral support to the first author during the course of his PhD.

Conflicts of Interest: The authors declare that they have no conflicts of interest to disclose.

References

1. Trueman, P.; Lowson, K.; Blighe, A.; Meszaros, A.; Wright, D.; Glanville, J.; Taylor, D.; Newbould, J.; Bury, M.; Barber, N.; et al. *Evaluation of the Scale, Causes and Costs of Waste Medicines Evaluation of the Scale, Causes and Costs of Waste Medicines*; YHEC/School of Pharmacy, University of London: London, UK, 2011; Volume 17.
2. PSNC. Disposal of Unwanted Medicines: PSNC Main site. Available online: https://psnc.org.uk/services-commissioning/essential-services/disposal-of-unwanted-medicines/ (accessed on 4 February 2019).
3. BMA. BMA-Dispensed But Unopened Medications. British Medical Association. Available online: https://www.bma.org.uk/collective-voice/committees/patient-liaison-group/resources/dispensed-but-unopened-medications (accessed on 4 February 2019).
4. Cauchi, R.; Berg, K. State Prescription Drug Return, Reuse and Recycling Laws. National Conference of State Legislatures. Available online: https://www.ncsl.org/research/health/state-prescription-drug-return-reuse-and-recycling.aspx (accessed on 9 January 2020).
5. GIVMED. Available online: https://givmed.org/en/ (accessed on 9 January 2020).
6. Mackridge, A.J.; Marriott, J.F. Returned medicines: Waste or a wasted opportunity? *J. Public Health* **2007**, *29*, 258–262. [CrossRef] [PubMed]
7. Bekker, C.L.; van den Bemt, B.J.F.; Egberts, A.C.G.; Bouvy, M.L.; Gardarsdottir, H. Patient and medication factors associated with preventable medication waste and possibilities for redispensing. *Int. J. Clin. Pharm.* **2018**, *40*, 704–711. [CrossRef] [PubMed]
8. Toh, M.R.; Chew, L. Turning waste medicines to cost savings: A pilot study on the feasibility of medication recycling as a solution to drug wastage. *Palliat Med.* **2017**, *31*, 35–41. [CrossRef] [PubMed]
9. Lenzer, J. US could recycle 10 million unused prescription drugs a year, report says. *BMJ* **2014**, *349*, g7677. [CrossRef] [PubMed]
10. Connelly, D. Should pharmacists be allowed to reuse medicines? *Pharm. J.* **2018**, *301*. [CrossRef]
11. Alhamad, H.; Patel, N.; Donyai, P. How do people conceptualise the reuse of medicines? An interview study. *Int. J. Pharm. Pr.* **2018**, *26*, 232–241. [CrossRef] [PubMed]
12. Kümmerer, K. *Why Green and Sustainable Pharmacy?* Springer: Berlin/Heidelberg, Germany, 2010. [CrossRef]

13. Paut Kusturica, M.; Tomas, A.; Sabo, A. Disposal of unused drugs: Knowledge and behavior among people around the world. In *Reviews of Environmental Contamination and Toxicology*; Springer: Cham, Germany, 2017; Volume 240, pp. 71–104. [CrossRef]
14. Bound, J.P.; Voulvoulis, N. Household disposal of pharmaceuticals as a pathway for aquatic contamination in the United Kingdom. *Environ. Health Perspect.* **2005**, *113*, 1705–1711. [CrossRef] [PubMed]
15. Bound, J.P.; Kitsou, K.; Voulvoulis, N. Household disposal of pharmaceuticals and perception of risk to the environment. *Environ. Toxicol. Pharm.* **2006**, *21*, 301–307. [CrossRef]
16. Guerrero-Preston, R.; Brandt-Rauf, P. Pharmaceutical residues in the drinking water supply: Modeling residue concentrations in surface waters of drugs prescribed in the United States. *Puerto Rico Health Sci. J.* **2008**, *27*, 236–240.
17. NHS. NHS Carbon Footprint Measuring Carbon Footprint NHS Requirements Sustainable Development Unit. Available online: https://www.sduhealth.org.uk/policy-strategy/reporting/nhs-carbon-footprint.aspx (accessed on 4 February 2019).
18. Xie, Y.; Breen, L. Who cares wins? A comparative analysis of household waste medicines and batteries reverse logistics systems: The case of the NHS (UK). *Supply Chain Manag.* **2014**, *19*, 455–474. [CrossRef]
19. NHS Business Services Authority. Help with NHS Prescription Costs. Available online: https://www.nhsbsa.nhs.uk/help-nhs-prescription-costs (accessed on 4 February 2020).
20. The Pharmaceutical Journal. Council Approves Use of Patient-Returned and Date-Expired Medicines in the Event of Pandemic Flu. Available online: https://www.pharmaceutical-journal.com/news-and-analysis/news/council-approves-use-of-patient-returned-and-date-expired-medicines-in-the-event-of-pandemic-flu/10036098.article (accessed on 4 February 2019).
21. Department of Health & Social Care. Update: EpiPen and EpiPen Junior (Adrenaline Auto-Injector Devices)–Supply Disruption. Available online: https://www.sps.nhs.uk/articles/shortage-of-epipen/ (accessed on 4 February 2019).
22. Department of Health & Social Care. A Guide to Managing Medicines Supply and Shortages. Available online: https://www.england.nhs.uk/wp-content/uploads/2019/11/a-guide-to-managing-medicines-supply-and-shortages-2.pdf (accessed on 4 February 2019).
23. McRae, D.; Allman, M.; James, D. The redistribution of medicines: Could it become a reality? *Int. J. Pharm. Pract.* **2016**, *24*, 411–418. [CrossRef] [PubMed]
24. Kotchen, M.; Kallaos, J.; Wheeler, K.; Wong, C.; Zahller, M. Pharmaceuticals in wastewater: Behavior, preferences, and willingness to pay for a disposal program. *J. Environ. Manag.* **2009**, *90*, 1476–1482. [CrossRef] [PubMed]
25. Persson, M.; Sabelström, E.; Gunnarsson, B. Handling of unused prescription drugs–knowledge, behaviour and attitude among Swedish people. *Environ. Int.* **2009**, *35*, 771–774. [CrossRef]
26. Ajzen, I. The theory of planned behavior. *Organ. Behav. Hum. Decis. Process.* **1991**, *50*, 179–211. [CrossRef]
27. Koger, S.M.; Winter, D.D.N.; Winter, D.D.N. *The Psychology of Environmental Problems: Psychology for Sustainability*, 3rd ed.; Psychology Press: London, UK, 2010.
28. de Leeuw, A.; Valois, P.; Ajzen, I.; Schmidt, P. Using the theory of planned behavior to identify key beliefs underlying pro-environmental behavior in high-school students: Implications for educational interventions. *J. Environ. Psychol.* **2015**, *42*, 128–138. [CrossRef]
29. Pakpour, A.H.; Zeidi, I.M.; Emamjomeh, M.M.; Asefzadeh, S.; Pearson, H. Household waste behaviours among a community sample in Iran: An application of the theory of planned behaviour. *Waste Manag.* **2014**, *34*, 980–986. [CrossRef]
30. Davis, G.; Morgan, A. Using the Theory of Planned Behaviour to determine recycling and waste minimisation behaviours: A case study of Bristol City, UK. *Aust. Community Psychol.* **2008**, *20*, 105–117.
31. Armitage, C.J.; Conner, M. Efficacy of the theory of planned behaviour: A meta-analytic review. *Br. J. Soc. Psychol.* **2001**, *40*, 471–499. [CrossRef]
32. Francis, J.; Eccles, M.P.; Johnston, M.; Walker, A.E.; Grimshaw, J.M.; Foy, R.; Kaner, E.F.S.; Smith, L.; Bonetti, D. *Constructing Questionnaires Based on the Theory of Planned Behaviour: A Manual for Health Services Researchers*; Centre for Health Services Research: Newcastle upon Tyne, UK, 2004; pp. 1–42. ISBN 9540161-5-7.
33. Hindi, A.; Parkhurst, C.; Rashidi, Y.; Ho, S.Y.; Patel, N.; Donyai, P. Development and utilisation of the medicines use review patient satisfaction questionnaire. *Patient Prefer. Adherence* **2017**, *11*, 1–10. [CrossRef]
34. Jöreskog, K.; Sörbom, D. *LISREL 8.72: A guide to the Program and Applications*; SPSS Inc.: Illinois, MS, USA, 2005.

35. Bansal, H.S.; Taylor, S.F. Investigating interactive effects in the theory of planned behavior in a service-provider switching context. *Psychol. Mark.* **2002**, *19*, 407–425. [CrossRef]
36. Powpaka, S. Factors affecting managers' decision to bribe: An empirical investigation. *J. Bus. Ethics.* **2002**, *40*, 227–246. [CrossRef]
37. The European Parlament and the Council of the European Union. Directive 2011/62/eu of the European Parliament and of the Council of 8 June 2011. *Off. J. Eur. Union* **2011**, *1*, 74–87.
38. Ajzen, I. The theory of planned behavior. In *Handbook of Theories of Social Psychology*; SAGE Publications: London, UK, 2012; Volume 1, pp. 438–454.
39. Bekker, C.; Van Den Bemt, B.; Egberts, T.C.G.; Bouvy, M.; Gardarsdottir, H. Willingness of patients to use unused medication returned to the pharmacy by another patient: A cross-sectional survey. *BMJ Open* **2019**, *9*, 1–5. [CrossRef] [PubMed]
40. Oluka, O.C.; Nie, S.; Sun, Y. Quality assessment of TPB-based questionnaires: A systematic review. *PLoS ONE* **2014**, *9*, 1–8. [CrossRef]

Publisher's Note: MDPI stays neutral with regard to jurisdictional claims in published maps and institutional affiliations.

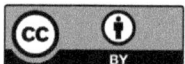

© 2020 by the authors. Licensee MDPI, Basel, Switzerland. This article is an open access article distributed under the terms and conditions of the Creative Commons Attribution (CC BY) license (http://creativecommons.org/licenses/by/4.0/).

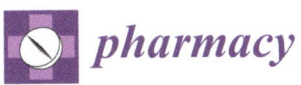

Article

Medicines as Common Commodities or Powerful Potions? What Makes Medicines Reusable in People's Eyes

Monica Chauhan [1], Hamza Alhamad [1,2], Rachel McCrindle [3], Terence K. L. Hui [3], R. Simon Sherratt [3] and Parastou Donyai [1,*]

1. Reading School of Pharmacy, University of Reading, Reading RG6 6AP, UK; monicachauhan15@hotmail.co.uk (M.C.); halhamad@zu.edu.jo (H.A.)
2. Department of Pharmacy, Zarqa University, Zarqa 132222, Jordan
3. Department of Biomedical Engineering, School of Biological Sciences, University of Reading, Reading RG6 6AY, UK; r.j.mccrindle@reading.ac.uk (R.M.); t.hui@reading.ac.uk (T.K.L.H.); r.s.sherratt@reading.ac.uk (R.S.S.)
* Correspondence: p.donyai@reading.ac.uk; Tel.: +44-118-378-4704; Fax: +44-118-378-4703

Abstract: Background: Medicines reuse involves dispensing quality-checked, unused medication returned by one patient for another, instead of disposal as waste. This is prohibited in UK community pharmacy because storage conditions in a patient's home could potentially impact on the quality, safety and efficacy of returned medicines. Our 2017 survey examining patients' intentions to reuse medicines found many favoured medicines reuse. Our aim was to analyse the qualitative comments to explore people's interpretations of what makes medicines (non-)reusable. Methods: Thematic analysis was used to scrutinize 210 valid qualitative responses to the survey to delineate the themes and super-ordinate categories. Results: Two categories were "medicines as common commodities" versus "medicines as powerful potions". People's ideas about medicines aligned closely with other common commodities, exchanged from manufacturers to consumers, with many seeing medicines as commercial goods with economic value sanctioning their reuse. Fewer of the comments aligned with the biomedical notion of medicines as powerful potions, regulated and with legal and ethical boundaries limiting their (re)use. Conclusion: People's pro-medicines-reuse beliefs align with perceptions of medicines as common commodities. This helps explain why patients returning their medicines to community pharmacies want these to be recycled. It could also explain why governments permit medicines reuse in emergencies.

Keywords: medicines; reuse; recycle; medicines reuse; attitudes

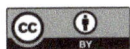

1. Introduction

Medicines reuse is the idea that quality-checked, unused, prescribed medication returned by one patient can be re-dispensed for another patient instead of disposal as waste. Medicines reuse is currently prohibited in the UK community pharmacy context, mainly because the storage conditions in a patient's home could potentially impact on the quality, safety and efficacy of returned medicines kept there, outside of the formal supply chain [1,2]. However, disregarding medicines reuse is not a sustainable position either. Firstly, a third of the cost of prescribed medicinal waste relates to medicines returned to community pharmacies for disposal [3], a problem which could arguably be addressed with the implementation of a safe medicines reuse programme. Secondly, unpredictable events such as pandemics [4] and drug shortages [5] continue to force the UK government to temporarily relax its rules on medicines reuse in any case, a situation which could be made safer with better investment and research into secure medicines reuse practices.

Internationally, doctors, academics and officials have been debating medicines reuse for many decades. Canadian doctors, for example, have called for the recycling of expensive cancer drugs for disadvantaged patients [6], and in the UK in 2012, even the then director of the NHS Sustainable Development Unit argued for research-informed debate on medicines reuse [7]. Indian academics have called for medicines reuse to be explored [8], and researchers from Italy have examined the pros and cons of donating returned medicines to organizations in Europe, Africa and Latin America against WHO's formal advice to withhold such donations [9]. However, it is also worth noting that research shows that underground medication exchange activities are already taking place among patients, for example with diabetes medication [10], which negates these "intellectual" arguments about medicines reuse. Another example is a study in Iran, reporting the frequent self-reuse of antibiotics by people who keep their medicines in places such as their fridge in case they are needed at a later time [11]. This type of "illicit" medicines reuse practice even extends to the scavenging and the onward recycling of medicines from waste disposal sites in some developing countries [12]. Thus, the concept of medicines reuse does not just remain relevant conceptually, it can also be considered an urgent public health issue because informally it already takes place, further warranting research.

The uncertainties about the quality, safety and efficacy of returned medicines relate to the chemical and physical properties of medicines, which can be affected by fluctuations in the environment in which medicines are kept in a patient's home, including changes in temperature, light, humidity, cleanliness and motion/agitation. It is consequently possible for the active ingredient of the medication to degrade, or the formulation to break down so that ultimately less of the medicine is available to treat the disease. Yet, some countries around the world have already instigated medicines reuse schemes but without sophisticated ways of checking for the potential impact of the storage conditions on the stability of the medication. For instance, in Athens, Greece, the GivMed programme allows people access to leftover medicines [13]. Similarly, in many states of the United States (US), medicines donation and reuse programmes exist to support those unable to afford medicines [14]. The practice also appears to have been taking place in the Kingdom of Brunei since 2006 [15]. In these schemes, donated medicines are checked by licensed pharmacists against specific criteria to allow their re-dispensing. However, these checks are largely visual and although they might prevent the re-entry of obviously damaged medicines into the system, they cannot realistically safeguard against physically or chemically degraded content being inadvertently accepted for reuse. This is because visual checks are a mere proxy marker of quality—they do not reveal the storage history of returned medicines nor the impact of that history on the contents within. Thus, for example, a product that requires cold storage could be brought back for reuse, having been kept at room temperature, without necessarily showing physical signs of damage. This is against a backdrop of research that shows, for example 58.3% of patients store their thermolabile medicines outside of the correct temperature recommendations [16].

In the UK, the COVID-19 pandemic caused the government to permit care homes and hospices to draw up standard operating procedures to enable medicines reuse if impacted by shortages [17]. However, here again, the quality checks relied on the visual inspection of any potential medicines rather than any in-depth safeguards, very similar to the protocol for the evaluation and redistribution of donated medicines used in a pilot medication recycling project in Singapore [18]. This type of practice exposes potential contradictions in the very conceptualization of returned medicines by those in positions of power—on the one hand, these are deemed potentially unsafe and must not be reused because their content might have degraded, and on the other, they are deemed safe on passing visual and expiry checks (as proxies for the potency of the active ingredient and formulated medicine inside).

When the public are asked about medicines reuse in formal studies, conflicting ideas about medicines are again highlighted. For example, people interviewed in an Australian study about medication waste questioned whether expired medicines are really totally worthless or could be somehow reused, while also referring to these as "cast-offs" [19]. In the UK too, the people we interviewed in 2016 juxtaposed the potential economic and environmental benefits of medicines reuse with stability and safety worries [20]. The latter was also a predominant feature of interviews conducted in the Netherlands in 2014/15, where the potential to prevent medication waste was set against a guarantee of product quality for any re-dispensed medication [21]. In 2017, we developed and validated a theory of planned behaviour-based medicines reuse questionnaire and used this to survey over a thousand people with at least one chronic health condition in the UK [22]. We showed that people could be encouraged to embrace medicines reuse via practical measures that illustrate the safety and quality assurance of reissued medicines, educational interventions that bolster beliefs about the pro-environmental benefits, and norm-based interventions, encouraging doctors and pharmacists to endorse the practice. Based on ours and others' work, it is certainly clear then that ordinary people, when questioned, also recognize the need for medicines to be quality-assured if they are to be reused. What remains unresolved, however, is whether people understand the nuanced way in which the quality of medication might degrade and, in turn, need to be assured, i.e., whether they recognize medicines as complicated entities worthy of a greater level of scrutiny than visual inspections alone if their safety and quality is to be checked. This is important for the success of wide-scale medicines reuse programmes which would rely on patient uptake. The topic is also important to help explain how medicines on the one hand are deemed potentially unsafe and not reusable by policy makers (because their content might have degraded), yet on the other, deemed safe on passing visual and expiry checks in emergencies and other cases. The core interest of this paper, therefore, is to study how people conceptualize medicines and the properties that make them reusable or not.

The specific aim was to thematically analyse the qualitative responses in our 2017 survey on medicines reuse [22] to explore people's interpretations of the properties of medicines that made them (non-)reusable in order to explore and study the presence of contradictions or conflicting ideas which both make medicines "reusable" and do not, in our participants' view.

2. Materials and Methods

The primary data for this study came from our 2017 survey that employed the medicines reuse questionnaire and was completed by 1003 people who had at least one chronic health condition [22]. It is important to highlight that a quantitative analysis of the survey responses has already been published elsewhere [22]. This survey itself was developed as part of the Ph.D. of one of the co-authors (H.A.) and the publication referenced above contains full details of the questionnaire items, their development and validation, the distribution of the survey as well as the demographics of the participants [22]. The survey had a representative number of participants from across the UK in terms of gender, ethnicity, geographical location and educational level and readers are again referred to the existing publication for the participant details [22].

Within the responses, there were 210 valid qualitative comments to analyse in response to the question "If you have any comments, or ideas regarding the concept of medication reuse, please share them here". These comments were extracted into an Excel spreadsheet for the analysis.

Thematic analysis was employed for the analysis [23]. This approach was used because it provided a way of organising the qualitative data in the form of themes: recurrent topics, ideas or statements identified across the corpus of data. P.D. reviewed all the qualitative comments to confirm that names or other information that might identify the participants had been removed. The comments were analysed manually by M.C. in consultation with P.D., according to the six phases described by Braun and Clarke [23]. The process involved familiarisation with the data, coding, searching for themes, reviewing themes, defining and naming themes, and writing up, as follows.

After familiarisation with the data, M.C. coded each comment and assigned initial "code names". These codes first reflected what made medicines "reusable" and what did not. Consider the following three examples:

Example 1. *"It is worth thinking about to save the NHS money..."*

Example 2. *"If they are sealed and none taken out the pack this would help the NHS save money."*

Example 3. *"Providing the products were in date, quality checked, safety checked, and original packing I would have no objections as it should save the NHS a huge amount of money."*

Example 1 was initially assigned the code "NHS saving" based on the essence of what was being communicated. Example 2 was also coded "NHS saving" but also with the codes "appearance" and "packaging". Finally, example 3 was given numerous codes, "quality", "expiry", "safety", "packaging", and "NHS savings". This process was completed for the entire list of 210 comments. This constituted what is known as first-order coding, the lowest level of coding where the aim is simply to organize and categorize the data by capturing chunks of ideas and giving them labels in a purely descriptive way with minimal interpretation.

Once all the initial codes had been generated, it was possible to group the codes according to recurrent topics or ideas by seeing the patterns in ideas from one quote to another. This second-level coding aimed to go beyond the simple description of the data to instead interpret the meaning of the words. Here, labels were devised which captured the meaning of larger segments of the data, thus reducing the number of codes by sorting ideas into broader and more encompassing categories. Thus, for example, the initial codes of "packaging", "expiry", and "appearance" were grouped according to the theme of "physical appearance". Here, the interpretive element is the description given to the category, that "the external features and overall physical appearance of a commodity are adequate to indicate what is held within. Therefore, intact sealed packaging of medicines suggests an authentic product of good quality inside".

The final stage of coding involved drawing out the overarching themes within the data. The aim of this third-order coding was to identify superordinate constructs that were more global so that larger-scale patterns could be identified. This was completed by continuing to check and compare the ideas, checking other relevant literature in the field and even standing back from the data so that more general concepts and patterns could be drawn out. Thus, for example, the theme of "physical appearance", identified above, was placed within the superordinate category of "medicines as common commodities" which encapsulates commonly held ideas about what makes medicines the same as any other commodity and therefore suitable for reuse. It was at this stage that the two superordinate categories, described more fully in the Results section below, were formed.

3. Results

Two super-ordinate categories encapsulated people's ideas about what made medicines "reusable" or not, each with four distinct themes. The categories and themes and their explanations are provided in Table 1 and further described in the text below.

The majority of people's views related to ideas and concepts that defined medicines as common commodities, sanctioning their reuse (Figure 1).

3.1. Medicines as Common Commodities

The four themes within this category relate to how people see medicines as similar to any common commodity. Most of the patient comments fell within these themes.

Table 1. The concepts developed after the analysis of medicines reuse beliefs, including the two main categories "medicines as common commodities" and "medicines as powerful potions" with their themes and explanations.

Medicines as Common Commodities	Medicines as Powerful Potions
This category encapsulates commonly held ideas about what makes medicines the same as any other commodity and therefore suitable for reuse.	This category describes what confers medicines their potency and special status distinct from ordinary commodities, thus cautioning against reuse.
Physical appearance	*The drug development process*
The external features and overall physical appearance of a commodity are adequate to indicate what is held within. Therefore, intact sealed packaging of medicines suggests an authentic product of good quality inside.	Drug discovery and development processes are time consuming, expensive and intricate. Numerous stages ensure stable and effective final formulations, making medicines complex compared to other commodities.
Social life of medicines	*Specially regulated products*
Medicines have metaphorical life stages, with a medicine's death (when consumed) resulting in its afterlife (internal effects) to restore, improve or maintain health. Failure to reuse unused medication therefore makes its existence meaningless.	Medicines are strictly regulated by authorities to illustrate quality, safety and efficacy before and after authorization. This includes giving expiry dates and storage conditions to maintain the shelf life.
Social and economic benefit	*Unique to an individual's health*
Here, medicines are standardized commercial goods with economic value, exchanged between manufacturers and consumers to meet their needs. Reusing medicines thus brings benefit by reducing medicines spending and waste.	Medicines are prescribed for specific individuals with the unique therapeutic effects dependent on the individual's circumstances. Medicines must not be reshared as their outcome in others cannot be guaranteed.
False analogy	*Handling to meet legal and practice guidelines*
This fallacy assumes that if two things are alike in one aspect, then they will be similar in another aspect too. Thus, if devices and appliances used to diagnose and treat health conditions can be reused, then so can medicines.	The sale or exchange of medicines (over the counter or via prescription) must adhere to legal protocols and accuracy and clinical checks. As powerful substances, their casual handling could cause harm to patients.

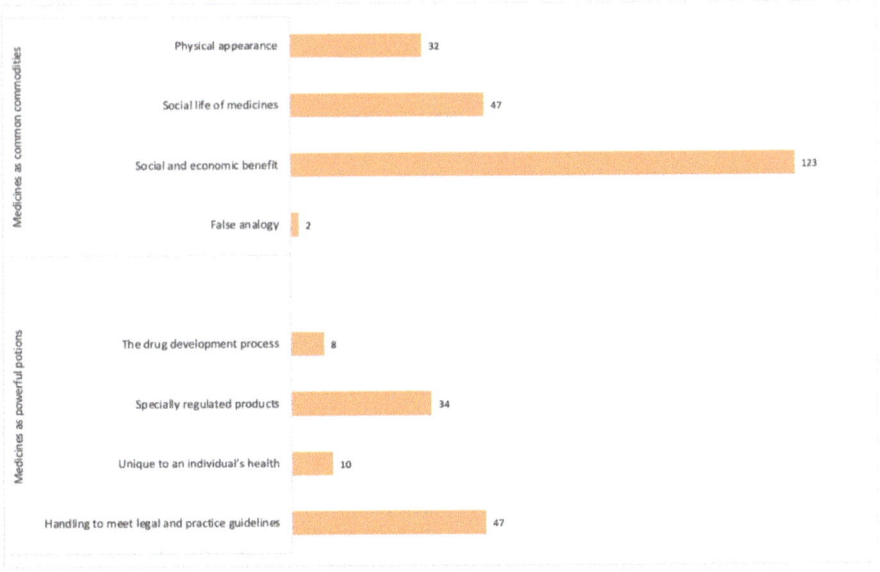

Figure 1. The number of times each theme was identified in the qualitative comments from the 210 survey participants. Note. Some comments were categorized according to two or more themes.

3.1.1. Physical Appearance

This theme encapsulates the idea that the external appearance of medicines, the packaging, neatness and overall visual state, are a strong indicator of the quality of what is held within. These superficial features thus, apparently, reflect the quality and function of the drug. Individuals made positive comments about the idea of reuse by relating to different physical features of the packaging as an indicator of quality. For example, the seal on the packaging was mentioned numerous times with the idea being that a sealed product would be suitable for reuse. The logic is that a blister pack that is presented with a seal and is completely labelled with no damage such as creases or torn edges would suggest the medicine inside is unchanged, safe, and appropriate to be reused. For example:

"When will the reuse of medication become legal? As long as it's sealed, I would be happy." (Participant 91).

"As long as medication is in sealed blister packs showing expiry date then it has to be a good thing." (Participant 23).

"No reason at all not to re-use medication that is sealed and labelled." (Participant 185).

3.1.2. Social Life of Medicines

This theme originates from studies within the field of medical anthropology, which position medicines as commodities with life stages, playing various roles in each stage to restore, improve and maintain health. The stage of medication death reflects the consumption and administration of medicines, with the afterlife where the desirable effects of medicines are produced within the human body. According to this concept, wasting and destroying medicines that are unused and unexpired, and not reusing them, results in a meaningless existence for the medicines themselves because they are not used to their complete potential. Thus, many regretted that medicines were being "wasted" and especially as it looked like "nothing was wrong" with them, where the outer appearance remained intact. For example:

"Please do it. I have had to return medication in the past just for it to be thrown away. It is wrong and wasteful when there is nothing wrong with it." (Participant 112).

"I think it is a brilliant idea. I have returned medication to the pharmacy in the past and thought it wasteful to destroy." (Participant 135).

"Having had to return medication from 2 people who died and had much surplus, it has always seemed to be to be such a waste." (Participant 177).

3.1.3. Social and Economic Benefit

Here, people see medicines as commercial goods. The exchange of medicines allows people to meet their health requirements, and businesses to meet their targets and profits. Within this theme, reusing medicines, i.e., the re-exchange of pharmaceuticals between pharmacies and patients, benefits the public and the NHS by reducing healthcare costs and medicinal waste. This was the most commonly occurring theme. Many individuals positively encouraged the reuse of medicines because, they postulated, this would help the economy, i.e., reduce NHS and patient expenses, reduce waste produced from the destruction of unused and unwanted medicines, and allow the environment to be kept cleaner by minimizing landfill waste. In general, patients expressed a clear link between reusing medicines and a reduction in healthcare costs. This suggests medicines are given an economic value, similar to other common commodities. For example:

"I am entirely in favour of reusing medication. Far too much is wasted at great expense to the NHS and thus the taxpayer." (Participant 10).

"Blisters go to landfill and cannot be recycled." (Participant 40).

"I believe that unused, unopened pills should be reused, instead of being destroyed. Even given free to places where medications are too expensive for people who are living in poverty." (Participant 191).

3.1.4. False Analogy

This theme draws upon people's current knowledge of the types of products that are currently reused within healthcare. The fallacy assumes that if two things are alike in one or more aspects, then they will also be alike in another aspect. Thus, because all pharmaceutical goods including medicines, appliances and devices are used with the intention to diagnose, treat or prevent diseases, reusing one product should mean that all others are also suitable for reuse. For example, if dressings and medical devices that have not been opened or tampered with can be reused, then so can medicines, including solid and liquid dosage forms. For example:

"(reuse) Applies to other things within NHS e.g., dressings, stoma products." (Participant 21).

"As long as medication/dressing etc. has not been tampered with, use and not waste them." (Participant 149).

3.2. Medicines as Powerful Potions

The four themes within this category relate to the special features of medication that set them apart from ordinary commodities. Less than a quarter of the comments reflected these themes.

3.2.1. The Drug Development Process

Drug discovery and development processes are time consuming, expensive and complex. There are many stages involved in producing highly stable and effective formulations of drugs, including pharmacological and pharmacokinetic testing, along with their manufacturing. Thus, the development and maintenance of medicines being complex, sets them apart from everyday commodities. A limited number of comments reflected this theme. Participants mentioned the need for scientific data, evidence, and published trials to evidence continued drug stability before proceeding with medicines reuse. Some thought that not all types of formulations would be suitable for reuse.

"Need to see published trials." (Participant 192).

"Only reuse quality medications not generics." (Participant 88).

"Adhesive on morphine patches not of best quality." (Participant 82).

3.2.2. Specially Regulated Products

This theme acknowledges the regulations of medicines by authorities such as the medicines and healthcare products regulatory agency (MHRA) to ensure quality, safety and efficacy standards are achieved and maintained before and after the licensing and marketing of medicines. This includes giving expiry dates and specifying storage conditions to preserve and maintain shelf life and prevent drug degradation. Although many of the participants expressed pro-medicines reuse intentions, some still commented on the potential impact of the storage environment on medicines and whether this would affect their quality. Concerns were also expressed on the safety and authenticity of drugs, as it is difficult to verify how and where medicines have been kept and handled. For example:

"Conditions under which it may have been stored are unknown e.g., insulin in fridge." (Participant 90).

"Many people will be afraid that re-using meds runs a risk of contamination." (Participant 36).

"Even though the medication would appear to be sealed in its original packaging you don't know how it has been stored, this could have an effect on it if stored in too hot or too cold temperatures." (Participant 66).

"Proof of stability is a big concern." (Participant 38).

3.2.3. Unique to an Individual's Health

This theme relates to the purposeful selection and prescribing of medicines to treat someone's health condition. Healthcare professionals will have carefully chosen a specific medicine, from a range of treatment options, to suit the individual's needs. The therapeutic effects and outcomes of a medicine, it follows, will be dependent on the patient's unique set of circumstances, as determined by the health professional. Accordingly, medicines should not be shared because their outcomes cannot be guaranteed under a different set of circumstances—instead, when no longer needed, medicines ought to be returned to the pharmacy for disposal. In this way, medicines are quite unlike ordinary commodities. The survey was completed by people with chronic health conditions. Many responded considering their own medicines, such as antidiabetics on which they rely to remain well. In addition, some comments conveyed a strong desire to adhere to advice given by health professionals, as the experts in their field. This theme highlights the complexity of medicines and the supervision that is needed alongside their usage. For example:

"I am type 1 diabetic and don't feel that reusing medication is for any diabetic." (Participant 203).

"I would reuse sealed medication only if my Dr said it was safe." (Participant 5).

3.2.4. Handling to Meet Legal and Practice Guidelines

According to this theme, the dispensing of prescription-only medicines (POMs) carried out by trained staff and checks by pharmacists must be accurate and follow protocols, such as standard operating procedures (SOPs) to maximize patient safety and care. This is because medicines are powerful and valuable and can be susceptible to misuse or cause harm if mishandled. This was a commonly occurring theme. Individuals cautioned against reusing medicines, highlighting negative repercussions if they are handled casually. Thus, quality checks by trained health professionals were deemed essential to assess the safety and appropriateness of medicines for use, central to patient care. A few participants also commented on the possibility of fake medicines entering the supply chain, which further necessitated the need for thorough checks. Thus, medicines are not the same as other commodities as there is a lot more at stake should they be mismanaged.

"I worry about fake medication." (Participant 28).

"Providing everything has been checked out by professionals and have long use by date." (Participant 96).

"There would need to be very strict guidelines in place to ensure patient safety." (Participant 130).

4. Discussion

This research is important because it unearths how people think about medicines and the properties that make them reusable or not. The category of "medicines as common commodities" encapsulates commonly held ideas about what makes medicines the same as any other commodity and therefore suitable for reuse, and the category of "medicines as powerful potions" describes what confers medicines their potency and special status, distinct from ordinary commodities thus cautioning against their reuse. These categories highlight the contradictory ways in which medicines can be viewed by different, and sometimes even the same people, and helps explain how medicines can be deemed both reusable and not reusable. The findings can help policy makers understand what makes people (even themselves) receptive to the idea of medicines reuse and importantly, how existing medicines reuse practices (e.g., visual inspections) might in fact be more in line with the everyday view of medicines as common commodities rather than the "powerful potions" view normally advocated by biomedicine.

A strength of this study is that the primary data came from a survey that captured views about medicines reuse from a representative sample of the UK patient population [22]. The sample was representative in terms of gender, ethnicity, geographical location and education level. As such, the data can be generalised to the wider population, and therefore displays some level of external validity. Additionally, as the data came from patients with chronic conditions who are more likely to be using medicines regularly, their opinions towards reuse would be expected to be more meaningful than if gathered from healthy volunteers. A weakness is that the study relied on the analysis of static comments written in an online survey where it was not possible to seek further information or justification to the answers provided. Another limitation of the study is that, although sufficient for a qualitative analysis, only 210 respondents made written comments on the questionnaire, which represented a fifth of the overall number of participants.

The majority of the comments from the survey belonged in the category of medicines as common commodities, with only a quarter reflecting medicines as powerful potions. Commodities are standardized goods or services enabling an exchange or sale between the manufacturers/providers and consumers; of economic value, commodities are primarily produced to meet market demand and satisfy individuals' needs [24]. Medical anthropologists' examination of medicines as commodities positions these with social, cultural and economic aspects far beyond their material (chemical) properties [25]. As such, medicines are commodities for exchange with social lives, and different life stages and roles as they move from one setting to another, i.e., from manufacturers to marketing, prescription by healthcare professionals, and dispensing by pharmacies for patients' use [26]. This notion of commodification contrasts with a biomedical understanding, where, in line with the category of powerful potions, medicines are classified according to potency, are restricted and regulated in their use and given specific directions for storage and administration, marking them as highly distinct from everyday commodities.

Dichotomous representations of medicines are not new. For example, in previous work, medication has been described as "marvellous medicines" versus "dangerous drugs" [27]. Similarly, when antipsychotics are prescribed in dementia, they are either "the lesser of two evils" or "medicines not smarties" [28]. In this study, the dichotomization explains what on the one hand permits the reuse of medicines but on the other inhibits it. The participants' notion of medicines as ordinary commodities was most commonly captured by the theme of social and economic benefits, followed by the themes of the social life of medicines and physical appearance. Thinking about medicines in terms of their economic value is not new and examining the literature, studies promoting medicines reuse, including our own [20], do tend to cite cost savings as a viable reason to explore the practice [29,30]. However, the economic argument is only part of the equation.

In their 1989 paper, Van der Geest and Whyte [31] argued that the "thinginess" of medicines makes them democratic; medicines are thought to contain the power of healing in themselves, thus anyone who "gains access to them can apply their power". This is what makes medicines transactable and subject to commoditization. However, Van der Geest and Whyte [31] also argued medicines are "enclaved commodities" because their biochemical properties necessitate in-depth knowledge about disease and people's functioning when they are handled; health professionals thus attempt to limit access to medicines to prevent waste, misuse or harm. This is despite countless strategies of diversion by people that include selling, stealing, smuggling, hoarding, forging, exchanging and using medicines as gifts [31]. Seen in this light, it could be argued that the category of medicines as "powerful potions" is in line with health professionals' view of them as "enclaved commodities", which explains why returned medicines are normally kept safe by pharmacists and sent away for disposal (so that further access to them is prevented). Indeed, the need to meet legal and practice guidelines, and being specially regulated products, were the main themes that distinguished medicines as powerful potions that needed special caution if to be reused. On the other hand, it could be argued that seeing medicines as "common commodities", in line with the notion of the democratization of medicines explains why so many patients returning their unwanted medicines to pharmacies voice a request for these to be reused. It also explains the illicit medicines reuse practices identified in the introduction to this paper.

Seeing medicines as both similar and different to other commodities at the same time is perhaps the key to why even government decision makers are willing to accept the notion of medicines reuse under certain circumstances even when this practice is normally unthinkable to them. For example, medicines reuse was permitted when the availability of medicines was threatened during the recent pandemic [17]—presumably because it was better to have a product available, albeit one that might be less potent, to meet market demand, than to have none at all. However, the dichotomization unearthed in this study does not actually justify this approach. After all, as argued earlier, the visual inspection of medicines cannot actually guarantee their safety. This is because it is possible that the active ingredient of the medication degrades, or the formulation breaks down so that ultimately less of the medicine is available to treat the disease, even if the packaging passes visual checks. Due to the plausible weaknesses in mere visual checks, we propose a more robust mechanism using the novel ReMINDS (www.reading.ac.uk/ReMINDS; accessed on 16 April 2021) ecosystem as a solution for reusing returned prescribed medicines. This system relies on active sensing technologies integrated with the Internet of Things platform to validate the quality and safety of the medicines while interconnecting the relevant stakeholders [32,33]. Such a system would acknowledge medicines as both "powerful potions" but also as transactable things, subject to commoditization. In this way, it would be possible to recognize the social and economic benefit of medicines reuse without relinquishing the biomedical principles that ensure the potency and special status of medicines. Future studies will aim to explore the use of such technologies in order to make medicines reuse a safe and effective process.

5. Conclusions

This study unearthed people's interpretations of the properties of medicines that make them reusable or not reusable. Two categories of "medicines as common commodities" and "medicines as powerful potions" were generated. Although these categories appear to contradict each other, they conceivably also provide the key as to why people want medicines reuse to take place on a wider scale and why even governments allow the practice in emergencies. Arguably, even health professionals and policy makers who advocate medicines reuse based on cursory visual checks are won over by the argument of medicines as common commodities in contrast with their biomedical training which normally safely posits medicines within the realm of "powerful potions". However, rather than compromising on quality and safety in order to meet market demands, developing and using active sensing technologies could be the key to ensuring a plausible medicines reuse practice in the future, allowing the value and social life of medicines to be fully realized while protecting the public from potential harm.

Author Contributions: Conceptualization, P.D. and M.C.; methodology, P.D., H.A. and M.C.; validation, P.D.; formal analysis, M.C.; data curation, M.C. and P.D.; writing—original draft preparation, M.C.; writing—review and editing, P.D., R.M., T.K.L.H., R.S.S. and H.A.; supervision, P.D.; project administration, P.D.; funding acquisition, H.A. All authors have read and agreed to the published version of the manuscript.

Funding: This research was part of a PhD project sponsored and funded by Zarqa University (under the regulation of the Jordanian Ministry of Higher Education).

Institutional Review Board Statement: This study was approved by the University of Reading's Research Ethics Committee through the School Exemptions process (reference number 30/15) with an amendment approved 2/2017.

Informed Consent Statement: The informed consent of all participants involved in the study was obtained by giving them study information and seeking their voluntary completion of the survey.

Data Availability Statement: The authors can be emailed for further information about the data.

Acknowledgments: We thank Zarqa University for the funding of the PhD project. We also thank the participants who answered the 2017 survey.

Conflicts of Interest: The authors declare no conflict of interest.

References

1. Department of Health [ARCHIVED CONTENT] Repeat Prescribing Systems: Department of Health—Publications. Available online: https://webarchive.nationalarchives.gov.uk/+/http://www.dh.gov.uk/en/Publicationsandstatistics/Publications/PublicationsPolicyAndGuidance/Browsable/DH_4892136 (accessed on 26 February 2021).
2. House of Commons—Public Accounts—Minutes of Evidence Supplementary Memorandum from the Department of Health 2009. Available online: http://www.publications.parliament.uk/pa/cm200809/cmselect/cmpubacc/99/8121708 (accessed on 16 April 2021).
3. Trueman, P.; Lowson, K.; Blighe, A.; Meszaros, A. *Evaluation of the Scale, Causes and Costs of Waste Medicines Evaluation of the Scale, Causes and Costs of Waste Medicines*; York Health Economics Consortium: York, UK, 2011; Volume 17.
4. Council approves use of patient-returned and date-expired medicines in the event of pandemic flu. *Pharm. J.* **2008**, *280*, 645.
5. Important Update—Extended Use of EpiPen® 300 mcg Adrenaline Auto-Injectors beyond Labelled Expiry Dates: PSNC Main Site. Available online: https://psnc.org.uk/our-news/important-update-extended-use-beyond-labelled-expiry-dates-for-select-lots-of-epipen-0-3mg-adrenaline-auto-injectors/ (accessed on 7 April 2021).
6. Doyle, S. Canada lags behind United States in drug return, reuse and recycling programs. *CMAJ.* **2010**, *182*, E197–E198. [CrossRef] [PubMed]
7. PRACTICE: Should Pharmacists Start Recycling Medicines? Available online: https://www.chemistanddruggist.co.uk/cpd-article/should-pharmacists-start-recycling-medicines (accessed on 10 April 2021).
8. Neelam, S.; Vipula; Monica, K.; Mohini, K. Reusing Medicines-An Unexplored Concept in India. *Indian J. Pharm. Pract.* **2014**, *7*, 1–6.
9. Nicoli, F.; Paudel, D.; Bresciani, G.; Rodi, D.; Siniscalchi, A. Donation programme of returned medicines: Role of donors and point of view of beneficiaries. *Int. Health* **2018**, *10*, 133–136. [CrossRef]
10. Litchman, M.L.; Oser, T.K.; Wawrzynski, S.E.; Walker, H.R.; Oser, S. The Underground Exchange of Diabetes Medications and Supplies: Donating, Trading, and Borrowing, Oh My! *J. Diabetes Sci. Technol.* **2019**, *14*, 1000–1009. [CrossRef]
11. Foroutan, B.; Foroutan, R. Household storage of medicines and self-medication practices in south-east Islamic Republic of Iran. *East. Mediterr. Health J.* **2014**, *20*, 547. [CrossRef]
12. Patway, M.A.; O'Hare, W.T.; Sarker, M.H. An illicit economy: Scavenging and recycling of medical waste. *J. Environ. Manag.* **2011**, *92*, 2900–2906. [CrossRef]
13. GIVMED. Available online: https://givmed.org/en/ (accessed on 9 January 2020).
14. Cauchi, R.; Berg, K. State Prescription Drug Return, Reuse and Recycling Laws. Available online: https://www.ncsl.org/research/health/state-prescription-drug-return-reuse-and-recycling.aspx (accessed on 9 January 2020).
15. Nurolaini, K.; Sultana, S.; Wai See, W. Medication Wastage and its Disposal Amongst Patients at Suri Seri Begawan Hospital in Brunei Darussalam. *Med. Health* **2016**, *11*, 139–150. [CrossRef]
16. Cuéllar, M.J.; Marco, J.L.; Pérez-Castelló, I.; Castelló Escrivá, A. Calidad en la conservación de los medicamentos termolábiles en el ámbito domiciliario. *Rev. Calid. Asist.* **2010**, *25*, 64–69. [CrossRef]
17. Donyai, P.; McCrindle, R.; Sherratt, R.S.; Hui, T.K.L. COVID-19 Pandemic Is Our Chance to Learn How to Reuse Old Medicines. Available online: https://theconversation.com/covid-19-pandemic-is-our-chance-to-learn-how-to-reuse-old-medicines-137671 (accessed on 22 February 2020).
18. Toh, M.R.; Chew, L. Turning waste medicines to cost savings: A pilot study on the feasibility of medication recycling as a solution to drug wastage. *Palliat. Med.* **2017**, *31*, 35–41. [CrossRef] [PubMed]
19. Kelly, F.; McMillan, S.; Spinks, J.; Bettington, E.; Wheeler, A.J. 'You don't throw these things out:' an exploration of medicines retention and disposal practices in Australian homes. *BMC Public Health* **2018**, *18*, 1–12. [CrossRef]
20. Alhamad, H.; Patel, N.; Donyai, P. How do people conceptualise the reuse of medicines? An interview study. *Int. J. Pharm. Pract.* **2018**, *26*, 232–241. [CrossRef]
21. Bekker, C.L.; Gardarsdottir, H.; Egberts, T.C.G.; Bouvy, M.L.; van den Bemt, B.J.F. Redispensing of medicines unused by patients: A qualitative study among stakeholders. *Int. J. Clin. Pharm.* **2017**, *39*, 196–204. [CrossRef] [PubMed]
22. Alhamad, H.; Donyai, P. Intentions to "Reuse" Medication in the Future Modelled and Measured Using the Theory of Planned Behavior. *Pharmacy* **2020**, *8*, 213. [CrossRef]
23. Braun, V.; Clarke, V. Using thematic analysis in psychology. *Qual. Res. Psychol.* **2006**, *3*, 77–101. [CrossRef]
24. Hashimzade, N.; Myles, G.; Black, J. Commodity. In *Oxford Reference*; Oxford University Press: Oxford, UK, 2017; ISBN 9780191819940.
25. van der Geest, S.; Hardon, A. Social and cultural efficacies of medicines: Complications for antiretroviral therapy. *J. Ethnobiol. Ethnomed.* **2006**, *2*, 48. [CrossRef]
26. De Boeck, F. On van der Geest and Whyte's Article 'The Charm of Medicines: Metaphors and Metonyms'. *Med. Anthropol. Q.* **1991**, *5*, 170–172. [CrossRef]
27. Prosser, H. Marvelous medicines and dangerous drugs: The representation of prescription medicine in the UK newsprint media. *Public Underst. Sci.* **2010**, *19*, 52–69. [CrossRef]

28. Gill, D.; Almutairi, S.; Donyai, P. "The Lesser of Two Evils" Versus "Medicines not Smarties": Constructing Antipsychotics in Dementia. *Gerontologist* **2019**, *59*, 570–579. [CrossRef] [PubMed]
29. Mackridge, A.J.; Marriott, J.F. Returned medicines: Waste or a wasted opportunity? *J. Public Health* **2007**, *29*, 258–262. [CrossRef] [PubMed]
30. Bekker, C.L.; Gardarsdottir, H.; Egberts, A.C.G.; Molenaar, H.A.; Bouvy, M.L.; van den Bemt, B.J.F.; Hövels, A.M. What does it cost to redispense unused medications in the pharmacy? A micro-costing study. *BMC Health Serv. Res.* **2019**, *19*, 243. [CrossRef] [PubMed]
31. Van Der Geest, S.; Whyte, S.R. The Charm of Medicines: Metaphors and Metonyms. *Med Anthr. Q.* **1989**, *3*, 345–367. [CrossRef]
32. Hui, T.K.L.; Donyai, P.; McCrindle, R.; Sherratt, R.S. Enabling Medicine Reuse Using a Digital Time Temperature Humidity Sensor in an Internet of Pharmaceutical Things Concept. *Sensors* **2020**, *20*, 3080. [CrossRef]
33. Hui, T.K.L.; Mohammed, B.; Donyai, P.; McCrindle, R.; Sherratt, R.S. Enhancing Pharmaceutical Packaging through a Technology Ecosystem to Facilitate the Reuse of Medicines and Reduce Medicinal Waste. *Pharmacy* **2020**, *8*, 58. [CrossRef] [PubMed]

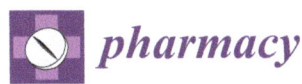

Article

Enhancing Pharmaceutical Packaging through a Technology Ecosystem to Facilitate the Reuse of Medicines and Reduce Medicinal Waste

Terence K. L. Hui [1], Bilal Mohammed [2], Parastou Donyai [2] and Rachel McCrindle [1] and R. Simon Sherratt [1],*

1. Department of Biomedical Engineering, School of Biological Sciences, University of Reading, Berkshire RG6 6AY, UK; t.hui@reading.ac.uk (T.K.L.H.); r.j.mccrindle@reading.ac.uk (R.M.)
2. School of Pharmacy, University of Reading, Berkshire RG6 6AP, UK; b.mohammed@student.reading.ac.uk (B.M.); p.donyai@reading.ac.uk (P.D.)
* Correspondence: r.s.sherratt@reading.ac.uk

Received: 6 March 2020; Accepted: 27 March 2020; Published: 31 March 2020

Abstract: Background: The idea of reusing dispensed medicines is appealing to the general public provided its benefits are illustrated, its risks minimized, and the logistics resolved. For example, medicine reuse could help reduce medicinal waste, protect the environment and improve public health. However, the associated technologies and legislation facilitating medicine reuse are generally not available. The availability of suitable technologies could arguably help shape stakeholders' beliefs and in turn, uptake of a future medicine reuse scheme by tackling the risks and facilitating the practicalities. A literature survey is undertaken to lay down the groundwork for implementing technologies on and around pharmaceutical packaging in order to meet stakeholders' previously expressed misgivings about medicine reuse ('stakeholder requirements'), and propose a novel ecosystem for, in effect, reusing returned medicines. **Methods**: A structured literature search examining the application of existing technologies on pharmaceutical packaging to enable medicine reuse was conducted and presented as a narrative review. **Results**: Reviewed technologies are classified according to different stakeholders' requirements, and a novel ecosystem from a technology perspective is suggested as a solution to reusing medicines. **Conclusion**: Active sensing technologies applying to pharmaceutical packaging using printed electronics enlist medicines to be part of the Internet of Things network. Validating the quality and safety of returned medicines through this network seems to be the most effective way for reusing medicines and the correct application of technologies may be the key enabler.

Keywords: reuse of medicines; reduce medicinal waste; intelligent pharmaceutical packaging; medicine re-dispensing; theory of planned behavior

1. Introduction

Medicinal waste has not only been a problem in the NHS (National Health Service) [1], but also a challenge in other countries in terms of public health, the environment and governmental expenditures [2–4]. Trueman et al. [5] reported that £300M of prescribed medicines are wasted every year mainly through medication non-adherence. Together with those unused, unwanted and unexpired medicines, they are major sources of preventable medicinal waste that can currently only be disposed of through managed (e.g., disposal centers at community pharmacies) and unmanaged methods (e.g., domestic sewage, public bins, etc.). One of the ways to tackle medicinal waste is to explore the idea of medicine reuse, which is currently not permitted in the UK [6,7]. A legally approved re-dispensing of medicines scheme has started to work in some areas of the world such as the *SIRUM (Supporting*

Initiatives to Redistribute Unused Medicine (https://www.sirum.org/)) originating from the California [8], the *Pharmaceutical donation and reuse programs* operating now in many states of the US [9], and the *GivMed* (https://givmed.org/en/) programme facilitating access to leftover medicines using a smartphone app in Greece [7]. However, there are restrictions to the types and the sources of medicines to be reused since the quality and safety of the returned medicines are not guaranteed [10]. Donating medicines to remote areas that lack resources is another way of reducing medicinal waste through recycling medicines. Nevertheless, the reusing of dispensed medicines is generally not allowed because a proper way of validating the quality of returned medicines is not yet available. Thus, prescribed medicines from individuals are usually not allowed to be donated abroad either [11,12]. A sustainable pharmaceutical supply chain (PSC) management may provide an alternative solution to reducing medicinal waste through the concept of reverse flows. Viegas et al. [13] classifies reverse flows into donation, Reverse Logistics (RL) and Circular Economy (CE), where CE illustrates a close loop supply chain paving the way to reuse returned medicines. The complicated communication flows between a large number of PSC stakeholders could be an obstacle blocking a smooth reverse flow implementation. Pharma 4.0, an extension of Industry 4.0 to pharmaceutical manufacturing, may help establish seamless connections between stakeholders through Internet of Things (IoT) technologies [14,15]; however, the big concern in managing and monitoring the quality of returned medicines still needs to be resolved.

The reuse of medicines is a behavior that can be studied using behavioral sciences [16,17]. Within this perspective, technologies are essential to facilitate attitude change by validating that the medicines returned back to pharmacies have maintained their quality and are safe to use [18,19]. The reuse of prescribed medicines, especially in the UK, is an underexplored research area and the corresponding technologies facilitating this action seem to be an uncharted territory. A structured literature review is reported in this paper to categorize the required technologies applicable to the design of pharmaceutical packaging facilitating the reuse of medicines and the reduction of medicinal waste. Pharmaceutical packaging provides much useful information about a medicine and its use. Additional data regarding its quality and safety which are critical for re-dispensing returned medicines can also be monitored when appropriate technology is applied [20].

Pharmaceutical packaging is regarded as the "key facilitator" for establishing a friendly patient-medication relationship through a patient-centered strategy [21], thus, embedding suitable technologies onto the packaging itself seems to be the best approach for developing the concept of medicine reuse. Manufacturers have already begun implementing technologies into pharmaceutical packaging in order to provide clear information to patients, to protect medicines from the environment, and to cope with changing government regulations and policies [22–25]. The main targets for applying embedded technologies to the packaging are normally focusing on supply chain management [21,26], anti-counterfeit enforcement [27,28], and quality and safety indications [29,30]. Static technologies dominate previous research on pharmaceutical packaging where the interaction with the package requires an external system such as a RFID (radio frequency identification) reader or barcode scanner using a one-way data transmission protocol. Some of these static technologies may require human interaction to identify their readings such as the TTI (time–temperature indicators) sensing devices extensively used in the food packaging industry [31]. Alternatively, active technologies provide a better package-to-human interaction based on the packaging itself. However, a higher degree of integration of latest digital technologies with the pharmaceutical packaging is required for communicating with the surrounding or remote computing devices. Connection to the Internet using the IoT concept is a new technological trend for telehealthcare empowering a ubiquitous communication with technology embedded pharmaceutical packaging based on cyber-physical systems (CPS) [15,32]. Intelligent packaging, a term extensively used in food packaging, has been implementing both passive and active technologies to inform consumers of the condition of the packaged food [33]. Many technologies used in intelligent food packaging, especially those related to sensing and reporting, can also be applied to pharmaceutical packaging. Emerging multidisciplinary research has enabled technologies to be more effectively applied to reduce medicinal waste through enhancing medication adherence, particularly those studies based on the analysis of human behaviors through a combination of psychology, medication and pharmacy [34,35]. Similarly, it could be argued that the application of technology could influence people to engage in medication reuse by addressing the relevant determinants of intentions to take part in such a scheme in the future. Qualitative studies, as well as the application of the theory of planned behavior (TPB) have previously analyzed intentions and actions towards the returning and re-dispensing of medicines [16–19], and there are technologies that can help shape user behaviors towards the goal of medicines reuse.

As a precursor to defining a medicine reuse ecosystem, this research conducts a structured literature survey and summarizes the technologies that can be applied to facilitating behavioral changes towards reusing returned medicines. The terms reuse, re-dispense and recycle of medicines are used interchangeably in the current article, distinguishing them from unwanted medicines that need to be disposed of or incinerated, and which will be treated via medicine disposal through waste management. Section 2 describes the structured literature review method used in the searching and screening of peer review papers from popular academic search engines, and how the definitions of inclusion and exclusion are made. The results are presented in Section 3 where a taxonomy of technologies are classified according to the different factors affecting human behaviors. Discussions are made in Section 4 with regard to how the technologies identified in this study can be used to facilitate reuse with their pros and cons further elaborated. A medicine reuse management ecosystem based on the result of the literature review is proposed from a technology perspective and Section 5 explains its structure. Finally, Section 6 concludes the present study and lays down future research directions.

2. Methods

A structured literature review was conducted to identify and categorize the available technologies that can help design pharmaceutical packaging to facilitate the reuse of returned prescribed medicines. A rapid scoping review approach based on the PRISMA (Preferred Reporting Items for Systematic reviews and Meta-Analyses) protocol was chosen for the literature survey using a single reviewer, but with awareness of the limitations of not conducting a full multiple-reviewer systematic review [36,37]. The current study focuses on examining a novel concept of implementing appropriate technologies to facilitate the shaping of human behaviors for medicine reuse. PRISMA protocol provided a structured, reproducible and transparent methodology to conduct the article search, and using a single reviewer enabled a rapid review approach which fit the purpose for laying down the groundwork for a future full systematic review of specific studies identified in the present research [38].

Understanding human behaviors is essential in providing healthcare to the general public. Continuous education and constant enhancement of services are essential to influence individual decisions towards planned directions [39]. Previous studies have shown that patients and stakeholders in the pharmaceutical sector generally accept the concept of reusing dispensed medicines as long as certain criteria are met. Bekker et al. [17] investigated patients' willingness to use recycled medicines, McRae et al. [18] looked at the same issue through the healthcare professionals' perspective, and Bekker et al. [16] went further to collect the views from all related stakeholders. A more systematic analysis of human behaviors for reuse of medicines in the UK was reported by Alhamad et al. [19], and the three beliefs based on the TPB were studied using a thematic analysis of the associated attitudes after interviewing the local community. The criteria from these empirical studies are similar and the technological requirements are summarized in Table 1.

Table 1. Technological Requirements for the Reuse of Medicines.

Requirements	Quality	Safety	Others
Patients' perspective [17]	(1) storage and handling conditions.	(1) tamper-proof packaging; (2) anti-counterfeit.	(1) patient incentive; (2) cost effectiveness.
Healthcare professionals' perspective [18]	(1) storage conditions (temperature, moisture and light); (2) contamination of package (stain, smell); (3) last dispensing date.	(1) tamper-proof packaging; (2) anti-counterfeit.	(1) cost effectiveness; (2) legal issues regarding pharmacist responsibility, medicine recall, paperwork, efficacy, and governmental regulations.
Stakeholders' perspective [16]	(1) monitor storage conditions (temperature, light, humidity, agitation, and lapsed expiration date).	(1) anti-counterfeit; (2) track and trace system to the packages for re-dispensed medicines.	(1) patients' incentive; (2) pharmacists' incentive; (3) cost benefits shared by stakeholders (patients, pharmacists and health insurance companies).
TPB Behavioral beliefs [19]	(1) storage conditions (temperature, humidity and cleanliness); (2) contaminated packaging.	(1) tamper-proof packaging; (2) errors introduced by patients or pharmacists; (3) anti-counterfeit.	(1) cost effectiveness.
TPB Normative beliefs [19]	Nil	Nil	(1) concern mostly on the social norm for reusing medicines.
TPB Control beliefs [19]	(1) monitor storage conditions (temperature, light, humidity, agitation, and lapsed expiration date).	(1) tamper-proof packaging; (2) anti-counterfeit.	(1) patient incentive; (2) on-site and off-site collection and distribution system.

Pharmaceutical packaging is not the only place for implementing technologies to facilitate the shaping of human behaviors towards reusing returned medicines, associated technologies working cohesively with the sensor embedded packaging are also essential in supporting related activities. Therefore, the literature review for the present study has focused on both the technologies implementable on the packaging and those that extend the embedded pharmaceutical packaging to the outside world such as the Internet in order to share the information with every stakeholder. Table 1 provides the requirements for shaping the stakeholders' behaviors for medicine reuse based on the qualitative research described previously, and Table 2 illustrates a consolidated version removing duplicates and converting the requirements into keywords for conducting the literature search.

Table 2. Keywords for literature search according to the requirements listed in Table 1.

Requirements	Technologies	Keywords for Search
Quality	(1) storage temperature monitoring (2) storage humidity monitoring (3) storage lighting monitoring (4) storage contamination monitoring (5) agitation monitoring (6) lapsed expiration date monitoring	(1) (intelligent OR smart OR monitor) AND packaging AND temperature (2) (intelligent OR smart OR monitor) AND packaging AND (humidity OR moisture) (3) (light OR optical OR UV) AND food AND packaging (4) packaging AND contamination (5) (vibration OR shock OR acceleration OR shake OR agitation) AND packaging (6) (report OR monitor OR detection) AND expiry
Safety	(1) tamper-proof packaging (2) anti-counterfeit (3) track & trace collecting and dispensing system (4) errors tracking from patients and pharmacists	(1) (evident OR resistant OR detection OR proof) AND tamper AND packaging (2–4) (pharmaceutical OR intelligent OR smart OR packaging) AND counterfeit

The scope of the current study is limited to the technologies applicable to meeting the quality and safety requirements which are common to all involved stakeholders. However, a brief discussion on how other requirements are tackled can be found in Section 4. Searching of technologies relies on the keywords derived from the requirements through a selection of popular search engines which provide comprehensive listings of journal articles from engineering, pharmacy, medical and psychological sciences. As the purpose of this survey is to lay down the groundwork for deeper systematic review of individual technologies that are appropriate for medicine reuse, the searching formulas were restricted to the titles of papers enabling a preliminary study of latest technologies on recycling medicines. Synonyms for keywords were used to expand the search to a wider area of study; however, the term "pharmaceutical" is not used in some formulas due to the fact that technological research on pharmaceutical packaging is not yet a major research topic for certain technologies. A zero result was obtained in many rounds of keyword searches when the term "pharmaceutical packaging" was in place, so the term was finally removed in some of the search formulas. The five chosen search engines for finding the literature in the present study are: Google scholar (https://scholar.google.com/), Scopus (https://www.scopus.com/), IEEE Xplorer digital library (https://ieeexplore.ieee.org/Xplore/home.jsp), Web of Science (https://wok.mimas.ac.uk/), and Pubmed (https://www.ncbi.nlm.nih.gov/pubmed/).

PRISMA flow was followed for screening and selecting the articles to be further studied in this paper, and Figure 1 depicts the selection process flow. The numbers of chosen articles for each process are also illustrated in the flow chart. Other than those academic papers retrieved from the search engines mentioned above, handpicked articles were also collected mainly based on the citations from the collected papers.

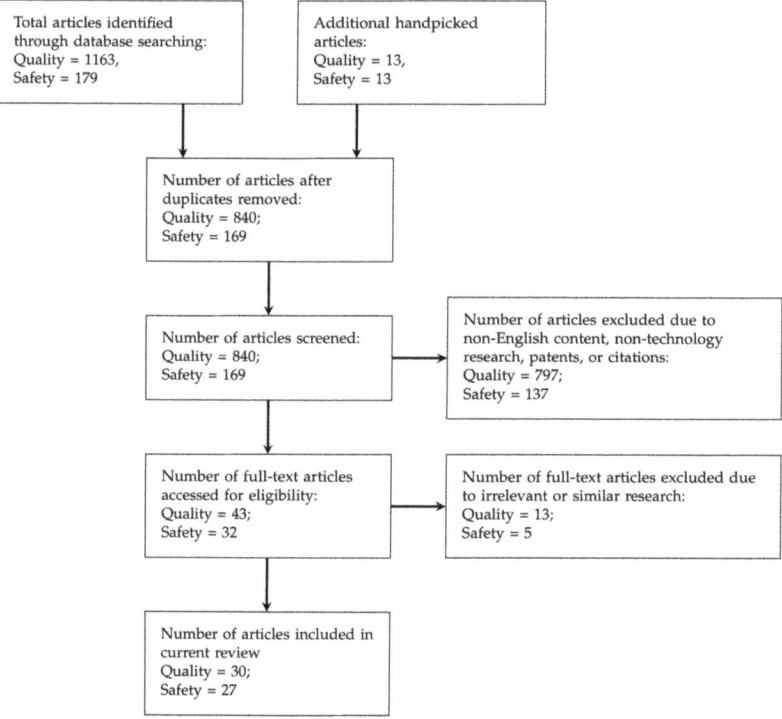

Figure 1. PRISMA [36] flow for screening literature (articles collected are classified into Quality and Safety requirements).

3. Results

The results of literature review show that the technologies, especially those embedded in pharmaceutical packaging, for reusing medicines returned from patients are still largely ignored by mainstream academic research. Legal issues could be one reason, but the lack of technologies to enable a comprehensive validation of the quality and safety of returned medicines may also be a big obstacle. Law makers, as well as other stakeholders in society, may be skeptical about re-dispensing returned medicines without proper validation [16]. This section describes how latest technologies collected from the literature review can enable the reuse of returned medicines according to the two groups of stakeholder requirements for quality and safety listed in Table 2.

Intelligent packaging has been a major research topic in the food industry and many of its technologies can also be applied in pharmaceutical packaging. The literature review suggests that the main purpose for intelligent food packaging focuses on monitoring the freshness of the food content rather than observing the storage condition of the medicines in pharmaceutical packaging [40]. Deterioration of the packaged food is basically the major concern in the food industry. Müller and Schmid [33] proposes that (i) environmental conditions, (ii) quality characteristics or quality indicator compounds, and (iii) data carriers are the three major concepts in intelligent food packaging. Application of technologies to these concepts, especially the environmental condition monitoring, is closely resembled to the pharmaceutical counterpart where the sensors are measuring the surroundings of pharmaceutical packaging rather than the space inside food packaging. Sensing technologies based on chemical, biological or physical sensors are the core components in intelligent food packaging enabling passive or active indications of the status of the packaged food to consumers [40,41]. Collection of articles was first focused on technologies applying directly to pharmaceutical packaging, but those that applied to food packaging were also chosen in this study when no relevant article was found in the pharmaceutical sector.

Before achieving economies of scale, the high cost of implementation in intelligent pharmaceutical packaging could restrict the application to high priced medicines. However, recycling of the packaging materials has become a trend in protecting the environment and reducing the overall costs in adding technological ingredients into smart packaging [42], thus, the integration of relatively high cost components can be justified.

3.1. Technologies for Quality Requirements

Sensors play a crucial part in pharmaceutical packaging for quality assurance of dispensed medicines. The requirements in Table 1 suggest the major quality indicators which detect and report the real-time status of the medicines. Indications include the storage environment (e.g., temperature, humidity, lighting), the handling methods (e.g., contamination, agitation, motion), and the expiration date.

Time–temperature indicators (TTI) are the most popular attachment to an intelligent package reporting the history of the temperature variation for a certain period of time [43]. Specific technologies contribute to the different implementation of the TTI sensing devices with various time scales and sensing technologies for detecting temperature of the storage environment [44] as well as the contents [45]. However, the physical indication of the TTI devices normally requires human intervention through visual inspection. Computer vision based on computational intelligence can replace the human judgment for TTI result recognition but a complicated setup is needed. Mijanur Rahman et al. [46] enhanced the TTI concept using biosensors enabling the detection of the sensing results through a digital interface.

Thin-film technologies through printed electronics or nanotechnology further improve the integration of the pharmaceutical packaging with information technology (IT). Quality assurance indication for the real-time storage conditions can then be shared with all connected stakeholders. Printed electronics allow key sensors such as temperature, humidity and ambient light to be printed on paper or plastic foil. Together with a printed RFID tag, an IT connected storage sensing structure can be built on pharmaceutical packaging [47–50]. Processing power for performing complicated logical operations is possible by combining prebuilt electronic modules (e.g., microprocessor, other sensors not available yet in printed electronics, etc.) with printed circuits through the hybrid printed electronics methodology [51,52]. Nanotechnology strengthens the thin-film technologies through depositing carbon nanotubes onto the packaging materials and further enhances the manufacturing time and increases the functionality of the embedded electronics for quality monitoring of medicines [53–55].

Contamination detection of the medicines inside the packaging is not trivial. Johnston et al. [56] suggested the usage of PT/GC/MS (Purge and Trap/Gas Chromatography/Mass Spectrometry) methods for detecting smoke contaminated packages, while Mielniczuk and Pogorzelska [57] used GC/MS to examine the microbial contaminants. Both proved to be effective, but they are not field-applicable since portable PT/GC/MS machines are not yet generally available. Computer vision could be an alternative for visual inspection of microbial contamination, perhaps under ultraviolet light. However, the resolution for handheld cameras such as those in smartphones may need to be upgraded allowing the general public to conveniently capture and analyze the small particle size of contaminants [58]. An indirect method suggested for identifying potential contamination was to look for visible damage on the packaging [59,60]. Thus, tamper-proof packaging can act as indirect protection from contamination.

Agitation and vibration of the pharmaceutical packaging may affect some medicines, such as insulin [61]. Monitoring of unexpected motions during transportation and storage is therefore necessary to validate the quality for specific types of medicines [62]. The literature search suggests that motion sensing for agitation or spinning applying particularly to pharmaceutical packaging is not being used. No article was found according to the formulas defined in Section 2. However, wearable motion sensors are an emerging topic undergoing extensive research in the personal healthcare sector. Many of them measuring human activities according to variations of the different axis of acceleration or direction can be applied to pharmaceutical packaging as long as they can be flexibly and unnoticeably attached to the packaging materials using thin-film technologies [63,64].

Artificial intelligence combined with image processing enables recognition of the expiry date. Gong et al. [65] illustrated the detection of expiration date on the packaging through a deep neural network, and Peng et al. [66] applied an enhanced "efficient subwindow search" algorithm to locate and recognize the expiry date details from an image of the packaging. QR (quick response) codes combined with SMS (short message service) can be an alternative but a smartphone is required and a predefined standard for QR codes becomes necessary [67]. A dynamic display on the pharmaceutical packaging showing all details of the medicines will be a better way to show all updated information to the patients, and an e-ink (electronic ink) display will be a good low-power (zero power when the display content is stable) method acting as a real-time visual indicator on the pharmaceutical packaging [68]. The flexible e-ink display not only shows the updated information of the medicine inside the packaging, a microprocessor driving the display can also report a real-time quality status according to the sensing results. An electrochromic (EC) display further improves the relatively high-power refresh cycles in e-ink technology during screen content update, and provides a promising alternative for printing a low-power thin-film dynamic display on paper [69,70].

3.2. Technologies for Safety Requirements

Safety of medicines is the next critical concern in the reuse process. Even if the returned medicines are quality assured through the technologies mentioned in the previous section, two safety requirements from the stakeholders must be met before medicines could be re-dispensed: tamper-proofing and anti-counterfeiting (see Table 1 for details). Tamper-evident technologies provide indications of whether medicines have been used or adulterated, and counterfeit protection technologies supply methods for authentication.

Tamper-evident pharmaceutical packaging is a mature concept now after the Tylenol tragedy in 1982 where seven patients died due to the intentional adulteration of the medicine [71]. Government regulations enforced the pharmaceutical industry after the incident to implement appropriate tamper-evident and tamper-resistant technologies particularly on pharmaceutical packaging protecting medicines from adulteration [72]. Since then, popular tamper-evident technologies have given indications on broken sealing of the packaging through (i) film wrapping; (ii) blister or strip packs; (iii) sealed pouches and sachets; (iv) tape seals; (v) bubble packs; (vi) heat shrink bands or wrappers; (vii) container mouth seals; (viii) breakable caps; (ix) tear-away caps; (x) sealed metal tubes; and (xi) laminated tubes [73]. Tamper-evident applies also to the external packaging during transportation using RFID embedded film wrap which prevents tampering for the whole pallet of medicines [74]. Tamper-proof packaging must be strong enough to prevent accidental breaking; however, also easy enough to use [75]. To enhance the manufacturability of tamper-proof pharmaceutical packaging in the factories, blow fill seal [23] and IML (in-mold lamination) [76] provide better ways to integrate the tamper-evident sealing into the medicine production process in a single flow but the cost may be higher.

Electronic interfaces allow tamper-proof technologies to be extended to the digital world for automatic recognition of intentional and unintentional tampering. Digital electronics interacting with tamper-evident technologies are still at an early stage, and research examples can be found in relation to blister packs which are the most popular pharmaceutical packaging for tablets by attaching an aluminum film on top of a thermoformed plastic tray [77]. Floerkemeier and Siegemund [78] illustrated the addition of a conductive wire matrix on top of the blister pack where the wires were broken when an individual medicine was removed. The broken wires then activated the built-in communication module to send a message to the patient's smartphone or a web server registering the usage status of the medicines. This technology is applied to track medication adherence but it can also be used in tamper-proofing. A more advanced tamper-proof solution was demonstrated by Gao et al. [79] who used a controlled delamination material (CDM) as a sealing layer covering the medicines. This CDM layer can be delaminated through activation by electrical power controlled by an RFID tag.

Tamper-proof technologies prevent the pharmaceutical packaging from malicious physical attacks, and also provide indications for potential contamination of the medicines. However, a tamper-evident sealing mechanism will not protect patients from falsified medicines whereas anti-counterfeit technologies can help fight against counterfeiting. Anti-counterfeiting relies on sharing information between suppliers, customers and governments where unique, traceable and unmodifiable identity of individual medicines must be shared on a single platform [80]. Overt technologies, such as holograms and color-shifting paints, usually apply to packaging surfaces allowing trained examiners or even consumers to do visual anti-counterfeiting authentication. These technologies, however, are easily replicated and normally do not last for long. Alternatively, covert technologies such as security taggants and micro-imaging, are basically invisible to naked eyes and require additional tools for examination. Therefore, authentication by normal consumers on covert anti-counterfeiting technologies are restricted. A combination of overt and covert methodologies have been adopted in pharmaceutical packaging to enhance the counterfeit protection strategy from outside of the packaging down to the surface of the medicine, or even inside the individual medicine [81,82].

Anti-counterfeiting technologies can be applied to the packaging materials. Different types of spectroscopy methods, such as Fourier Transform Infrared (FT-IR) or Near Infrared (NIR) spectroscopy can be used to examine the texture of the packaging materials to authenticate the medicine identity [83]. The use of mathematical modeling using discrete Fourier transforms is also possible to perform the authentication by analyzing the texture of the packaging material through an image [84]. Simske et al. [85] proposed a fully variable data printing method applying inks with different visibility under various light spectrums to reject counterfeit medicines.

Tagging technology applicable to anti-counterfeiting has evolved by adding micro-scale taggants directly onto medicines, especially those in the form of tablets or capsules. Printings on the irregular surfaces of the tablets combined with the random minor alignment differences create fingerprints for an individual tag associated with each tablet. A database of these fingerprints can be used as an authentication tool [86]. A biodegradable micro-scale QR code label was proposed by Fei and Liu [87] where the label was attached to the tablet with the code being readable by a smartphone. The QR code can also be debossed on the tablet's surface through a laser but the depth and the surface materials may affect the reading sensitivity [88]. A microtaggant technology further enhances tagging techniques by using micro-meter scale polymer microbeads with QR tags for on-dose authentication [89]. Reading of the tags may be a destructive process if the reader needs to examine the code on individual tablets, thus, a better reading method should be used for non-destructive examination. Raman spectroscopy provides a non-invasive alternative allowing the recognition of the tags even from the outside of the pharmaceutical packaging [90–92].

A proper track and trace system of the medicines from manufacturers to the patients, or multiple patients in case of medicine reuse, is a better way to protect from counterfeiting. A call-in numeric token printed on the packaging can be used to register the medicine once it is used the first time [93], but this method may not help authenticate a reused medicine. Al-Bahri et al. [94] proposed a complete track and trace system based on a central server on the Internet allowing each medicine to be treated as a digital object with unique identity. This DOA (digital object architecture) realizes a shared platform for all stakeholders to retrieve dedicated information when enough cybersecurity is properly implemented. The open and distributed ledger process of blockchain technology enables tracking of medicines registering every transaction among manufacturers, suppliers, pharmacists and patients. The open ledger blockchain can also register the multiple recycling actions between patients [95–97].

The Falsified Medicines Directives (FMD) [98] operating in Europe since February 2019 may force the implementation of anti-counterfeiting on pharmaceutical packaging through the addition of QR codes and tamper-proof sealing. However, the certification system may need to be adjusted to fit for a re-dispensing process for medicines reuse.

4. Discussion

Technologies for tackling quality and safety requirements can be found from contemporary research but most of them are passive in nature where interaction of medicines with the digital world is missing. The literature review in Section 3 is summarized in Table 3 illustrating a taxonomy of technologies classified according to individual applications and stakeholders' requirements. Sharing real-time information about medicines between stakeholders is important to maintain a complete medicine reuse system. Storage conditions can be digitally sensed, reported and analyzed dynamically through embedded microprocessors or via cloud computing services. A decision for returning and re-dispensing can be displayed directly on the packaging or indirectly through the smartphone or any surrounding smart devices. A judgment on re-dispensing returned medicines relies on a safety authentication process where the validation of unopened, undamaged and genuine medicines can be performed at pharmacies using dedicated analyzers. Active technologies together with network connectivity empower smart pharmaceutical packaging for the reuse of returned, unused, and unexpired medicines. IoT provides such a platform for sharing information of the medicines through the Internet for every stakeholder, and the concept of a smart object comprising a pharmaceutical packaging with the medicines inside acts as an IoT edge device with digital sensing and network connection [99]. A cloud computing service enables the exchange of information between the smart devices and the stakeholders through wearables, smartphones or full featured computers [100].

Table 3. Latest technologies for reusing returned medicines.

Requirements	Technologies
Quality	(i) storage temperature monitoring: passive TTI [43–45] (ii) storage temperature monitoring: active TTI with digital interfaces [46] (iii) thin-film technology: printed sensors and RFID tags [47–50] (iv) thin-film technology: hybrid printed circuits [51,52] (v) thin-film technology: nanotechnology [53–55] (vi) contamination detection: PT/GC/MS methodology [56,57] (vii) contamination detection: computer vision [58] (viii) contamination detection: tamper-evident check [59,60] (ix) motion detection: wearable sensors [63,64] (x) expiry date detection: visual inspection [66] (xi) expiry date detection: QR codes and smartphones [67] (xii) on packaging display: e-ink displays [68] and EC displays [69,70]
Safety	(i) tamper-proof: tamper-evident and tamper-resistance on packaging [71–73,75] (ii) tamper-proof: tamper-evident for transportation [74] (iii) tamper-proof: implementation during production [23,76] (iv) tamper-proof: built-in digital interfaces [77,78] (v) anti-counterfeit: overt/covert indications [80–82] (vi) anti-counterfeit: packaging materials inspection [83–85] (vii) anti-counterfeit: tagging on label, on medicine and on-dose [86–89] (viii) anti-counterfeit: readers for mini-size tags [90–92] (ix) anti-counterfeit: track and trace systems through Internet [93,94] (x) anti-counterfeit: open ledger based on blockchain [95–97]

A similar structure to that discussed above can be found in a smart medicine box which is an emerging research topic integrating digital sensors and networking capability so that they can monitor normal medicines put inside the box. Additional technologies can be applied to the surroundings of the smart medicine box as well for facilitating an electronic reminder for medication adherence [101], an in-house track and trace system [102], or an interaction with remote servers for telehealthcare [103,104]. Embedding IoT technologies into pharmaceutical packaging allows normal packages of medicines to become intelligent packaging [105–107], thus, the requirements for reusing medicines are met where an extension of the real-time information to cloud computing empowers all stakeholders to share data on a single platform. However, three other critical technologies may need to be further investigated to realize an intelligent pharmaceutical packaging for medicines reuse:

(i) Thin-film technologies

Printed electronics and nanotechnology mentioned previously provide methods to place electronic circuits on packaging materials. However, these technologies are still not common and complicated circuitry such as wireless modules and high-power microprocessors are still not directly printable onto the packaging surface.

(ii) Energy harvesting

RFID is normally used to provide power to read a passive tag but a continuous power supply for maintaining the regular sensing and the network connection is required. Technology for printed batteries is still in an early stage [108], energy harvesting techniques such as extracting ambient energy could be an alternative [109], and wireless charging can also be a good candidate supplying continuous power to the embedded electronics from a distance [110]. However, all these technologies are not yet mature enough for immediate implementation onto intelligent pharmaceutical packaging.

(iii) Flexible display

Flexible displays using e-ink or EC technology show a promising way to use minimum energy to sustain a dynamic changing electronic display mounted on existing flat or curved pharmaceutical packaging. Although no power is required for maintaining e-ink screen contents, the irregular updates still require a significant amount of electrical power to align the color pigments. Electrochromism technology reduces the energy for updating EC displays but a regular refresh process is required to keep the screen content visible. New low cost, low energy and printable technologies for pharmaceutical packaging are required.

Other than the two main groups of requirements discussed in Section 3, there are other concerns from the stakeholders in Table 1 to be resolved before an action for reusing medicines can be taken, and they are summarized as below:

(a) patients' incentive for returning unwanted medicines,
(b) pharmacists' incentive for extra workload in re-dispensing medicines,
(c) cost effectiveness monitoring of reusing medicines,
(d) legal issues such as legislation on re-dispensing medicines and professional standards for pharmacists,
(e) social norm for promoting medicine reuse,
(f) on-site and off-site collection and distribution system.

Items (a) to (e) are not directly related to technology. However, technologies may help quantify the data (e.g., immediate cost saving for recycling certain medicines, calculation and distribution of incentives to related stakeholders, etc.) or support information exchange in a social networks on the Internet. Social networking may also gather supporting power to influence government decisions on changing policies. Item (f) may make use of the IoT platform to collect, register, authenticate and re-dispense using a proven track and trace system through the IoT networks.

5. ReMINDS Ecosystem

Based on the qualitative research within pharmacy practice and the concept of technology integration for pharmaceutical packaging, a group called ReMINDS (Reuse of Medicines through Informatics, Networks and Sensors) has recently been established in the University of Reading with the aim of promoting the reuse of medicines in the UK. ReMINDS is driven by a multidisciplinary team with members coming from pharmacy, computer science and biomedical engineering.

The reuse of medicines is not purely a technical issue since (i) it creates legal concerns involving changes in policies by governments, (ii) it affects commercial decisions involving changes in financial performance for pharmaceutical companies, (iii) it requires voluntary actions involving changes in patient behaviors through patient beliefs, and (iv) it increases extra workloads and risks involving changes in the code of conduct for pharmacists. Previous research suggests that every stakeholder in society contributes part of the responsibility to recycle returned and unused medicines where an ecosystem is apparently established by itself. A novel ReMINDS ecosystem for reusing dispensed medicines through a technology perspective is proposed and Figure 2 depicts the relationship between each party in the hypothesized ecosystem for medicine reuse. The concept of ReMINDS ecosystem can be one of the solutions for reusing dispensed medicines and reducing medicinal waste, and it is built on top of the IoT where seamless connections between medicines and the related stakeholders is the key for success.

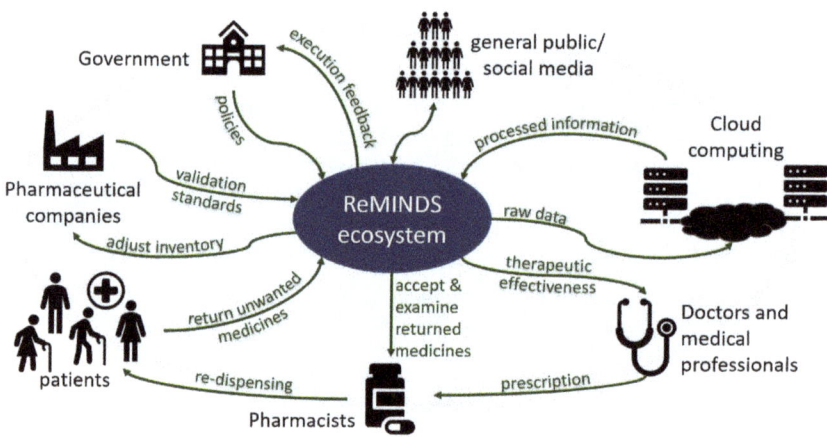

Figure 2. An ecosystem for the reuse of medicines from a technology perspective.

Patients and pharmacists are not the only groups in society responsible for taking actions in returning and re-dispensing medicines, other stakeholders in society as a whole play different but crucial roles in maintaining a sustainable ecosystem for reusing medicines. Patients may be the first decision maker to return unused medicines back to the recycle centers, and technologies can provide indications for when and where the medicines are reused or disposed. Pharmacists accept and examine the returned medicines, and technologies enable them to validate the usable conditions before re-dispensing. Raw data of the types, quantity and quality of returned medicines are uploaded to a cloud server empowering an off-site analysis, different entities can retrieve information using various analytical methods. Doctors and healthcare professionals write the prescriptions to the patients but they may not be directly involved in the whole return and re-dispense process; however, technologies allow them to investigate the therapeutic effectiveness based on the information collected and analyzed through cloud computing. Pharmaceutical companies provide standards to pharmacists for validation of the usable conditions for returned medicines, for examples, the duration and limits for out-of-range storage temperature or humidity. Government is a key stakeholder who can set or change the policies enabling and governing related activities, the lawmakers may require specific information from the cloud server to monitor and adjust the execution of policies. As well as playing a role in returning unused medicines, the general public also act as a supporting role through online social networks by influencing the government and establishing a norm for the recycling of medicines.

6. Conclusions

A literature survey of latest technologies facilitating the design of intelligent pharmaceutical packaging for reusing medicines is reported. A taxonomy of the reviewed technologies is suggested according to the requirements for shaping human behaviors to take appropriate actions. Through a technology perspective, a novel ReMINDS ecosystem as a suggested solution for reusing returned prescribed medicines based on the literature review is proposed. Active sensing technologies integrated with the IoT platform indicate how a combination of informatics, networks and digital sensors facilitate society to make possible the reuse of medicines.

Technologies provide the tools to directly or indirectly meet the various requirements from each stakeholder. Embedded sensing and reporting electronics on the pharmaceutical packaging help validate the quality and safety of the medicines. Network connectivity helps connect the intelligent packaging globally to all stakeholders in the ReMINDS ecosystem. However, intelligent packaging for reusing medicines is still not mainstream research and more studies in thin-film technologies, energy harvesting, flexible low-power display are essential to empower the technologies on pharmaceutical packaging to become the key enabler for reusing returned prescribed medicines and reducing medicinal waste. Further research on developing and applying appropriate technologies onto and around the pharmaceutical packaging for establishing the hypothesized ReMINDS ecosystem will be one of the aims for the ReMINDS team.

Author Contributions: T.K.L.H. conceived and conducted the literature review and prepared the manuscript. B.M. prepared the initial article, reviewed and revised the manuscript. P.D. critically reviewed and revised the manuscript from a pharmaceutical perspective. R.M. critically reviewed and revised the manuscript from an informatics perspective. R.S.S. critically reviewed and revised the manuscript from a biomedical engineering perspective and funding acquisition. All authors have read and agreed to the published version of the manuscript.

Funding: This research was funded through the University of Reading Research Endowment Trust Fund (RETF), the Building Outstanding Impact Support Programme (BOISP), and an EPSRC summer studentship.

Conflicts of Interest: All authors declare no conflict of interest.

References

1. Hazell, B.; Robson, R. Pharmaceutical waste reduction in the NHS. *Rep. Version* **2015**, *1*, 1–24.
2. Opar, A. Rising drug costs prompt new uses for old pills. *Nat. Med.* **2006**, *12*, 1333. [CrossRef] [PubMed]
3. Toh, M.R.; Chew, L. Turning waste medicines to cost savings: A pilot study on the feasibility of medication recycling as a solution to drug wastage. *Palliat. Med.* **2017**, *31*, 35–41. [CrossRef] [PubMed]
4. Bekker, C.L.; Gardarsdottir, H.; Egberts, A.C.G.; Molenaar, H.A.; Bouvy, M.L.; van den Bemt, B.J.F.; Hövels, A.M. What does it cost to redispense unused medications in the pharmacy? A micro-costing study. *BMC Health Serv. Res.* **2019**, *19*, 243. [CrossRef]
5. Trueman, P.; Taylor, D.; Lowson, K.; Bligh, A.; Meszaros, A.; Wright, D.; Glanville, J.; Newbould, J.; Bury, M.; Barber, N.; et al. *Evaluation of the Scale, Causes and Costs of Waste Medicines. Report of DH Funded National Project*; York Health Economics Consortium and The School of Pharmacy, University of London: London, UK; 2010.
6. Bekker, C.; Gardarsdottir, H.; Egberts, A.; Bouvy, M.; van den Bemt, B. Worldwide initiatives to decrease medication wastage: A cross-national survey. In Proceedings of the 44th ESCP International Symposium on Clinical Pharmacy Medicines Information: Making Better Decisions, Lisbon, Portugal, 30 October 2015; Volume 38, p. 591.

7. Connelly, D. Should pharmacists be allowed to reuse medicines. *Pharm. J.* **2019**. [CrossRef]
8. Kaldy, J. Program Turns Discarded Drugs Into Lifesavers for Needy. *Caring Ages* **2015**, *16*, 9. [CrossRef]
9. Cauchi, R.; Berg, K. State Prescription Drug Return, Reuse and Recycling Laws. Available online: http://www.ncsl.org/research/health/state-prescription-drug-return-reuse-and-recycling.aspx (accessed on 10 November 2019).
10. Crews, J. *Prescription Drug Reuse and Recycling*; Taylor & Francis: Abingdon, UK, 2019. [CrossRef]
11. WHO. *Guidelines for Drug Donations*; World Health Organization: Geneva, Switzerlnad, 1999; Volume 20.
12. Gotink, M.H.; Ralitapole, D.K. Inter Care: Help for rural African hospitals. *Br. Med J.* **1988**, *297*, 1402. [CrossRef]
13. Viegas, C.V.; Bond, A.; Vaz, C.R.; Bertolo, R.J. Reverse flows within the pharmaceutical supply chain: A classificatory review from the perspective of end-of-use and end-of-life medicines. *J. Clean. Prod.* **2019**, *238*, 117719. [CrossRef]
14. Trappey, A.J.C.; Trappey, C.V.; Fan, C.Y.; Hsu, A.P.T.; Li, X.K.; Lee, I.J.Y. IoT patent roadmap for smart logistic service provision in the context of Industry 4.0. *J. Chin. Inst. Eng.* **2017**, *40*, 593–602. [CrossRef]
15. Ding, B. Pharma Industry 4.0: Literature review and research opportunities in sustainable pharmaceutical supply chains. *Process. Saf. Environ. Prot.* **2018**, *119*, 115–130. [CrossRef]
16. Bekker, C.L.; Gardarsdottir, H.; Egberts, T.C.G.; Bouvy, M.L.; van den Bemt, B.J.F. Redispensing of medicines unused by patients: A qualitative study among stakeholders. *Int. J. Clin. Pharm.* **2017**, *39*, 196–204. [CrossRef] [PubMed]
17. Bekker, C.; van den Bemt, B.; Egberts, T.C.G.; Bouvy, M.; Gardarsdottir, H. Willingness of patients to use unused medication returned to the pharmacy by another patient: A cross-sectional survey. *BMJ Open* **2019**, *9*, 1–5. [CrossRef] [PubMed]
18. McRae, D.; Allman, M.; James, D. The redistribution of medicines: Could it become a reality? *Int. J. Pharm. Pract.* **2016**, *24*, 411–418. [CrossRef] [PubMed]
19. Alhamad, H.; Patel, N.; Donyai, P. How do people conceptualise the reuse of medicines? An interview study. *Int. J. Pharm. Pract.* **2018**, *26*, 232–241. [CrossRef]
20. Black, G. Reuse of medicine: it's not about the money!: From my Little Black Book of pharmacy practice: Practice matters. *SA Pharm. J.* **2011**, *78*, 51–53.
21. Lorenzini, G.C.; Mostaghel, R.; Hellstrom, D. Drivers of pharmaceutical packaging innovation: A customer-supplier relationship case study. *J. Bus. Res.* **2018**, *88*, 363–370. [CrossRef]
22. Munzel, J. Pharmaceutical packaging: Technology and design requirements are on the rise. *J. Med Mark.* **2007**, *7*, 136–145. [CrossRef]
23. Zadbuke, N.; Shahi, S.; Gulecha, B.; Padalkar, A.; Thube, M. Recent trends and future of pharmaceutical packaging technology. *J. Pharm. Bioallied Sci.* **2013**, *5*, 98–110. [CrossRef]
24. Sehgal, S.; Jaithliya, T.; Khan, M.; Devi, A.N.; Banoo, J.; Tiwari, A. Recent trends and future of pharmaceutical packaging technology: An overview. *Eur. J. Biomed. Pharm. Sci.* **2018**, *5*, 957–966.
25. Madhusudan, P.; Chellukuri, N.; Shivakumar, N. Smart packaging of food for the 21st century—A review with futuristic trends, their feasibility and economics. *Mater. Today Proc.* **2018**, *5*, 21018–21022. [CrossRef]
26. Hara, L.; Guirguis, R.; Hummel, K.; Villanueva, M. More Than Bar Codes: Integrating Global Standards-Based Bar Code Technology Into National Health Information Systems in Ethiopia and Pakistan to Increase End-to-End Supply Chain Visibility. *Glob. Health Sci. Pract.* **2017**, *5*, 678–685. [CrossRef] [PubMed]
27. Lavorgna, A. The online trade in counterfeit pharmaceuticals: New criminal opportunities, trends and challenges. *Eur. J. Criminol.* **2015**, *12*, 226–241. [CrossRef]
28. Degardin, K.; Guillemain, A.; Klespe, P.; Hindelang, F.; Zurbach, R.; Roggo, Y. Packaging analysis of counterfeit medicines. *Forensic Sci. Int.* **2018**, *291*, 144–157. [CrossRef]
29. Patel, R.P.; Patel, Y.B.; Prajapati, B.G.; Borkhataria, C.H. Outline of Pharmaceutical Packaging Technology. *Int. Res. J. Pharm.* **2010**, *1*, 105–112.
30. Janjarasskul, T.; Suppakul, P. Active and intelligent packaging: The indication of quality and safety. *Crit. Rev. Food Sci. Nutr.* **2018**, *58*, 808–831. [CrossRef]
31. Selman, J.D. Time-temperature indicators. In *Active Food Packaging*; Springer US: Boston, MA, USA, 1995; pp. 215–237. [CrossRef]

32. Usak, M.; Kubiatko, M.; Shabbir, M.S.; Viktorovna Dudnik, O.; Jermsittiparsert, K.; Rajabion, L. Health care service delivery based on the Internet of things: A systematic and comprehensive study. *Int. J. Commun. Syst.* **2020**, *33*, e4179. [CrossRef]
33. Müller, P.; Schmid, M. Intelligent packaging in the food sector: A brief overview. *Foods* **2019**, *8*, 16. [CrossRef]
34. Kleppe, M.; Lacroix, J.; Ham, J.; Midden, C. A dual-process view on medication adherence: The role of affect. *J. Health Psychol.* **2017**, *24*, 1033–1042. [CrossRef]
35. Martin, L.R.; Feig, C.; Maksoudian, C.R.; Wysong, K.; Faasse, K. A perspective on nonadherence to drug therapy: Psychological barriers and strategies to overcome nonadherence. *Patient Prefer. Adherence* **2018**, *12*, 1527–1535. [CrossRef]
36. Swartz, M.K. The PRISMA Statement: A Guideline for Systematic Reviews and Meta-Analyses. *J. Pediatr. Health Care* **2011**, *25*, 1–2. [CrossRef]
37. Waffenschmidt, S.; Knelangen, M.; Sieben, W.; Bühn, S.; Pieper, D. Single screening versus conventional double screening for study selection in systematic reviews: A methodological systematic review. *BMC Med. Res. Methodol.* **2019**, *19*, 132. [CrossRef] [PubMed]
38. Munn, Z.; Peters, M.D.J.; Stern, C.; Tufanaru, C.; McArthur, A.; Aromataris, E. Systematic review or scoping review? Guidance for authors when choosing between a systematic or scoping review approach. *BMC Med. Res. Methodol.* **2018**, *18*, 143. [CrossRef] [PubMed]
39. Hubley, J. Understanding Behaviour: The Key to Successful Health Education. *Trop. Dr.* **1988**, *18*, 134–138. [CrossRef] [PubMed]
40. Yousefi, H.; Su, H.M.; Imani, S.M.; Alkhaldi, K.M.; Filipe, C.D.; Didar, T.F. Intelligent Food Packaging: A Review of Smart Sensing Technologies for Monitoring Food Quality. *ACS Sensors* **2019**, *4*, 808–821. [CrossRef]
41. Kuswandi, B.; Wicaksono, Y.; Jayus; Abdullah, A.; Heng, L.Y.; Ahmad, M. Smart Packaging: Sensors for monitoring of food quality and safety. *Sens. Instrum. Food Qual. Saf.* **2011**, *5*, 137–146. [CrossRef]
42. Vanderroost, M.; Ragaert, P.; Devlieghere, F.; De Meulenaer, B. Intelligent food packaging: The next generation. *Trends Food Sci. Technol.* **2014**, *39*, 47–62. [CrossRef]
43. Pavelková, A. Time temperature indicators as devices intelligent packaging. *ACTA Univ. Agric. Silvic. Mendel. Brun.* **2013**, *61*, 245–251. [CrossRef]
44. Wang, S.; Liu, X.; Yang, M.; Zhang, Y.; Xiang, K.; Tang, R. Review of Time Temperature Indicators as Quality Monitors in Food Packaging. *Packag. Technol. Sci.* **2015**, *28*, 839–867. [CrossRef]
45. Pereira, V.A., Jr.; de Arruda, I.N.Q.; Stefani, R. Active chitosan/PVA films with anthocyanins from Brassica oleraceae (Red Cabbage) as Time-Temperature Indicators for application in intelligent food packaging. *Food Hydrocoll.* **2015**, *43*, 180–188. [CrossRef]
46. Mijanur Rahman, A.T.M.; Kim, D.H.; Jang, H.D.; Yang, J.H.; Lee, S.J. Preliminary study on biosensor-type time-temperature integrator for intelligent food packaging. *Sensors* **2018**, *18*, 1949. [CrossRef]
47. Maslik, J.; Andersson, H.; Forsberg, V.; Engholm, M.; Zhang, R.; Olin, H. PEDOT: PSS temperature sensor ink-jet printed on paper substrate. *J. Instrum.* **2018**, *13*, C12010. [CrossRef]
48. Maiellaro, G.; Ragonese, E.; Gwoziecki, R.; Jacobs, S.; Marjanović, N.; Chrapa, M.; Schleuniger, J.; Palmisano, G. Ambient light organic sensor in a printed complementary organic TFT technology on flexible plastic foil. *IEEE Trans. Circuits Syst. Regul. Pap.* **2013**, *61*, 1036–1043. [CrossRef]
49. Feng, Y.; Xie, L.; Chen, Q.; Zheng, L. Low-Cost Printed Chipless RFID Humidity Sensor Tag for Intelligent Packaging. *IEEE Sensors J.* **2015**, *15*, 3201–3208. [CrossRef]
50. Javed, N.; Habib, A.; Amin, Y.; Loo, J.; Akram, A.; Tenhunen, H. Directly Printable Moisture Sensor Tag for Intelligent Packaging. *IEEE Sensors J.* **2016**, *16*, 6147–6148. [CrossRef]
51. Zhang, X.; Shan, X.; Wei, J. Hybrid flexible smart temperature tag with NFC technology for smart packaging. In Proceedings of the 19th Electronics Packaging Technology Conference, Singapore, 6 December 2017; pp. 1–5. [CrossRef]
52. Falco, A.; Salmerón, J.F.; Loghin, F.C.; Lugli, P.; Rivadeneyra, A. Fully printed flexible single-chip RFID tag with light detection capabilities. *Sensors* **2017**, *17*, 534. [CrossRef]
53. Kuswandi, B., Nanotechnology in Food Packaging. In *Nanoscience in Food and Agriculture*; Springer: Berlin/Heidelberg, Germany, 2016; pp. 151–183. [CrossRef]
54. Feng, Y.; Xie, L.; Mäntysalo, M.; Chen, Q.; Zheng, L. Electrical and humidity-sensing characterization of inkjet-printed multi-walled carbon nanotubes for smart packaging. *Sensors IEEE* **2013**, 1–4. [CrossRef]

55. Rahimi, R.; Zhou, J.; Jiang, H.; Soleimani, T.; Ziaia, B. Facile fabrication of low-cost passive wireless humidity sensor for smart packaging via all-laser processing of metalized paper. In Proceedings of the Solid-State Sensors, Actuators and Microsystems Workshop, Hilton Head Island, SC, USA, 2018; pp. 326–329. [CrossRef]
56. Johnston, J.J.; Wong, J.P.; Feldman, S.E.; Ilnicki, L.P. Purge and Trap/Gas Chromatography/Mass Spectrometry Method for Determining Smoke Contamination of Foods and Packaging Materials. *J. Agric. Food Chem.* **1994**, *42*, 1954–1958. [CrossRef]
57. Mielniczuk, Z.; Pogorzelska, Z. Detection of microbial contamination of packaging for foodstuffs by gas chromatography-mass spectrometry method. *Packag. Technol. Sci.* **2002**, *15*, 47–51. [CrossRef]
58. Tretola, M.; Di Rosa, A.R.; Tirloni, E.; Ottoboni, M.; Giromini, C.; Leone, F.; Bernardi, C.E.M.; Dell'Orto, V.; Chiofalo, V.; Pinotti, L. Former food products safety: Microbiological quality and computer vision evaluation of packaging remnants contamination. *Food Addit. Contam. Part A* **2017**, *34*, 1427–1435. [CrossRef]
59. Troja, D.; Shabani, L.; Troja, R. Packaging systems influence on the microbial contamination of common pharmaceutical products. *J. Hyg. Eng. Des.* **2014**, *6*, 142–146.
60. White, K.; Lin, L.; Dahl, D.W.; Ritchie, R.J.B. When do consumers avoid imperfections? Superficial packaging damage as a contamination cue. *J. Mark. Res.* **2016**, *53*, 110–123. [CrossRef]
61. Akbarian, M.; Ghasemi, Y.; Uversky, V.N.; Yousefi, R. Chemical modifications of insulin: Finding a compromise between stability and pharmaceutical performance. *Int. J. Pharm.* **2018**, *547*, 450–468. [CrossRef] [PubMed]
62. Hii, M.S.Y.; Courtney, P.; Royall, P.G. An Evaluation of the Delivery of Medicines Using Drones. *Drones* **2019**, *3*, 52. [CrossRef]
63. Jing, Q.; Xie, Y.; Zhu, G.; Han, R.P.S.; Wang, Z.L. Self-powered thin-film motion vector sensor. *Nat. Commun.* **2015**, *6*, 8031. [CrossRef]
64. Yamamoto, Y.; Harada, S.; Yamamoto, D.; Honda, W.; Arie, T.; Akita, S.; Takei, K. Printed multifunctional flexible device with an integrated motion sensor for health care monitoring. *Sci. Adv.* **2016**, *2*, e1601473. [CrossRef]
65. Gong, L.; Yu, M.; Duan, W.; Ye, X.; Gudmundsson, K.; Swainson, M. A Novel Camera Based Approach for Automatic Expiry Date Detection and Recognition on Food Packages. In *Artificial Intelligence Applications and Innovation. IFIP Advances in Information and Communication Technology*; Springer: Cham, Switzerland, 2018; pp. 133–142. [CrossRef]
66. Peng, E.; Peursum, P.; Li, L. Product Barcode and Expiry Date Detection for the Visually Impaired Using a Smartphone. In Proceedings of the International Conference on Digital Image Computing Techniques and Applications (DICTA), Perth, Australia, 3 Decemebr 2012; pp. 1–7. [CrossRef]
67. Ramalingam, M.; Puviarasi, R.; Zakaria, N.D.A.B. Developing mobile application for medicine expiry date detection. *Int. J. Pure Appl. Math.* **2018**, *119*, 3895–3900.
68. Blankenbach, K.; Duchemin, P.; Rist, B.; Bogner, D.; Krause, M. Smart Pharmaceutical Packaging with E-Paper Display for improved Patient Compliance. In *SID Symposium Digest of Technical Papers*; Wiley: Hoboken, NJ, USA, **2018**; Volume 49, pp. 271–274.
69. Kai, H.; Suda, W.; Ogawa, Y.; Nagamine, K.; Nishizawa, M. Intrinsically Stretchable Electrochromic Display by a Composite Film of Poly(3,4-ethylenedioxythiophene) and Polyurethane. *ACS Appl. Mater. Interfaces* **2017**, *9*, 19513–19518. [CrossRef]
70. Brooke, R.; Edberg, J.; Crispin, X.; Berggren, M.; Engquist, I.; Jonsson, P.M. Greyscale and Paper Electrochromic Polymer Displays by UV Patterning. *Polymers* **2019**, *11*. [CrossRef]
71. Kumbhar, M.S.; Choudhary, N.H.; Dighe, D.A.; Singh, M.C. Tamper Evident Pharmaceutical Packaging - Needs and Advances. *Int. J. Pharm. Sci. Rev. Res.* **2012**, *13*, 141–153.
72. CPG. *Compliance Policy Guide Sec. 450.500 Tamper-Resistant Packaging Requirements for Certain Over-the-Counter Human Drug Products MAY 1992*; Federal Register; US Food and Drug Administration: Washington, DC, USA, 2015; Volume 63, pp. 59463–59471.
73. Kumar, A.K.; Gupta, N.V.; Lalasa, P.; Sandhil, S. A review on packaging materials with anti-counterfeit, tamper-evident features for pharmaceuticals. *Int. J. Drug Dev. Res.* **2013**, *5*, 26–34.
74. O'Connor, M.C. Packaging Maker Offering Tamper-Evident RFID Film. *RFID J.* Available online: https://www.rfidjournal.com/articles/view?2959 (accessed on 24 March 2020).
75. Jo, C.L.; Ambs, A.; Dresler, C.M.; Backinger, C.L. Child-resistant and tamper-resistant packaging: A systematic review to inform tobacco packaging regulation. *Prev. Med.* **2017**, *95*, 89–95. [CrossRef] [PubMed]

76. Naitove, M. In food packaging, peelable IML serves as tamper-evident seal. *Plast. Technol.* **2018**, *64*, 14–16.
77. Mayberry, J. Make your mark: Tamper-evident packaging remains invaluable for safety-conscious consumers. *Pharm. Process.* **2013**, *28*, 36–37.
78. Floerkemeier, C.; Siegemund, F. Improving the effectiveness of medical treatment with pervasive computing technologies. In Proceedings of the UbiHealth: The 2nd International Workshop on Ubiquitous Computing for Pervasive Healthcare Applications, Seattle, WA, USA, 12 October, 2003.
79. Gao, J.; Pang, Z.; Chen, Q.; Zheng, L.R. Interactive packaging solutions based on RFID technology and controlled delamination material. In Proceedings of the RFID 2010: International IEEE Conference on RFID, Orlando, FL, USA, 16 April 2010; pp. 158–165. [CrossRef]
80. Choi, J.B.; Rogers, J.; Jones, E.C. The impact of a shared pharmaceutical supply chain model on counterfeit drugs, diverted drugs, and drug shortages. In Proceedings of the Portland International Conference on Management of Engineering and Technology (PICMET), Portland, OR, USA, 2–6 August 2015; pp. 1879–1889. [CrossRef]
81. Shah, R.Y.; Prajapati, P.N.; Agrawal, Y.K. Anticounterfeit packaging technologies. *J. Adv. Pharm. Technol. Res.* **2010**, *1*, 368–373. [CrossRef] [PubMed]
82. Bansal, D.; Malla, S.; Gudala, K.; Tiwari, P. Anti-Counterfeit Technologies: A Pharmaceutical Industry Perspective. *Sci. Pharm.* **2013**, *81*, 1–14. [CrossRef]
83. Andria, S.E.; Fulcher, M.; Witkowski, M.R.; Platek, S.F. The Use of SEM/EDS and FT-IR Analyses in the Identification of Counterfeit Pharmaceutical Packaging. *Am. Pharm. Rev.* **2012**, *15*, 62.
84. Li, Y.; Li, J. The Intelligent Texture Anti-counterfeiting Algorithm Based on DFT. In Proceedings of the Ninth International Conference on Intelligent Information Hiding and Multimedia Signal Processing, Beijing, China, 16 October 2013; pp. 590–593. [CrossRef]
85. Simske, S.; Mucher, P.; Martinez, C. Using variable data security printing to provide customized package protection. *Int. Conf. Digit. Prod. Print. Ind. Appl. Final. Program Proc.* **2005**, *3*, 112–113.
86. Ishiyama, R.; Takahashi, T.; Makino, K.; Kudo, Y.; Kooper, M.; Abbink, D. Medicine Tablet Authentication Using "Fingerprints" of Ink-Jet Printed Characters. In Proceedings of the International Conference on Industrial Technology (ICIT), Melbourne, Australia, 15 February 2019; pp. 871–876. [CrossRef]
87. Fei, J.; Liu, R. Drug-laden 3D biodegradable label using QR code for anti-counterfeiting of drugs. *Mater. Sci. Eng.* **2016**, *63*, 657–662. [CrossRef]
88. Ludasi, K.; Jójárt-Laczkovich, O.; Sovány, T.; Hopp, B.; Smausz, T.; Regdon, G., Jr. Comparison of conventionally and naturally coloured coatings marked by laser technology for unique 2D coding of pharmaceuticals. *Int. J. Pharm.* **2019**, *570*, 118665. [CrossRef]
89. Han, S.; Bae, H.J.; Kim, J.; Shin, S.; Choi, S.; Lee, S.H.; Kwon, S.; Park, W. Lithographically encoded polymer microtaggant using high-capacity and error-correctable QR code for anti-counterfeiting of drugs. *Adv. Mater.* **2012**, *24*, 5924–5929. [CrossRef]
90. Platek, S.F.; Ranieri, N.; Batson, J. Applications of the FDA's Counterfeit Detection Device (CD3+) to the Examination of Suspect Counterfeit Pharmaceutical Tablets and Packaging. *Microsc. Microanal.* **2016**, *22*. [CrossRef]
91. Kwok, K.; Taylor, L.S. Analysis of the packaging enclosing a counterfeit pharmaceutical tablet using Raman microscopy and two-dimensional correlation spectroscopy. *Vib. Spectrosc.* **2012**, *61*, 176–182. [CrossRef]
92. Eliasson, C.; Matousek, P. Noninvasive Authentication of Pharmaceutical Products through Packaging Using Spatially Offset Raman Spectroscopy. *Anal. Chem.* **2007**, *79*, 1696–1701. [CrossRef]
93. Nilsson, E.; Nilsson, B.; Järpe, E. A pharmaceutical anti-counterfeiting method using time controlled numeric tokens. In Proceedings of the International Conference on RFID-Technologies and Applications, Sitges, Spain, 15 March 2011; pp. 343–347. [CrossRef]
94. Al-Bahri, M.; Yankovsky, A.; Kirichek, R.; Borodin, A. Smart System Based on DOA & IoT for Products Monitoring & Anti-Counterfeiting. In Proceedings of the 4th MEC International Conference on Big Data and Smart City (ICBDSC): Muscat, Oman, 15–16 January 2019; pp. 1–5. [CrossRef]
95. Garankina, R.Y.; Zakharochkina, E.R.; Samoshchenkova, I.F.; Lebedeva, N.Y.; Lebedev, A.V. Blockchain Technology and its Use in the Area of Circulation of Pharmaceuticals. *J. Pharm. Sci. Res.* **2018**, *10*, 2715–2717.
96. Pashkov, V.; Soloviov, O. Legal implementation of blockchain technology in pharmacy. In Proceedings of the 7th International Interdisciplinary Scientific Conference: Society, Health, Welfare, Rīga Stradiņš University (RSU), Rīga, Latvia, 10–12 October 2018; Volume 68, pp. 1–8. [CrossRef]

97. Shi, J.; Yi, D.; Kuang, J. *Pharmaceutical Supply Chain Management System with Integration of IoT and Blockchain Technology*; Smart Blockchain; Qiu, M., Ed.; Springer International Publishing: Berlin/Heidelberg, Germany, **2019**, pp. 97–108.
98. Ogden, J. Implementing the EU Falsified Medicines Directive. *Prescriber* **2019**, *30*, 30–33 [CrossRef]
99. Nowakowski, W. The Internet of Things: From smart packaging to a world of smart objects? *Elektronika* **2016**, *10*, 70–75. [CrossRef]
100. Suganya, G.; Premalatha, M.; Anushka, S.; Muktak, P.; Abhishek, J. IoT based Automated Medicine Dispenser for Online Health Community using Cloud. *Int. J. Recent Technol. Eng.* **2019**, *7*, 1–4.
101. Thakkar, H.; Trivedi, V.; Jolapara, U.; Chauhan, J. MED-IoT: A Medicine Confirmation System. In Proceedings of the International Conference on Smart City and Emerging Technology (ICSCET), Mumbai, India, 5 January 2018; pp. 1–5. [CrossRef]
102. López-Nores, M.; Pazos-Arias, J.J.; García-Duque, J.; Blanco-Fernández, Y.; Ramos-Cabrer, M. Introducing smart packaging in residential networks to prevent medicine misuse. In Proceedings of the IEEE International Symposium on Consumer Electronics, Las Vegas, NV, USA, 9 January 2008; pp. 1–3. [CrossRef]
103. Srinivas, M.; Durgaprasadarao, P.; Raj, V.N.P. Intelligent medicine box for medication management using IoT. In Proceedings of the 2nd International Conference on Inventive Systems and Control (ICISC), JCT College of Engineering and Technology, Tamil Nadu, India, 19–20 January 2018; pp. 32–34. [CrossRef]
104. da Silva, D.V.; Gonçalves, T.G.; Pires, P.F. Using IoT technologies to develop a low-cost smart medicine box. In Proceedings of the 25th Brazillian Symposium on Multimedia and the Web, WebMedia 2019, Espírito Santo, Brazil, 26 October 2019; pp. 97–101. [CrossRef]
105. Yang, G.; Xie, L.; Mantysalo, M.; Zhou, X.L.; Pang, Z.B.; Xu, L.D.; Kao-Walter, S.; Chen, Q.; Zheng, L.R. A Health-IoT Platform Based on the Integration of Intelligent Packaging, Unobtrusive Bio-Sensor, and Intelligent Medicine Box. *IEEE Trans. Ind. Inform.* **2014**, *10*, 2180–2191. [CrossRef]
106. Pang, Z.; Tian, J.; Chen, Q. Intelligent packaging and intelligent medicine box for medication management towards the Internet-of-Things. In Proceedings of the 16th International Conference on Advanced Communication Technology, PyeongChang, Korea, 16 February 2014; Volume 2, pp. 352–360. [CrossRef]
107. Farahani, B.; Firouzi, F.; Chang, V.; Badaroglu, M.; Constant, N.; Mankodiya, K. Towards fog-driven IoT eHealth: Promises and challenges of IoT in medicine and healthcare. *Future Gener. Comput. Syst.* **2018**, *78*, 659–676. [CrossRef]
108. Kumar, R.; Shin, J.; Yin, L.; You, J.M.; Meng, Y.S.; Wang, J. All-Printed, Stretchable Zn-Ag2O Rechargeable Battery via Hyperelastic Binder for Self-Powering Wearable Electronics. *Adv. Energy Mater.* **2017**, *7*, 1–8. [CrossRef]
109. Garg, N.; Garg, R. Energy harvesting in IoT devices: A survey. In Proceedings of the International Conference on Intelligent Sustainable Systems (ICISS), SCAD Institute of Technology at Palladam, Tirupur, India, 7–8 December 2017; pp. 127–131. [CrossRef]
110. Meile, L.; Ulrich, A.; Magno, M. Wireless Power Transmission Powering Miniaturized Low Power IoT devices: A Review. In Proceedings of the 8th International Workshop on Advances in Sensors and Interfaces (IWASI), Otranto, Italy, 14 June 2019; pp. 312–317. [CrossRef]

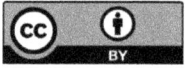

© 2020 by the authors. Licensee MDPI, Basel, Switzerland. This article is an open access article distributed under the terms and conditions of the Creative Commons Attribution (CC BY) license (http://creativecommons.org/licenses/by/4.0/).

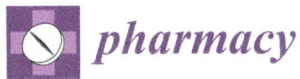

Article

The Effect of Quality Indicators on Beliefs about Medicines Reuse: An Experimental Study

Yasmin Lam [1], Rachel McCrindle [2], Terence K. L. Hui [2], R. Simon Sherratt [2] and Parastou Donyai [1,*]

[1] Reading School of Pharmacy, University of Reading, Reading RG6 6AP, UK; yasmin.lam@hotmail.co.uk
[2] Department of Biomedical Engineering, School of Biological Sciences, University of Reading, Reading RG6 6AY, UK; r.j.mccrindle@reading.ac.uk (R.M.); t.hui@reading.ac.uk (T.K.L.H.); r.s.sherratt@reading.ac.uk (R.S.S.)
* Correspondence: p.donyai@reading.ac.uk; Tel.: +44-118-378-4704; Fax: +44-118-378-4703

Abstract: Background: A number of studies have examined beliefs about medicines reuse. Although the practice is prohibited in UK community pharmacy, it does take place elsewhere in the world where it relies on visual checks of returned medicines as an indicator of their quality. One proposal is to integrate sensor technology onto medication packaging as a marker of their quality instead. Our aim was to gauge people's beliefs about medicines reuse, in an experiment, with or without sensor technology and with or without the promise of visual checks completed by a pharmacist, as experimental conditions, should the practice be sanctioned in the UK in the future. Methods: A between participant study was designed with two independent factors testing the hypothesis that sensors and visual checks would increase pro-medicines-reuse beliefs. A questionnaire was used to measure medicines reuse beliefs and collect qualitative comments. Results: Eighty-one participants took part. Attitudes toward medication offered for reuse, participants' perceived social pressure to accept the medication, and their intention to take part in medicines reuse all increased with the presence of sensors on packaging and with the promise of pharmacist visual checking, with the former causing a greater increase than the latter, and the combination of both making the greatest increase. People's qualitative comments explained their concerns about medicines reuse, validating the findings. The use of sensors on medication packaging warrants further investigation if regulators are to consider approving medicines reuse in the UK.

Keywords: medicines; sensors; pharmacist; medicines reuse; attitudes

Citation: Lam, Y.; McCrindle, R.; Hui, T.K.L.; Sherratt, R.S.; Donyai, P. The Effect of Quality Indicators on Beliefs about Medicines Reuse: An Experimental Study. *Pharmacy* **2021**, *9*, 128. https://doi.org/10.3390/pharmacy9030128

Academic Editor: Jon Schommer

Received: 8 April 2021
Accepted: 7 July 2021
Published: 21 July 2021

Publisher's Note: MDPI stays neutral with regard to jurisdictional claims in published maps and institutional affiliations.

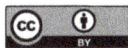

Copyright: © 2021 by the authors. Licensee MDPI, Basel, Switzerland. This article is an open access article distributed under the terms and conditions of the Creative Commons Attribution (CC BY) license (https://creativecommons.org/licenses/by/4.0/).

1. Introduction

A number of studies have examined people's views about the idea of medicines reuse, a practice that involves re-dispensing quality-checked, unused, prescribed medication for other patients instead of disposal as waste [1–4]. This is important because a strong body of evidence shows that inappropriate disposal of unwanted medicines (e.g., disposal via domestic waste and the sewage system), in a host of countries, contributes to the contamination of soil and groundwater with a multitude of drug substances which can even make their way into drinking water [5,6]. Medicines reuse offers a potential solution to minimizing this problem, by encouraging people to return their unwanted medicines to the pharmacy, either for safe disposal or for re-dispensing to other patients [3]. Of course, there are other much more significant ways of reducing environmental contamination from medicinal products, including better research and manufacturing processes at the pharmaceutical industry level, and more responsible prescribing and dispensing practices within the community level [5]. However, medicines reuse, by encouraging people to return their medicines to the pharmacy, also has the potential to help reduce the stockpiling of medicines within patients' homes, something that can otherwise lead to accidental poisoning and inappropriate self-administration of medicines for undiagnosed conditions [7]. It is also important to remember the financial impact of medication waste, considered in detail elsewhere [8,9]. Finally, there is the potential for medicines reuse to help with the supply of medicines under special circumstances, for example when there are drug shortages or affordability gaps.

Indeed medicines reuse is permitted in some countries such as Greece [10] and the United States [11], mainly for benevolent reasons—the idea being, briefly, that suitable medicines can re-enter the supply chain and be reissued to others in need. However, medicines reuse is prohibited in the UK. The same is true for most other European counties too. A snapshot report on the fate of unused pharmaceuticals in a number of European countries, published in 2013 pointed to a promising recycling scheme in Hungary named Recyclomed [12]. However, on inquiring about the scheme the authors of this paper were recently informed, via email, that for drug safety reasons drug manufacturers opposed both the reuse of medicines as well as any recycling of the packaging via that scheme. Thus, in Hungary, the UK and most other countries in Europe, the main intervention for addressing the inappropriate disposal of unwanted medicines is to offer formal waste collection services for the sole purpose of incineration [12]. The exception is a scheme offered in Portugal named Valormed, which although does not support medicines reuse, does separate collections into elements to be incinerated and packaging components to be recycled [12].

UK officials often cite uncertainties about the quality, safety and efficacy of returned medicines kept in patients' homes, outside of the formal supply chain, as the reason to oppose the practice of medicines reuse [13–15]. These risks are also recognized by members of the public who would not want to receive poor-quality, harmful or incorrect medication as a result of medicines reuse [3]. Thus, the re-use or recycling of another patient's medicine is not normally recommended by the UK's Department of Health and Social Care (DHSC). This stance also has to be viewed within the context of a reliable, national healthcare service that has no cause to risk compromising patient safety, theoretically or materially, for any potential benefit that might be gained from sanctioning medicines reuse. However, as we have argued elsewhere, a persistent objection to the idea of medicines reuse is unrealistic because unpredictable events such as pandemics [16] and drug shortages [17] result in temporary U-turns in the UK Government's position on medicines reuse in any case, but in a space devoid of sufficient investment and research. Thus, a reasonable stance might be to recognize the risks associated with medicines reuse and try to ameliorate these with potential solutions. To this end, we propose a robust mechanism for validating the quality and safety of medicines kept within and outside of the formal supply chain, using the novel ReMINDS (www.reading.ac.uk/ReMINDS, Accessed on 17 July 2021) ecosystem. This system relies on active sensing technologies integrated with the Internet of Things platform to indicate the 'reusability' of medicines while interconnecting the relevant stakeholders [18,19]. The availability of such a system should make medicines reuse, whether a temporary measure or not, a much safer practice in the future. Regardless, engaging people in medicines reuse, should the practice be sanctioned by medicines regulators in the future, will still rely on their voluntary participation in such a scheme. For example, the recent proposal to permit care homes and hospices in the UK to draw up standard operating procedures to enable medicines reuse if impacted by shortages due to the pandemic, still required active consent from people affected by such a scheme (donating and receiving) [20].

The studies that have examined people's views about medicines reuse in countries such as the UK and the Netherlands are clear that the practice would be acceptable to many people provided the quality and safety of the medicines can be guaranteed [1–4]. For example, in the Netherlands, 61.2% of survey respondents were willing to use medication returned unused to the pharmacy by another patient as long as the quality of these medicines was somehow verified [1]. In the UK too, we found 54.5% of our respondents intended to, wanted to (56.5%) or expected to (56.5%) reuse medication in the future [4]. What-is-more, the findings from our theory-driven study [21] highlight the importance of creating conditions that will illustrate to people that medicines reuse would not expose them to additional medication-related risks [4].

The current way in which returned medicines are screened for reuse relies on the judgement of the pharmacist [22] or another registered health professional [20]. However, as we have argued elsewhere, these methods currently only use history-checking and visual checks, and do not uncover the actual prior storage conditions of returned medicines nor the impact of that storage on the contents within—thus act as proxy measures of quality only. The gap in the market, in our view, is for technologies, for example sensors to measure and track the interaction of the storage conditions (e.g., temperature, light, humidity) with the medicinal pack when kept outside of the formal pharmacy supply chain [18,19]. Sensors that work in this way could reassure people, and reasonably regulators, about the continued quality of reused medicines. Indeed, this is the basis of our proposed ReMINDS ecosystem.

To test these ideas with the public, whose participation in medicines reuse would be key to its success in a hypothesized future scenario, we designed a simple two-factor experiment to gauge people's responses to the idea of medicines reuse, with or without the presence of a sensor to monitor storage conditions and with or without assurances about a pharmacist's involvement in visual checking the candidate medicine. We imagined that participants would view medicines reuse more favourably with the presence of a sensor and if given specific information about a candidate medicines having been visually checked by a pharmacist.

2. Materials and Methods

2.1. Design

A between-participants design was used. One independent variable was the presence of a sensor on the medication box (we chose a standard levothyroxine calendar pack) to monitor the storage environment of the medication presented to the participants. This had two conditions, one condition where the packaging was presented without the sensor and one where it was shown with the sensor accompanied by the researcher reading out the following script: "There is a sensor monitoring the storage conditions of this medication box. This means the temperature and humidity is monitored." The other independent variable was visual checking. This also consisted of two conditions, one condition where no additional information on visual checking was given and one where additional information was provided, that a pharmacist had been involved in visual checking the medicine, with the following script read out: "The pharmacist has performed quality and safety checks before giving this medication to you". The combination of the different conditions is shown in Table 1.

Table 1. The experimental combinations.

Experiment	Sensor on Packaging	Pharmacist Visual Check
Scenario 1	No	No
Scenario 2	Yes	No
Scenario 3	No	Yes
Scenario 4	Yes	Yes

The dependent variable was medicines reuse beliefs. This was measured by asking the participants to complete a short questionnaire after being shown the medication box for their specific scenario.

To control for any differences in the participants, the scenarios were allocated at random. In addition, some basic demographic data about the participants were collected in order to check for any substantial differences in the four groups. To control for potential experimenter effects, the researcher was careful to give the experimental instructions in a standard way each time, not favouring a certain outcome, nor giving away any verbal/non-verbal cues that would unduly influence the participants. To control for any other differences in the way the medication was perceived, the boxes of levothyroxine tablets presented were totally identical (apart from the presence of the sensor where appropriate).

2.2. Hypothesis

Our hypothesis was that participants would give more positive responses to questions about medicines reuse with the presence of the sensor on the packaging compared to without. We also tested another hypothesis that the addition of a statement about the pharmacist's involvement in the visual checking of the medication would also result in more positive responses to questions about medicines reuse compared to without.

2.3. Materials

Two identical calendar packs of levothyroxine 100 mcg tablets, which usually requires storage at room temperature, were used to represent the medication under consideration. The box containing the 'sensor' (used in Experiments 2 and 4) was fitted with a temperature indicator which was a Timestrip® Plus sticker (Figure 1) and a photo-reduced version of an SCS humidity indicator (available from https://staticcontrol.descoindustries.com/ Accessed on 17 July 2021). Both indicators were non-functioning and used for theoretical purposes in order to simulate the monitoring of temperature and humidity, respectively, via a sensor.

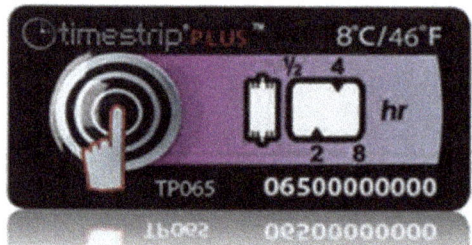

Figure 1. Timestrip® Plus temperature indicator (available from https://timestrip.com/ accessed on 17 July 2021).

The questionnaire was based on an existing, already-validated medicines reuse questionnaire developed using Ajzen's theory of planned behaviour (TBP) model [23], published fully elsewhere [4] (see Figure 2).

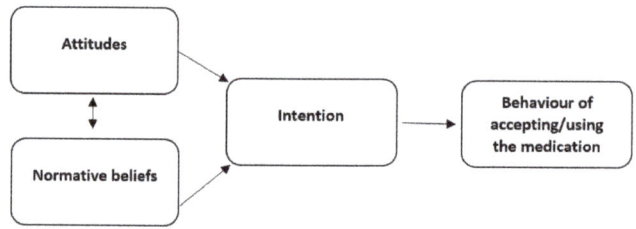

Figure 2. The theory of planned behavior model applied to reusing medication.

The questionnaire composed of three sections. Section 1 consisted of demographic questions on gender, age, level of education and ethnicity. Section 2 listed 11 statements, each with a five-point Likert response scale to indicate agreement/disagreement with the statements, from strongly disagree to strongly agree. The statements were categorised into three clusters: (a) attitude toward reusing the medicine; (b) normative beliefs/social pressure to accept the medication for reuse; (c) intention to accept the medication (see Table 2). A third section invited the participants to add any comments by hand.

Table 2. The 11 statements categorized according to the theory of planned behaviour (TPB) model. For the analysis, the mean score for 'attitude' for each individual was calculated from responses to Questions 1–5, for 'normative beliefs/social pressure' from Questions 6–9, and for 'intention' from Questions 10 and 11.

TPB Category	Statement
Attitude toward reusing the medication	1. This medication would be safe to use 2. This medication would be harmful 3. This medication would be of low quality 4. This medication would be good 5. It would be satisfying to accept this medication
Normative beliefs/social pressure to accept the medication for reuse	6. My family would believe I should accept this medication 7. My close friends would believe I should accept this medication 8. My doctor would believe that I should accept this medication 9. My pharmacist would believe that I should accept this medication
Intention to accept the medication	10. I would accept this medication 11. I would want to use this medication

2.4. Procedure

Participants from the University of Reading's Whiteknights Campus were approached and consented via an information leaflet. Each participant was shown a standard empty levothyroxine medication box and allocated at random to receive one of four scenarios all with the same information about medicines reuse; with or without the presence of the sensor, and with or without the visual-check information involving the pharmacist (see Table 1). At the experiment's start, a standard script was followed for all of the participants:

"This research project is about re-using medicines, which is when a pharmacist gives medication that has been brought back to their pharmacy by one patient, for another patient to use. Currently, in the UK this is not allowed. Imagine you need to collect some medication for yourself from the pharmacy. You are told that the pharmacist had previously given this particular box of medication to another patient (shows participants the medication box, according to scenario and reads out the additional information for Scenarios 2, 3, and 4 as appropriate). That patient did not need this box of medication, so they returned it to the pharmacy a month later. The box is unopened, is the original packaging and the anti-tampering sticker is still attached to it. The medication is also well within the expiry date. This box of medication is then given to you for your own use. Do you have any questions so far? Based on this information, please fill out the questionnaire."

All participants then completed the questionnaire. The participants were finally debriefed about the aims of the study and asked if they had any questions.

Data from questionnaires were transferred to SPSS® (version 25). The scores from the negatively phrased statements (2, 3) were reversed. The data were then analysed using analysis of variance (ANOVA) with the mean attitude toward the medication, mean perceived social pressure (normative beliefs) to accept the medication, and mean intention to accept the medication, as the dependent variables. The presence of the sensor and inclusion of pharmacist visual-check information were the independent variables.

2.5. Participants

Eighty-one participants took part in this experiment. Participants were either staff or students present on the Whiteknights Campus of the University of Reading in November or December 2019. They were approached opportunistically and recruited with an information letter and consent form. There were 41 females, 39 males and 1 who preferred not to disclose their gender. The participants were aged between 18 and 64. There was an even distribution of gender, age, educational qualification and ethnicity across the different experimental scenarios as shown in Table 3.

Table 3. The socio-demographic information of the participants according to the experimental scenarios.

Characteristics	Scenario 1 (n = 20) (%)	Scenario 2 (n = 20) (%)	Scenario 3 (n = 21) (%)	Scenario 4 (n = 20) (%)	Total (n = 81) (%)
Gender					
Female	11 (55.0)	10 (50.0)	12 (57.0)	8 (40.0)	41 (50.6)
Male	9 (45.0)	10 (50.0)	8 (38.0)	12 (60.0)	39 (48.1)
Prefer not to say	0 (0.0)	0 (0.0)	1 (5.0)	0 (0.0)	1 (1.2)
Age					
18–24	12 (60.0)	7 (35.0)	11 (52.0)	9 (45.0)	39 (48.1)
25–34	4 (20.0)	9 (45.0)	5 (24.0)	4 (20.0)	22 (27.2)
35–44	2 (10.0)	1 (5.0)	1 (5.0)	5 (25.0)	9 (11.1)
45–54	1 (5.0)	1 (5.0)	3 (14.0)	1 (5.0)	6 (7.4)
55–64	1 (5.0)	2 (10.0)	1 (5.0)	1 (5.0)	5 (6.2)
Highest qualification					
GCSE	1 (5.0)	3 (15.0)	4 (19.0)	4 (20.0)	12 (14.8)
A level	8 (40.0)	3 (15.0)	4 (19.0)	7 (35.0)	22 (27.2)
Bachelor's degree	7 (35.0)	7 (35.0)	7 (33.0)	4 (20.0)	25 (30.9)
Master's degree	3 (15.0)	2 (10.0)	4 (19.0)	2 (10.0)	11 (13.6)
PhD	1 (5.0)	0 (0.0)	0 (0.0)	2 (10.0)	3 (3.7)
Other	0 (0.0)	4 (20.0)	2 (10.0)	1 (5.0)	7 (8.6)
Prefer not to say	0 (0.0)	1 (5.0)	0 (0.0)	0 (0.0)	1 (1.2)
Ethnicity					
English/Welsh/Scottish	8 (40.0)	9 (45.0)	12 (57.0)	8 (40.0)	37 (45.7)
Any other white background	4 (20.0)	0 (0.0)	0 (0.0)	2 (10.0)	6 (7.4)
White and black Caribbean	0 (0.0)	1 (5.0)	0 (0.0)	2 (10.0)	3 (3.7)
White and Asian	0 (0.0)	0 (0.0)	1 (5.0)	0 (0.0)	1 (1.2)
Other mixed	0 (0.0)	0 (0.0)	2 (9.0)	0 (0.0)	2 (2.6)
Indian	1 (5.0)	3 (15.0)	1 (5.0)	0 (0.0)	5 (6.2)
Pakistani	0 (0.0)	2 (10.0)	3 (14.0)	3 (15.0)	8 (9.9)
Bangladeshi	0 (0.0)	1 (5.0)	0 (0.0)	0 (0.0)	1 (1.2)
Chinese	2 (10.0)	1 (5.0)	0 (0.0)	0 (0.0)	3 (3.7)
Other Asian background	2 (10.0)	0 (0.0)	1 (5.0)	0 (0.0)	3 (3.7)
African	1 (5.0)	2 (10.0)	1 (5.0)	2 (10.0)	6 (7.4)
Caribbean	1 (5.0)	1 (5.0)	0 (0.0)	2 (10.0)	4 (4.9)
Other ethnic group	1 (5.0)	0 (0.0)	0 (0.0)	1 (5.0)	2 (2.5)

Forty participants received a scenario (2,4) where the sensor was attached to the packaging and 41 received a scenario (3,4) which informed them that a pharmacist had completed visual checks on the product.

2.6. Qualitative Analysis

The qualitative comments left on the questionnaires were also analysed using thematic analysis [24]. This approach was used because it provided a way of organising the qualitative data in the form of themes: recurrent topics, ideas or statements identified across the corpus of data. The comments were analysed manually by YL in consultation with PD, according to the six phases described by Braun and Clarke [24]. The process involved familiarisation with the data, coding, searching for themes, reviewing themes, defining and naming themes, and writing up. After familiarisation with the data, YL coded each comment and assigned initial 'code names'. The codes were then grouped together under common themes and the themes in turn were grouped according to two higher-order categories.

3. Results

In terms of people's 'attitude' toward the medication, the F ratios were calculated to be as follows; for the effect of the presence of the 'sensor', $F(1, 77) = 7.09$, $p < 0.01$, the provision of information about visual-checking by the 'pharmacist', $F(1, 77) = 9.63$, $p < 0.005$, and the interaction between sensor and pharmacist, $F(1, 77) = 0.001$, $p = 0.974$ (see Figure 3).

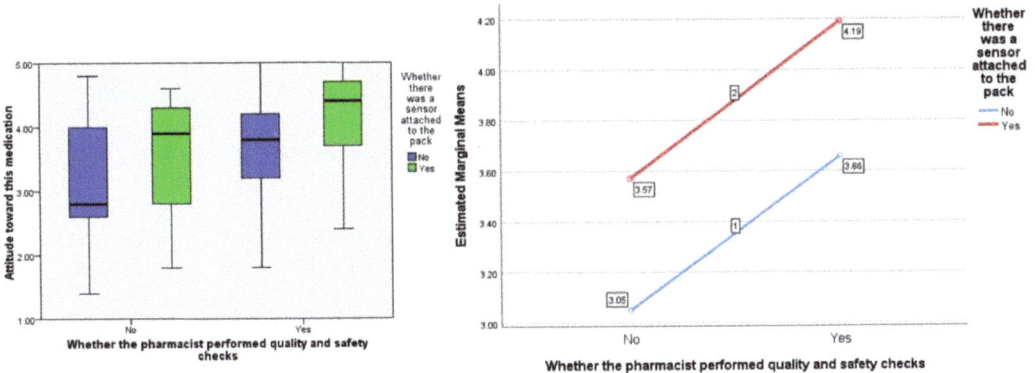

Figure 3. Box plot showing the effect of the independent variables on the 'attitude' score (highlighting median values) and, separately, the estimated marginal means plotted against each other to show any interaction (none in this instance).

In terms of people's perceived 'social pressure' to accept the medication, the F ratios were calculated to be as follows; for the effect of the presence of the 'sensor' $F(1, 77) = 7.99$, $p < 0.01$, the provision of information about visual-checking by the 'pharmacist', $F(1, 77) = 7.55$, $p < 0.01$, and the interaction between sensor and pharmacist $F(1, 77) = 0.02$, $p = 0.887$ (see Figure 4).

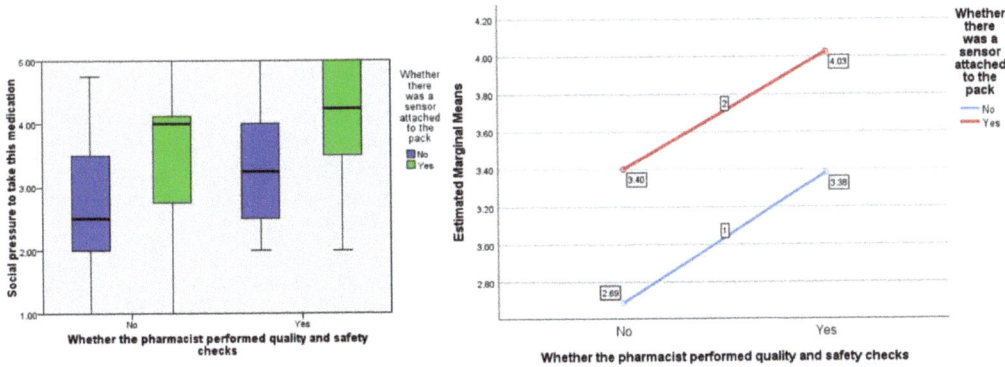

Figure 4. Box plot showing the effect of the independent variables on the 'social pressure' score (highlighting median values) and, separately, the estimated marginal means plotted against each other to show any interaction (none in this instance).

In terms of people's 'intention' to accept the medication, the F ratios were calculated to be as follows; for the effect of the presence of the 'sensor', $F(1, 77) = 5.21$, $p < 0.05$ the provision of information about visual-checking by the 'pharmacist', $F(1, 77) = 10.71$, $p < 0.005$, and the interaction between sensor and pharmacist, $F(1, 77) = 0.018$, $p = 0.903$ (see Figure 5).

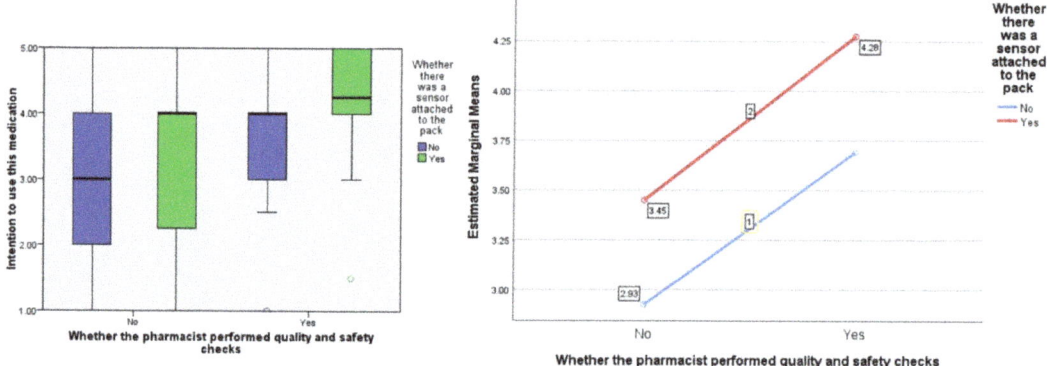

Figure 5. Box plot showing the effect of the independent variables on the 'intention' score (highlighting median values) and, separately, the estimated marginal means plotted against each other to show any interaction (none in this instance).

3.1. Qualitative Comments

The two super-ordinate categories identified are shown below along with their themes.

3.2. Participants' Expectations of Medicines Reuse

The four themes within this category relate to people's expectations of medicines reuse.

3.2.1. Physical Characteristics of Re-Dispensed Medicines

Regardless of the scenario, participants wondered whether the medication packaging had been previously opened and wanted factors such as anti-tampering stickers and pharmacist checks to improve their confidence about the authenticity of any reused medication. For example:

- "If you told me it's been unopened and you can tell by the antitampering sticker, it is fine to take." (45–54-year-old male, Scenario 1)
- "If tampered then I would give more uncertainty but if checks are in place and come back fine, I would have no issue. (18–24-year-old female, Scenario 4)

3.2.2. Process of Checking for Quality

Participants in Scenarios 3 and 4 were told that a pharmacist had checked the medication for quality and safety. Many thought that a pharmacist was the right professional to be trusted to perform quality and safety checks of returned medicines. Moreover, for some participants in Scenario 4, the presence of a sensor was thought to enhance the pharmacist's ability to confirm the safety of the medicine. For example:

- It is safe to take as long as pharmacist has checked it (18–24-year-old female, Scenario 3).
- Happier to receive re-used medication that contains a sensor than without due to it aiding the pharmacist with their safety checks. (18–24-year-old male, Scenario 4).

3.2.3. Logistics of Medicines Reuse

In Scenarios 3 and 4, some participants were concerned about the potential burden on pharmacists performing the quality and safety checks of returned medicines due to the additional workload that would be involved. A number of participants in Scenario 3 were uncertain about effectiveness of the checks performed by the pharmacist. For example:

- In theory would reduce medicines wastage however safety cannot be guaranteed even with checks and would be an extra workload on community pharmacists. (25–34-year-old female, Scenario 3).

3.2.4. Incentives to Engage in Medicines Reuse

A number of participants would only engage in medicines reuse under specific conditions. For example:

- I would only take it if there was an incentive e.g., no others available and if it was cheaper/free of charge. (18–24-year-old male, Scenario 1).
- If I was in desperate need of the medication, I would believe that it was safe for me. But I would still be a little cautious when taking it. People can open and re-seal. (18–24-year-old female, Scenario 4).

3.3. Understanding the Consequences of Medicines Reuse
3.3.1. Potential Disadvantages of Re-Dispensing Medicines

Some participants expressed uncertainties over the quality and safety of medicines, once handled by other people. Further, some expressed that re-dispensed medicines could be unsafe due to contamination. For example:

- I don not trust where a stranger has put the box. It could change the medication quality. (18–24-year-old, female, Scenario 1).
- I do not like the idea of someone else other than a healthcare practitioner being in handle of my medication. (18–24-year-old female, Scenario 2).
- The packaging could be infected with unidentified bacteria, so taking a risk could be potentially dangerous. (18–24-year-old, Scenario 3).

3.3.2. Potential Advantages of Medicines Reuse

Some participants also mentioned the economic and environmental benefits of reusing medicines. Several participants stated that medicines reuse could aid the NHS in minimizing costs. For example:

- I think if it's safe and good to use and it would help reduce cost to the NHS. (35–44-year-old female, Scenario 4).
- I think this is a very good idea and will stop wasting the medication. (55–64-year-old female, Scenario 3).
- Re-using unopened medication is a good idea. It could help prevent a shortage of specific medications that are needed. (18–24-year-old female, Scenario 4).

4. Discussion

As hypothesized, participants gave more positive responses to questions about medicines reuse with the presence of the sensor on the packaging compared to without. This was across all three domains of attitude toward the medication, social pressure to accept it, and intention to do so. Participants also gave more favourable responses on hearing about the pharmacist's involvement in the visual checking of the medication compared to without. What-is-more, consistently, the inclusion of the sensor on the packaging resulted in better (more pro-medicines-reuse) responses compared to the visual-checking statement, with the inclusion of both conditions giving the highest scores across attitude toward the medication, social pressure to accept it, and intention to do so. The study provides important evidence about the potential for sensors that measure and track the interaction of the storage conditions with the medicinal pack to reassure people about medicines reuse and encourage them to engage with such a scheme in the future should this be sanctioned by regulators.

A strength of this study is the use of the experimental method. Experiments allow researchers to manipulate the independent variables so that causal inference can be made in terms of the desired outcomes. Thus, through the design of our experiment, we were able to introduce the phenomenon of a sensor and visual-checking information in a controlled manner and then study the impact on people's pro-medicines-reuse beliefs. This provides a good degree of confidence about the cause-effect of the relationships that we were investigating. A potential weakness is that our participants' age and education were not representative of the general population or a hypothesized 'average' pharmacy customer. While education levels could influence decisions, the likely impact of age on risky decisions is less clear [25]. In addition, because of capacity constraints, each of the four scenarios was tested with only 20 people. Nonetheless, because of the large effect sizes between the different conditions, the study was evidently sufficiently powered to illustrate the statistically significant differences in the outcome measures. Another strength of the study is the accompanying qualitative analysis which provided added explanation to bolster the findings.

The comments from the questionnaire related either to people's expectations about medicines reuse or illustrated their understanding of the consequences of medicines reuse. In this way, the qualitative comments helped validate the main findings as the participants explained their concerns about the quality of re-dispensed medicines and highlighted how a sensor as well as the involvement of the pharmacist might help increase their confidence in such a product. The comments made by the participants also aligned well with other ideas about medicines reuse found in research elsewhere [1,3,4], for example its role in waste prevention, medicines shortages, its potential impact on pharmacist time and the idea of patient incentives to engage with the practice. One of the most significant outcomes of the current study, however, is the findings that the presence of sensors has a greater impact on people's pro-medicines reuse beliefs compared with the provision of information about pharmacist checks. Although it makes logical sense to trust technology that can provide objective proof about the storage conditions of medication, over and above the visual checks that a pharmacist might provide, this study adds evidence to the ideas proposed in our ReMINDS ecosystem as a publicly-acceptable solution for reusing returned, prescribed medicines [18,19]. This system relies on active sensing technologies on packaging, integrated with the Internet of Things platform to validate the quality and safety of the medicines while interconnecting the relevant stakeholders [11,12].

Smart packaging concepts are new to medication packs but have been around in the food industry for a number of years [26]. This is not to deny the other sophisticated features of pharmaceutical packaging, which is advanced and well researched [27]. However, the use of technology to enable reuse of medicines is not common and the corresponding research is not at all mainstream [18]. It is important to highlight that smart packaging in that industry consists of more than temperature/humidity sensors, extending to such things as integrity indicators, freshness indicators, and even radiofrequency identification (RFID) tags to identify and locate the product [28]. The current paper only tested the idea of one type of sensor, in a small experiment. Another learning point from the food industry is to consider the environmental impact of the packaging itself against the potential for it to reduce product waste [29]. Therefore, the attachment of sensor technology to medication packaging will not necessarily solve the overall problem of waste created by medication, unless shown to be carbon neutral. While the current paper makes a small contribution to understanding the public's attitude towards medicines reuse, research on smart packaging within the food industry also offers a wealth of more nuanced information about the impact of such technology on consumer perceptions [30]. For example, a recent review in the food industry unearths not only the functional value of smart packaging (e.g., protecting the content) but also communication value (e.g., perception of safer product), social value (e.g., societal trends towards sustainable living), emotional value (e.g., feeling more confident about the product), and so on [30]. There can also be barriers to the use of smart packaging, such as value barrier (e.g., increased price of final product) and tradition barrier (e.g., getting used to a new type of behavior) discussed in detail elsewhere [30].

It is worth noting that the sensors attached to the medication box (Timestrip® Plus sticker and a downsized version of an SCS humidity indicator) used in the experiments were non-functioning and used for theoretical purposes only in order to mimic the monitoring of temperature and humidity, respectively. More investigations should be undertaken in the future with appropriate indicators, specifically designed to function for medicines reuse schemes. These studies could probe consumer responses in more detail, to examine other potential values and barriers to the use of smart packaging for medication packs.

5. Conclusions

This study suggests that the addition of sensors to the packaging of medicines combined with visual quality and safety checks carried out by pharmacists create a more positive response about medicines reuse, compared to their absence. The use of sensors on medication packaging forms the basis of our proposed ReMINDS ecosystem, which warrants further investigation.

Author Contributions: Conceptualization, P.D. and Y.L.; methodology, P.D. and Y.L.; validation, P.D.; formal analysis, Y.L.; data curation, Y.L. and P.D.; writing—original draft preparation, Y.L.; writing—review and editing, P.D., R.M., T.K.L.H., R.S.S.; supervision, P.D.; project administration, P.D. All authors have read and agreed to the published version of the manuscript.

Funding: Not applicable.

Institutional Review Board Statement: This study has been subject to ethical review by the University of Reading's Research Ethics Committee and was approved through the in-school exceptions route (Study Number 54/19) on 2 December 2019.

Informed Consent Statement: All potential participants were given an information sheet describing the purpose of the study, what their participation would involve and any data protection measures. Consent forms were then completed by each participant.

Data Availability Statement: The authors can be emailed for further information about the data.

Acknowledgments: We thank the study participants.

Conflicts of Interest: The authors declare no conflict of interest.

References

1. Bekker, C.; Van den Bemt, B.; Egberts, T.C.G.; Bouvy, M.; Gardarsdottir, H. Willingness of patients to use unused medication returned to the pharmacy by another patient: A cross-sectional survey. *BMJ Open* **2019**, *9*, e024767. [CrossRef] [PubMed]
2. Bekker, C.L.; Gardarsdottir, H.; Egberts, T.C.G.; Bouvy, M.L.; Van den Bemt, B.J.F. Redispensing of medicines unused by patients: A qualitative study among stakeholders. *Int. J. Clin. Pharm.* **2017**, *39*, 196–204. [CrossRef] [PubMed]
3. Alhamad, H.; Patel, N.; Donyai, P. How do people conceptualise the reuse of medicines? An interview study. *Int. J. Pharm. Pract.* **2018**, *26*, 232–241. [CrossRef] [PubMed]
4. Alhamad, H.; Donyai, P. Intentions to "Reuse" Medication in the Future Modelled and Measured Using the Theory of Planned Behavior. *Pharmacy* **2020**, *8*, 213. [CrossRef] [PubMed]
5. Toma, A.; Crişan, O. Green Pharmacy—A Narrative Review. *Med. Pharm. Rep.* **2018**, *91*, 391–398. [CrossRef] [PubMed]
6. Kümmerer, K. *Why Green and Sustainable Pharmacy?* Springer: Berlin/Heidelberg, Germany, 2010; ISBN 9783642051982.
7. Alhamad, H.; Patel, N.; Donyai, P. Towards Medicines Reuse: A Narrative Review of the Different Therapeutic Classes and Dosage Forms of Medication Waste in Different Countries. *Pharmacy* **2020**, *8*, 230. [CrossRef] [PubMed]
8. Abou-Auda, H.S. An economic assessment of the extent of medication use and wastage among families in Saudi Arabia and Arabian Gulf countries. *Clin. Ther.* **2003**, *25*, 1276–1292. [CrossRef]
9. Trueman, P.; Lowson, K.; Blighe, A.; Meszaros, A. *Evaluation of the Scale, Causes and Costs of Waste Medicines. Report of DH Funded National Project*; York Health Economics Consortium and The School of Pharmacy, University of London: London, UK, 2011; Volume 17, pp. 1–106.
10. GIVMED. Available online: https://givmed.org/en/ (accessed on 9 January 2020).
11. Cauchi, R.; Berg, K. State Prescription Drug Return, Reuse and Recycling Laws. Available online: https://www.ncsl.org/research/health/state-prescription-drug-return-reuse-and-recycling.aspx (accessed on 9 January 2020).
12. Health Care without Harm. *Unused Pharmaceuticals Where Do They End Up? A Snapshot of European Collection Schemes*; Health Care without Harm: Brussels, Belgium, 2013.
13. Department of Health. Repeat Prescribing Systems. Available online: https://webarchive.nationalarchives.gov.uk/+/http://www.dh.gov.uk/en/Publicationsandstatistics/Publications/PublicationsPolicyAndGuidance/Browsable/DH_4892136 (accessed on 26 February 2021).
14. House of Commons. Public Accounts. *Minutes of Evidence Supplementary Memorandum from the Department of Health*. 2009. Available online: https://publications.parliament.uk/pa/cm200809/cmselect/cmpubacc/99/8121708.htm (accessed on 16 July 2021).
15. Connelly, D. Should pharmacists be allowed to reuse medicines. *Pharm. J.* **2019**, *301*, 20–23. [CrossRef]
16. Council approves use of patient-returned and date-expired medicines in the event of pandemic flu. *Pharm. J.* **2008**, *280*, 645.

17. Adrenaline auto-injectors: Recent action taken to support safety. *Drug Safety Update* **2019**, *13*, 4. Available online: https://www.gov.uk/drug-safety-update/adrenaline-auto-injectors-recent-action-taken-to-support-safety (accessed on 20 July 2021).
18. Hui, T.K.L.; Mohammed, B.; Donyai, P.; McCrindle, R.; Sherratt, R.S. Enhancing Pharmaceutical Packaging through a Technology Ecosystem to Facilitate the Reuse of Medicines and Reduce Medicinal Waste. *Pharmacy* **2020**, *8*, 58. [CrossRef] [PubMed]
19. Hui, T.K.L.; Donyai, P.; McCrindle, R.; Sherratt, R.S. Enabling Medicine Reuse Using a Digital Time Temperature Humidity Sensor in an Internet of Pharmaceutical Things Concept. *Sensors* **2020**, *20*, 3080. [CrossRef] [PubMed]
20. Donyai, P.; McCrindle, R.; Sherratt, R.S.; Hui, T.K.L. COVID-19 Pandemic Is Our Chance to Learn How to Reuse Old Medicines. Available online: https://theconversation.com/covid-19-pandemic-is-our-chance-to-learn-how-to-reuse-old-medicines-137671 (accessed on 22 February 2020).
21. Alhamad, H.; Donyai, P. The Validity of the Theory of Planned Behaviour for Understanding People's Beliefs and Intentions toward Reusing Medicines. *Pharmacy* **2021**, *9*, 58. [CrossRef] [PubMed]
22. SafeNetRX.org. Available online: https://safenetrx.org/ (accessed on 23 March 2021).
23. Ajzen, I. The theory of planned behavior. In *Handbook of Theories of Social Psychology: Volume 1*; SAGE Publications: Thousand Oaks, CA, USA, 2012; ISBN 9781446249215.
24. Braun, V.; Clarke, V. Using thematic analysis in psychology. *Qual. Res. Psychol.* **2006**, *3*, 77–101. [CrossRef]
25. Mata, R.; Josef, A.K.; Samanez-Larkin, G.R.; Hertwig, R. Age differences in risky choice: A meta-analysis. *Ann. N. Y. Acad. Sci.* **2011**, *1235*, 18–29. [CrossRef] [PubMed]
26. Kuswandi, B.; Wicaksono, Y.; Jayus, J.; Abdullah, A.; Lee, Y.H.; Ahmad, M. Smart Packaging: Sensors for monitoring of food quality and safety. *Sens. Instrum. Food Qual. Saf.* **2011**, *5*, 137–146. [CrossRef]
27. Zadbuke, N.; Shahi, S.; Gulecha, B.; Padalkar, A.; Thube, M. Recent trends and future of pharmaceutical packaging technology. *J. Pharm. Bioallied Sci.* **2013**, *5*, 98–110. [CrossRef] [PubMed]
28. Fuertes, G.; Soto, I.; Carrasco, R.; Vargas, M.; Sabattin, J.; Lagos, C. Intelligent Packaging Systems: Sensors and Nanosensors to Monitor Food Quality and Safety. *J. Sens.* **2016**, *2016*, 4046061. [CrossRef]
29. Wikström, F.; Williams, H.; Verghese, K.; Clune, S. The influence of packaging attributes on consumer behaviour in food-packaging life cycle assessment studies—A neglected topic. *J. Clean. Prod.* **2014**, *73*, 100–108. [CrossRef]
30. Young, E.; Mirosa, M.; Bremer, P. A Systematic Review of Consumer Perceptions of Smart Packaging Technologies for Food. *Front. Sustain. Food Syst.* **2020**, *4*, 63. [CrossRef]

MDPI
St. Alban-Anlage 66
4052 Basel
Switzerland
Tel. +41 61 683 77 34
Fax +41 61 302 89 18
www.mdpi.com

Pharmacy Editorial Office
E-mail: pharmacy@mdpi.com
www.mdpi.com/journal/pharmacy

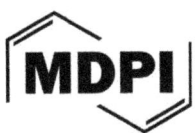

www.ingramcontent.com/pod-product-compliance
Lightning Source LLC
LaVergne TN
LVHW070712100526
838202LV00013B/1074